Dear Thomas C. Shevory

with compliments

Rihito Kimura

Advance Directives and Surrogate Decision Making in Health Care

Advance Directives and Surrogate Decision Making in Health Care

United States, Germany, and Japan

Edited by
Hans-Martin Sass
Robert M. Veatch
and Rihito Kimura

The Johns Hopkins University Press
Baltimore & London

Printed in the United States of America on
acid-free recycled paper

9 8 7 6 5 4 3 2 1

The Johns Hopkins University Press
2715 North Charles Street
Baltimore, Maryland 21218-4363
The Johns Hopkins Press Ltd., London
www.press.jhu.edu

Library of Congress Cataloging-in-Publication
Data will be found at the end of this book.
A catalog record for this book is available from
the British Library.

ISBN 0-8018-5831-3

Contents

Contributors

Rihito Kimura, J.D., L.L.M., is director of the Asian Bioethics Program at the Kennedy Institute of Ethics (Georgetown University, Washington, D.C.). He is also professor of bioethics and law at Waseda University, in Tokyo, Japan.

Dr. jur. Hans-Georg Koch is a member of the Max-Planck-Institut für ausländisches und internationales Strafrecht, in Freiburg, Germany.

Joanne Lynn, M.D., M.A., is director of the Center to Improve Care of the Dying at George Washington University (Washington, D.C.).

Alan Meisel, J.D., is a professor at the University of Pittsburgh School of Law.

Dr. med. Johannes Meran is a professor in the Department of Hematology and Oncology at the Hannover University Medical School (Germany).

Prof. Dr. Gen Ohi, M.D., Ph.D., M.P.H., is professor and chair of the Department of Ethics and Anthropology at the School of International Health (University of Tokyo).

Prof. Dr. Hubert Poliwoda is a professor in the Department of Hematology and Oncology at the Hannover University Medical School (Germany).

Prof. Dr. Hans-Martin Sass is a professor at the Institut für Philosophie at Ruhr Universität (Bochum, Germany) and director of the European Bioethics Program at the Kennedy Institute of Ethics (Georgetown University, Washington, D.C.).

Joan Teno, M.D., M.S., is co-director of the Center to Improve Care of the Dying at George Washington University (Washington, D.C.).

Dr. Tomoaki Tsuchida is a professor in the Department of International Cultural Studies at Nanzan University (Nagoya, Japan).

Robert M. Veatch, Ph.D., is professor of medical ethics and former director of the Kennedy Institute of Ethics (Georgetown University, Washington, D.C.) and a professor in the Department of Philosophy.

Introduction

Advancements in clinical treatment and in life-sustaining technologies have furthered a debate about whether the use of the full range of biomedical capabilities is warranted, mandated, or rather questionable from an ethical standpoint. Extraordinary or morally expendable treatment once was defined by many people as an intervention that, according to clinical experience and scientific prognosis, inevitably fails. Now, however, it is also defined in individual and patient-oriented terms, making those interventions expendable that do not produce more benefit than burden from the point of view of the personal values, visions, and wishes of the individual patient. Personal convictions, family traditions, religious values and visions, and variations in ethical reasoning, which were taken into account for centuries by classical philosophical and religious traditions and medical attitudes by certain theological thinkers, have been rejected by medical institutions and individual physicians who have felt strongly that they should do "everything possible" to prolong life whatever the circumstances as long as adequate technology is available.

Medical cases such as those of Karen Quinlan or Nancy Cruzan have become famous as court cases and also have become essential readings in teaching ethics. No reasonable arguments have been made that medical professionals shall make final decisions about how long a patient shall live. But, then, who shall make those decisions? Should a professional culture, whether medical or legal, have the final word in making crucial decisions, and to what extent can the law ever have an effective steering function in areas of highly technical decision making and judgment?

Traditional physician ethics of beneficence mandated that the beneficent expert combine ethics and expertise in the craft, making life-and-death decisions without burdening others, particularly the patient, with conflicts in decision making. Such a position made much sense in times when medical possibilities were limited and views of life and death were more or less uniform within the community. But in modern societies, rich with diverse values and wishes manifest in individual expressions and convictions, there is no longer a uniform, general answer to the question of when life-supporting medical interventions should cease. The answer the physician might give if only his or her convictions mattered is not necessarily the answer for the patient, who most likely will have other religious beliefs, visions, personal expectations, hopes, and fears. What is true for postmodern multicultural societies is even more true for the diversity of attitudes among different traditions, cultures, religions, and attitudes in the global village.

All cultures and traditions accept that individuals should not be treated against their will, that is, without giving consent. Weaker and stronger concepts of "informed consent" principles have made it into the textbooks of ethics and medicine and the paragraphs of law books and court decisions. But what about those who cannot give consent because of infirmity, anxiety, dementia, coma, or incompetence? Who shall decide for them, the physicians, the family, or procedural standards set up by providers or payees of medical services? Here is where advance health care planning and surrogates for health care decision making come in. The following question also arises: How much self-determination and power to direct care and treatment decisions can be entrusted to those who are no longer competent in the strict legal sense?

Although advance care documents are legally accepted in the United States and widely recognized clinically, in the legal and clinical settings in other countries such as Japan and Germany it would be very unusual to base clinical decisions on a patient's previous oral or written statements or for family members to go to court over medical treatment they consider unfit or futile based on their understanding of the patient's prospective preferences or their own understanding of futile versus beneficial treatment.

Moral reasoning in support of advance directive legislation and the clinical recognition of the validity of advance directives is based primarily on the concept of autonomy (i.e., the patient's or prospective patient's right to self-determination based on his or her own life plan). Therefore, in cultures where self-determination and individual autonomy and choice play a primary role in day-to-day life, competent and risk-aware adults will favor the execution of medical care directives in advance just as they write wills and employ other strategies, legal and nonlegal, to reduce future risk that their wishes will not be carried out. But thinking about death and dying, suffering, and one's own future incompetence is often so unpleasant or uncomfortable that many people postpone thinking and making decisions about future health care. It is interesting that denial of one's own mortality and the possibility of one's own future suffering occurs in those cultures and individuals who place a strong emphasis on staying in control. Public culture and individual attitudes in Germany seem to represent such a denial of dealing with one's own future dependence, weakness, pain, and suffering. On the other hand, individuals and public culture are characterized by high degrees of self-determination in most all other areas of life. In the older generation, at least, there is a more traditional understanding of the individual person as a part of the family and community, and therefore self-determination must be defined within the constraints and borders of family and community. In such a system, there is less motivation to make advance oral or written statements, as the family or community or the trusted medical professional is customarily trusted to "do the right thing."

However, advance medical directives and the designation of health care representatives are important not only when the principle of autonomy is ranked high. They are also useful to achieve other equally valid principles in good clinical practice such as the facilitating individualized patient-oriented treatment that integrates the patient's values, preferences, and visions into clinical decision making. For example, such principles demand that persons be respected and that treatment be individualized and personal even under the most conservative conceptions of paternalistic benevolence in physicians' ethics. How can a health care provider accurately determine prognosis and therapy if decisions are based solely on clinical and laboratory data and not also on nontechnical personal data of the "patient as a person"?

The contributors to this volume discuss the role and the validity of advance directives in medicine in a transcultural and interdisciplinary debate. First, the legal situations in the three countries—the United States, Germany, and Japan—are different. In the United States, living will forms have been well known for over two decades, the Patient Self-determination Act passed by the U.S. Congress requires hospitals to initiate discussions about advance directives with all patients upon admission, and all but a handful of states have enacted living will statutes (Meisel). There is no such law in Japan, reflecting a general reluctance to legislate issues of professional conduct and responsibility (Kimura). In Germany, various attempts to change the penal code to allow for physician-assisted suicide or euthanasia in terminal cases have been rebuffed. The clouds of Nazi Germany's so-called euthanasia program still weigh heavy on any discussion of end-of-life medical intervention and the withholding of treatment from incompetent persons. Recent court decisions, however, in Germany as well as in Japan have spelled out conditions under which physicians and clinical teams have to recognize preferences and directives previously expressed by the patient (Kimura, Koch). It remains to be seen how much those singular events in the field of law might influence the professional clinical culture or the layperson's willingness to accept advance care documents.

But different cultural and legal traditions are not the only differences that underlie the state of advanced health care planning in the United States, Germany, and Japan. There is also tension between the different professional cultures (such as medicine and law) as well as between professional and individual lay cultures. These tensions are manifest in attitudes toward health and disease, pain and suffering, and death and dying. One may also note distinctions in the extent of lay and professional acceptance of the practice of imposing one's own values on a future dying process, the weight placed on dignity in dying, and the role of medical intervention at the crossroads of life and death.

These differences provide the background for the project that has given rise to this volume. The project resulted from a collaboration among three research centers that focus on legal, ethical, and public policy problems in medicine, including advance planning for terminal illness. The design of the project was to form interdisciplinary research teams in each country drawing on the disciplines of medicine, law, and ethics. For the first phase, the teams from each country would conduct research necessary to provide an account of the medical, legal, and ethical milieu in their country that was shaping the country's attitudes, policies, and practices regarding advanced health care planning for terminal illness. This volume is the result of that research.

Three contributions each from each country—the United States, Germany, and Japan—present the clinician's (Lynn and Teno, Meran and Poliwoda, Ohi), legal expert's (Meisel, Koch, Kimura), and bioethicist's (Veatch, Sass, Tsuchida) review of the respective debate in the author's country. The authors give different, often contrasting, accounts of the role that advance care documents and the recognition of patient autonomy play in the clinical setting in each country.

The chapters also stress the role of law as a prospective instrument to promote "better," more patient-oriented treatment and to prevent senseless and unnecessary life-prolonging suffering at the end of life. As these authors point out, legal forces might also protect vulnerable individuals from being left alone or killed in violation of their human and civil rights and in sharp contrast to the tradition in physician ethics to protect life rather than to take it. In some countries, like Japan, the realm of unwritten law and regulation, rarely of written constructs, for cultural reasons has traditionally been the prime instrument for conflict resolution. At the opposite extreme, a country like the United States turns very readily to the courts and lawyers to solve conflicts of public and professional relations. It is a culture of litigation and rights' claims in which laypeople contemplating their future dying are increasingly willing to put their wishes in legal-sounding documents that are designed to force physicians as a matter of law to conform to the layperson's wishes.

We found Germany often filling an intermediate position, also reflecting the tradition of rights and law, but, at least at this point, not as quick to produce legal documents and litigation as the United States, relying instead on more private communications between health professional and layperson. On the other hand, Germans are not as reluctant as Japanese to convert more traditional approaches into public legal dispute.

We found a similar continuum on the underlying philosophical and ethical principles that provide the foundation for these legal and public policy positions. Japan is a traditional culture still oriented to patterns of familial loyalty and proper status relations. As described so movingly by Tsuchida, the well-being of the patient is the focus, with a community of familial and professional caregivers collaborating in the pursuit of the patient's well-being. Although the patient may not be consulted and certainly has not, at least until very recently, been seen as one demanding his or her rights, all seem to understand that they are in pursuit of a common communal goal.

Again at the opposite extreme, the United States is a country lacking an ancient common culture. In this highly pluralistic mix of people from various religions, cultures, and ideas, the individual has long been given a much more prominent place in the social structure. Liberal individualism, epitomized by the frontier mentality, provides the background for the rise of self-determination, autonomy, and tolerance of diversity as central cultural themes. The replacement of benevolent paternalism with liberal individualism gives rise to a moral system radically different from that of Japan.

Once again, Germany's ethical and philosophical commitments seem intermediary between the two extremes. The concepts of human dignity and self-determination are firmly based in an understanding of right and wrong or, more precisely, in the authoritative powers of systematic law, but notions of respect for traditional professional authority temper the affirmation of individual rights with a lingering reverence for beneficent involvement of health professionals and family in decisions about terminal care planning.

In all three countries there appears to be a shift from traditional nonverbal authority- and trust-based physician beneficence and the blind patient and family compliance toward more open interactions and even written documentation. This includes an increase in the incidence of forms that present rejection of certain treatments under certain conditions. This shift toward an acceptance of such written refusals also includes the designation of trusted proxies to supervise, direct, or refuse expert intervention. It remains to be seen whether generational attitudes will change from more traditional trust and compliance toward autonomy and contractual relationships with legal bindingness as their objective.

The objective of this transnational, transdisciplinary study was not to predict the future. Much less was it to determine which culture has the best legal, public policy, and ethical systems. Rather, it was to understand the systems—their similarities and differences—and their implications for shaping the public policies that will shape the legal and medical world to come.

A common understanding seems to be developing that highly advanced medical technologies cannot and should not be employed without integrating ethical reflections into clinical and public policy decision making. These will rely on instruments of the types that are the focus of this study: uniform, standard living wills that reject terminal illness life support as well as more complex and individualized instructional directives. They will also include directives in which proxy decision makers are named to act for incompetent dying patients and directives that combine instructional and proxy-naming functions. The appendix here includes samples of different forms of advance care planning and directing, from general to specific instructional forms to proxy models, value history schemes, narrative approaches to solicit patients' wishes and preferences, and combination forms. This multicultural review of advance directive forms suggests that there is not and will not be one single best model to morally, medically, or legally ensure that patients are not treated against their interests, values, or visions. Different professional cultures and lay attitudes have shaped and will continue to shape different models. The transdisciplinary and multicultural exchange on the perceived advantages and disadvantages of advance care instruments and of clinical decision making in crucial situations shed some light on the behavior of experts and laypeople in critical professional and lay decision making in medicine and the roles law will play in dealing with issues of death and dying and the care of the incompetent dying patient.

The methods of this research included not only the individual research of the team members included in this volume, but also intense collaboration over a three-year period. The drafts of the chapters were circulated to a team of approximately twenty research participants who met at the Kennedy Institute of Ethics in 1994. Portions of the team met in Tokyo at Waseda University and in Göttingen as guest of Hans-Ludwig Schreiber, president of Göttingen University, for second gatherings later that year, and then in Bochum, Germany, in the summer of 1995 for a final assessment of this phase of the project.

The second phase, which is being presented in various professional medical, legal, and philosophical journals in the English, German, and Japanese languages, is designed to move beyond the clinical, legal, and philosophical studies of the individual countries represented in this volume. That work is being conducted in nine teams that cross both disciplinary and national boundaries. The teams are examining six specific conditions (end-stage renal disease, cancer, HIV, dementias of elderly persons, amyotrophic lateral sclerosis [ALS], as well as healthy people) and the dimensions of the law-medicine relation. This second phase forces the research team to move beyond the national disciplinary perspectives that are analyzed here. This work is published in the *Jahrbuch für Recht und Ethik* (Annual Review of Law and Ethics), vol. 4 (1996). Additional publications will appear in clinical, legal, and philosophical journals.

This research was supported by a grant from the Volkswagen Foundation in the program area on law and attitude. We take this opportunity gratefully to acknowledge the generous support of the Volkswagen Foundation. Many people worked as part of this team. We would especially like to thank Laura Baker, Susanne Eschen, Ashley Fernandes, Moheba Hanif, Naoko Kakee, Arndt May, Kathy McMahon, Isao Morikawa, Hiroto Nagaoka, Kier Olsen, Gudrun Sikora, Katja Stiegel, and Sr. Marcia Uddoh for their vital participation in various phases of the project.

Part 1

United States

1

A Care Provider Perspective on Advance Directives and Surrogate Decision Making for Incompetent Adults in the United States

JOANNE LYNN, M.D., M.A., M.S.
JOAN TENO, M.D., M.S.

Characteristic Cases

Advance care planning and surrogate decision making for incompetent adults raise issues in a wide variety of clinical settings. We introduce the issues with two cases that are difficult and common and with two other cases that are quite rare but also illuminating. The common cases include one concerning an incompetent patient with a standard form of living will and one concerning an initially competent patient declining into a predictable state of incompetence with inadequate communication in advance. Both of these cases involve considerations of the appropriate role of the family. The third case involves a patient in a persistent vegetative state with a standard living will, in which an issue arises over tube feeding. The fourth case portrays the problem of discerning when others should overrule a written advance directive. The brief discussion after each case highlights important elements. References to empirical information in the literature are included in the second section.

The Case of the Living Will

Mr. P., a 76-year-old man living at home with his wife of many years, had gradually become quite forgetful, cognitively disabled, immobile, and dysarthric (unable to speak clearly) from the effects of severe supranuclear palsy (a form of neurological impairment related to Parkinson's disease, but with more severe cognitive disability). His awareness and ability to communicate fluctuated, such that sometimes he was able to enjoy family visits and to articulate that he knew he was dying and that he was a burden to his wife (which she countered with claims that he was still her joy and gave her life meaning). He had no understanding of his illness or decisions about his living arrangements. Ten years ago, he and his wife completed standard form living wills obtained at a meeting at their Catholic church. Two days ago, he had a most unusual bowel movement, being a dark maroon color with an unusual odor and consistency. His wife also felt that he was less attentive and called the home care nurse to evaluate him. An initial assessment revealed that he was having lower gastrointestinal tract bleeding, had developed a substantial but not critical anemia, and had no other obvious abnormalities on his chemistry tests and chest X-rays, which were taken at home. He was comfortable, without abdominal pain or shortness of breath.

The physician recommended hospitalization for evaluation and transfusion. The home care nurse discussed the options with Mrs. P., who was reticent to go against the physician's advice but was also uncomfortable with the prospect of having Mr. P. go to the hospital. On the basis of past experience, she pointed out that he often had done quite poorly in hospitals (and so had she). She claimed tearfully that hospitals "are just death houses with no one caring." She also asked what good it would do, for "surely he is going to die soon: why should he have to go through hospitalization on top of what he already faces?"

Then she noted that he had already signed a paper that should make his views clear. She couldn't remember exactly what it said, but she was sure she could find it. They hadn't talked about it since the day they signed their set of papers. It took many hours of looking through old papers, but she did find the old living will with its standard language: "If . . . the situation should arise in which there is no reasonable expectation of my recovery from extreme physical or mental disability, I direct that I be allowed to die and not be kept alive by medications, artificial means or heroic measures."

The next day, the home care nurse noted that the wife had seemed ambivalent about what to do before finding this old and nearly forgotten paper but now seemed more resolved not to allow hospitalization. The nurse called the physician and discussed the situation. The physician was annoyed and talked with Mrs. P. on the phone. He laid out the likely situation that the source of bleeding could be found and treated, returning Mr. P. to his comfortable existence until the supranuclear palsy led to some fatal complication. Mrs. P. said that it just did not make sense to put him through all this, that he was going to die anyway, and that he would not want anything done and had said so in this paper he had signed.

The physician pointed out that it was not clear that the paper addressed this situation, since it was not clear that he was terminally ill or that the diagnostic procedures and treatments that would be needed could be what was meant by "artificial means." Furthermore, the physician replied that Mr. P. could hardly have foreseen the situation ten years ago, when he was not even diagnosed with a serious illness. In sum, the physician contended that the living will was irrelevant. Mrs. P. was almost worn down but asked to think about it overnight.

At about ten o'clock, Mr. P. had a seizure, which terrified his wife. She could not reach the physician or the home care nursing service right away, so she called the emergency medical service. They found him obtunded, called the physician, and transported him to the hospital.

At the hospital emergency room his obtundation cleared, but his usual cognitive dysfunction remained. The physician insisted that he be hospitalized, and Mrs. P. did not object. However, she did insist on showing the house staff her husband's living will. The admitting resident wrote an order to forgo resuscitation (Do Not Resuscitate, or DNR) and noted in the medical record that "Patient is DNR because he has a living will."

The attending physician was furious when he reviewed the medical record, saying that the living will had nothing to do with a DNR order. The DNR order was rescinded, still without conversation with patient or family. After two weeks of hospitalization with various complications, Mr. P. was sent home. He was weaker, more confused, and less mobile. There was no clarification of the meaning of his living will and no development of a coherent plan for his care as he worsened.

DISCUSSION. In most settings, less than one-quarter of seriously ill or elderly persons complete formal advance directives. Those who do usually have no more insight and counsel than did Mr. and Mrs. P. Thus, there is routinely a gap between the intent of the patient and what is instructed within the written document, and another gap between what is written and the patient's actual situation.

When serious and progressively fatal illness arises, caregivers sometimes interpret the presence of a living will in seriously incorrect ways—either as irrelevant to decision making about resuscitation or as determinative that resuscitation should not be tried, for example. All too commonly, decision making proceeds without the active involvement of the patient or family, with or without a written directive. In fact, the decision to forgo resuscitation is most commonly made in the last few days before death, without direct communication with the patient, and often without knowledgeable communication with the family or surrogate.

A DNR order seems to function within our health care rituals just as last rites once did—as a marker of the fact that all concerned now see death as unavoidable. Its function as a tool of advance care planning is often quite trivial.

In comparison to its symbolic importance this case illuminates the ordinary mix of merit and uncertainty surrounding the use of formal advance directives and the inadequacies of the usual decision-making practices in ordinary cases.

The Case of Opportunities Lost

Miss R. came to the emergency room after her first seizure at age 38. A work-up disclosed minor but persistent focal neurological deficits, and a CT scan disclosed a neoplasm affecting the right frontal lobe. Surgery found a poorly differentiated astrocytoma that could not be completely removed. Radiation was undertaken in due course, and her functioning and symptoms remained tolerably good for many months. However, the tumor eventually began to cause progressively worse headaches, neurological dysfunctions, and sometimes diminished alertness. She developed severe side effects from steroids given to alleviate these symptoms. Her family was somewhat alienated by her discomfort and troubling appearance. Seizures recurred and became very worrisome, requiring drugs with substantial side effects in order to maintain some control.

After about a year, she became completely disabled and spent most of the days in bed. She seemed fairly comfortable, usually (but not always) recognized family, and often was able to point out immediate needs (bedpan, water to drink, repositioning, and so forth). The physician raised the question of whether it would be helpful to enroll her in a hospice program. After some investigation of the funding and services, her parents, who had become her primary caregivers, decided that a hospice program would be an advantage. The physician then informed them that enrolling in hospice required having a DNR order as well as his certifying that she had less than six months to live. This was the first time that they had heard the prognosis so clearly, and the first time that a DNR order had been discussed. However, they listened and did not object, and hospice services began.

When she began to be unable to swallow reliably, her parents called the hospice nurse anxiously wanting a feeding tube placed (being familiar with these devices from caring for an elderly relative who used one after a stroke). They were quite disconcerted to find that the hospice nurse felt that no artificial feeding was warranted. In fact, she pointed out that not being able to take steroids would probably accelerate death, which would be a good thing. The parents went along with the advice, though they were not clearly in accord with it. At this point, the parents noted that it would be much easier to make these decisions if they could only be more confident that Miss R. would have agreed with their choices. Miss R. died three weeks later at home.

Never in the course of her illness did the patient ask for, or did the physician offer, a prognosis about survival or about the course of functional decline. Never did her parents or physician ask about her preferences, her view of what characterized a good dying process, or even about what she would most like to avoid. The course of the illness was fairly predictable, and the care given would seem to be generally acceptable. However, there is no way to know whether the choices made reflected the patient's preferences, or even whether she preferred her parents to make them once she became incompetent. Moreover, her parents made treatment decisions largely through mere acquiescence to the physician's and nurse's recommendations.

DISCUSSION. Even with a predictably fatal illness that almost always robs the patient of mental competence for a substantial period before death, it is uncommon for advance plans to be made regarding the care to be implemented when key decisions arise later. As this patient came to terms with the recurrence of her illness and the effects of treatment, it would have been fairly easy to engage her in conversation about what she feared most, what she thought would happen, and what she hoped for. The responses would have provided the framework of an ongoing discussion that would have enabled her to offer direction regarding which parts of the course of her care were of particular importance to her, both contemporaneously and prospectively.

This guidance from the patient might have been determinative just by being understood by the physician and family, might also have been documented by the physician in the medical record, or might even have been written in a formal advance directive. How to ensure adherence to her views is a question that turns on the patient's preferences for control, the degree to which choices are unusual (and therefore the degree to which they are likely to be challenged), the prevailing medical practices and state law, and the availability of more formal methods of specifying preferences. However, a well-understood patient choice about a course of care should be able to be implemented without any formal documentation.

The Case of Persistent Coma and Tube Feeding

Mrs. C. was 48 years old when she had an apparent heart attack on the subway and was brought to a hospital emergency room, awake, scared, and uncomfortable. An electrocardiogram suggested the diagnosis of acute anterior wall myocardial infarction. The patient's heart went into ventricular fibrillation, and she was eventually resuscitated but not until after twenty minutes of chest compressions.

Although the other complications of the resuscitation and the underlying heart attack were resolved over the ensuing three weeks, her consciousness never returned. A neurologist diagnosed her as being in a persistent vegetative state, and her family was informed as to the likely course of her health and the dismal prognosis for any recovery of cognition or sentience. Mrs. C. was transferred to a nursing home in the fifth hospital week. She was fed by feeding tube, had a permanent tracheostomy, and required total care. Some family members still thought that she was aware, but her husband had gradually accepted the physician's opinion.

After two months, Mr. C. asked the physician now attending her at the nursing home what would happen if the feeding tube or the tracheostomy were removed. He was told that removing the tracheostomy tube had been shown to lead to coughing and severe wheezing, but that removing the feeding tube would probably just result in gradual wasting away, since she could not swallow, thereby leading to her death. Mr. C. felt that this latter course offered the best available outcome. He did some reading in the library about more well-known cases like that of Nancy Cruzan and talked with family members. Then he asked the physician to remove the feeding tube and let her die.

The physician felt that this was an acceptable course, especially now that it was almost six months since her cardiac arrest and there had been no return of neurological function. However, he and Mr. C. soon found an array of formidable forces opposing the proposed course of removing the feeding tube. The nurses and aides at the nursing home included many who opposed, based on such grounds as their lack of belief that the patient was actually insentient, their sense that not feeding her was outrageous and inhumane, and their conviction that there were many others in their nursing home who were in far poorer shape and would be at risk of the same treatment plan. The nursing home called its corporate lawyer who pointed out that this could cause adverse publicity and that state law might be read to require that the patient herself had requested this course before it could be implemented. In fact, the lawyer contended that the husband might have to become the court-appointed guardian in order to have any authority at all (despite the fact that his decisions had been accepted throughout her care, including consent to tracheostomy, to endoscopic placement of the feeding tube, and to institutionalization in the nursing home).

Eventually, Mr. C. had to take his case to court; he obtained guardianship but was denied the authority to withdraw the feeding tube because he could not show that Mrs. C. would clearly have preferred this withdrawal. Very frustrated, he spoke out in the media, often in direct opposition to her nursing home caregivers. An old friend saw this on local television and realized that she might have some helpful information. She called Mr. C. to relate that she and Mrs. C. had gone to a Ladies' Circle at church at which formal advance directives were discussed and that both of them had filled out living wills. She offered to help go through papers to see if a copy could be found. Mrs. C. had never mentioned this event to Mr. C., others in her family, or her physician. However, it turned out that she had mentioned it to a few coworkers over lunch one day, saying that she "hoped never to end up like that poor Quinlan girl." The living will was not found until years later (when it was discovered that she had inexplicably drawn a line through a standard phrase about forgoing artificial feeding if permanently unconscious), but the statements of the witnesses were enough to convince a judge that the initial denial of authority to withdraw the feeding tube had been in error. Mr. C. was granted the authority to withdraw the feeding tube after nearly a year of court-induced delay.

At this juncture, Mr. C. tried to move her to some other institution whose staff was less opposed to withdrawing the feeding tube and discovered that no such institution would come forward. After nearly another year, he decided to take her home, found a hospice nurse who was willing to help, and cared for her at home until she died about ten days later.

DISCUSSION. Persistent vegetative state is quite rare, probably affecting fewer than ten thousand persons a year in the United States (PCEMR 1983). However, it is a uniquely illuminating and troubling conceptual conundrum. The patient is alive but without any further experience. In a sense, the patient's own interests are comparable to what they would be if the patient were dead: reasonably dignified treatment, respect for the memory of the patient, disposition of estate, and concern for well-being of kith and kin. Most court cases and commentators see little reason to treat such patients in order to extend life. However, implementing such a plan can be quite difficult, as is shown in this case.

The role of the family is quite troubling in these cases. The families do, unavoidably, feel the impact of the costs of care, the prolonged limbo of having neither a death nor a life, the uncertainty over the guilt in "causing" a death if treatment is forgone, and the need to evidence allegiance to the severely disabled loved one. However, many of these issues are marginalized or unacceptable in the usual decision-making process, which is structured around advancing the interests of the patient (who has no such interests in a case of persistent vegetative state). Although the courts have the power to intervene and to rule on the issue, they usually cannot be sensitive to the issues that most of the community feels have become important—the interests and roles of the family.

Furthermore, the fragility and lack of clarity of evidence about the patient's wishes is common, even though these preferences are taken to be so important. Living wills are incomplete, uncounseled, lost, or otherwise difficult to apply. Recollections of witnesses are at risk of being shaped by a desire to bring about certain outcomes of situations. Was some of the recollection of the witnesses shaped by what they thought was at stake? Under the Cruzan ruling (*Cruzan* 1990), the courts can require a "clear and convincing" standard of evidence, rather than the more usual probate standard of "preponderance of the evidence." This might preclude forgoing tube feeding when the patient's own views are not well established, though the merits of that policy have been the subject of much dispute.

Many states have made a special issue of the choice to use or forgo feeding tubes, sometimes requiring that this issue be addressed specifically by the patient in a written advance directive; otherwise withdrawal is prohibited. This is problematic, since avoiding withdrawal prolongs some unwarranted suffering. These laws also have the effect of causing decisions not to initiate for fear that withdrawal at a later point will prove to be difficult.

The Case of a Potentially Erroneous Advance Directive

Mrs. B. was hospitalized with an apparently serious stroke. Her daughter came with her to the emergency room and presented a written living will that said that she did not want "artificial means" used to "prolong life." She had handwritten on the preprinted page the following instructions: "I want everything possible done to keep me alive as long as possible, except that I do not ever want to be put on a breathing machine or oxygen or forced feeding." The daughter interpreted this to mean that her mother would not want attempts at resuscitation but would want anything else that might enhance the chances for survival. However, when she saw that the emergency room staff had put her mother on oxygen and were preparing to intubate her (to protect the airway), she objected: "My mother specifically prohibited that!"

The physician in charge managed to have the daughter escorted away and proceeded to intubate and otherwise to stabilize the patient's medical situation. Then the physician talked with the now-distraught daughter. Wisely, the conversation was initiated with a validation of the daughter's role and importance and the possibility of reversing the treatments already initiated if doing so seemed warranted after clarifying the patient's own preferences. The physician asked the daughter to describe her mother's life and its recent course, then asked her to explain the living will and how it had come to be. It turned out that the patient had bought the living will form at a stationery store, apparently just noticing it while waiting to pay for something else. The daughter remembered her mother writing in the extra line after having seen a television movie that led her to feel that this would be a good idea. As far as the daughter knew, her mother had never talked with anyone about what she meant or what she thought the completed living will would achieve.

The physician pointed out that some of the instructions were in conflict (everything to prolong life in direct contradiction to the preprinted "no artificial means to extend life" language and the specific prohibition of a breathing machine). At least one request was difficult to make into a reasonable directive (forgoing oxygen). The admonition to refuse "forced feeding" seemed ambiguous—neither the daughter nor the physician could know if she meant to emphasize the coercion aspects or whether the patient had meant to include all artificial feeding. The daughter gradually saw the difficult position that the uncounseled advance directive form had created for those responsible for her mother's treatment. She proposed that all concerned proceed with making decisions as if the form did not exist. The physician modified this to say that he and the daughter would collaborate in making all decisions and that they would use whatever insights they could from the form or any other evidence of the patient's preferences.

This worked well for the initial treatment. After a few days, it was clear that the patient was not going to be able to swallow safely, though whether this was permanent or temporary was unclear. The patient's mentation had cleared a little, but she could not speak and seemed to have substantial expressive aphasia (confusion over language) as well as dysarthria (inability to speak clearly). The daughter and physician decided that they simply had to disregard whatever might have been meant by the admonition to avoid forced feeding. The patient fought the tube insertion and fretted with the tube all the time. She wriggled out of it from time to time. However, it could not be clear whether she really objected or just responded to momentary annoyances.

At this point, the daughter noted that the patient had converted to the Christian Scientist faith in the last few years, more recently than the date on her living will. The daughter was not sure whether this would mean that her mother would not want any medical treatment utilized.

DISCUSSION. Courts and commentators have contended that written advance directives are of substantially greater weight than are less formally communicated decisions and preferences. Nevertheless, a written advance directive must be susceptible to being overruled in some circumstances. In this case, multiple rationales exist for overruling the written directive: incoherence of the instructions, possible incompatibility of the instructions with later preferences, unreasonableness of the directive, and uncertainty about the intention behind the directive. The procedures for overruling apparently valid advance directives are quite unclear. A judge can always hear arguments and, in light of the particular circumstances, rule as to the degree to which the directive should be followed. However, most cases are not going to allow the time, financial costs, and public spectacle entailed in formal adjudication.

Discussion has begun about the proper procedures and justifications for a less formal framework for advance directives, within which there is room for interpretation or overruling. Clearly, mere irregularities in the formal execution (improper witnesses, not dated, etc.) should not be held to invalidate the advance directive. However, incoherent instructions usually warrant invalidation. Lack of conformity to the patient's long-held values or to statements by the patient documented in other ways should raise a concern, but the weight of the evidence will have to be assessed. Thoroughly unreasonable advance directives probably can be ignored, but one must be careful about the standard for unreasonableness. The directive would have to offend the sensibilities of almost everyone or otherwise be so aberrant that virtually no reasonable person could envision circumstances in which it would make sense.

Review of the Literature: Advance Directives

Ethics consultants attending the 1991 meeting of the Society of Bioethics Consultants answered a survey about life-sustaining treatment of patients in a persistent vegetative state. Fox and Stocking (1993), reporting on the results, note a "surprising" lack of consensus on treatment decisions for seven scenarios in which the instructions in an advance directive and family agreement with the directive varied. For example, when the directive stated that the person did not desire life-sustaining treatment and the family wanted "everything to be done," consultants were split evenly as to whether to honor the patient's preferences. This division occurred despite several prestigious organizations having released guidelines on decision making for incompetent persons in a persistent vegetative state that emphasize respecting the patient's views as expressed by an advance directive (President's Commission 1983; Council on Scientific Affairs of AMA 1990; Hastings Center 1987; Institute of Medical Ethics 1991). Does this lack of accord imply inadequacy of the dominant ethics model for medical decision making (which ignores family preference), a dysfunction of the consultants (who do not always defend the patient's interests), or some other concern?

Over the latter half of this century, the fundamental claim of American medical ethics has been that optimal medical decisions are those that are expected to achieve the best possible outcome as judged by the patient (Hastings Center 1987; Lynn and DeGrazia 1991). In the stirring words of Justice Cardozo (*Schloendorff* 1914), "Every human being of adult years and sound mind has a right to determine what shall be done with his body." Especially for decisions at the end of life, patient preferences are important because reasonable persons will differ on the desirability of various outcomes correlative to different care plans. Indeed, some persons view certain outcomes as states worse than death. For example, many people prefer death over the use of life-sustaining treatment that causes or prolongs suffering.

Most adults are not "of sound mind" when decisions about life-sustaining treatments are utilized, foregone, or withdrawn. Over the past three decades, this society has struggled with how decision making should proceed for a previously competent patient for whom a fairly serious decision must be made. The resulting standard calls on caregivers, family, and sometimes the courts to reconstruct the patient's likely decision (Coordinating Council 1991). That is, the decision for the person in a persistent vegetative state should be the one that the patient would choose if he or she could miraculously awaken and state his or her preferences and values. Varying with the scope and certainty of evidence as to what the now incompetent patient would want, Buchanan and Brock (1989) advise that decision making for those with impaired decision-making capacity should be guided by (1) the advance directive principle (when the patient has spoken about the issue clearly), (2) the substituted judgment principle (when there is good evidence as to what the patient would have wanted based on previous statements and values but not a clear advance directive), or (3) the best interests principle (when too little individuating evidence about this particular patient is available). We examine the empirical evidence that addresses the application of these principles to surrogate decision making for incompetent patients. Our discussion focuses on the implications of current empirical research for the theory and practice of decision making for incompetent adults, both those with and those without a written advance directive.

Use of the Advance Directive Principle

Advance directives arose out of the public outcry against the employment of burdensome medical technology. Luis Kutner (1969) proposed the "living will" in response to the case of a son who fatally shot his cancer-stricken mother who requested his aid in dying. A living will is the most common kind of instructional advance directive; it allows a person to state treatment preferences in advance of a period of incompetence. The living will started as a document that stated preferences to forgo life-sustaining treatments if the person writing the document were in a permanent state of unconsciousness or suffering from a terminal illness. The other major form of written advance directives names a proxy who is authorized to act as a surrogate decision maker for the patient. Examples include the standard durable power of attorney and the health care proxy, who is specifically authorized only to make health care decisions. One document can both provide instruction and name a decision maker. Recent directives have sometimes encouraged patients to indicate treatment preferences given hypothetical scenarios, for example, the medical directive (Emanuel and Emanuel 1992), or to provide detailed documentation of preferences and values, such as the values history (Gibson 1990), which provides advice for the named proxy about what the patient would choose if he or she were able to do so.

Determining how best to make decisions for persons who cannot voice their own views has been problematic, since we are rightly suspicious of anyone's authority to speak on behalf of another. For the now incompetent patient, an advance directive attempts to re-create the moral authority of contemporaneous decision making accorded to a competent patient by having that person state preferences in advance. If this can be achieved, it would be wise to encourage the widespread use of written directives, because it would directly and neatly clarify how decisions should be made for incompetent persons. Indeed, the Patient Self-determination Act (PSDA) mandated that all patients admitted to acute care hospitals, long-term care facilities, health maintenance organizations, and home care programs must be informed of their rights under state law to participate in medical decisions and to formulate written directives.

Empirical Evidence Required to Support the Advance Directive Principle

Good policy not only is based on sound theoretical reasoning but must also rely on effective implementation, which would require evidence that the following claims are true.

1. Individuals desire to participate in discussions about future medical decisions and are willing to write advance directives.
2. These individuals will be willing to communicate with surrogates and providers so that preferences and values are clearly stated (whether written or oral).
3. Preferences noted in the documents are valid, enduring, and important in shaping medical decision making.
4. Treatment decisions can reflect these preferences.
5. Achieving the above will end up benefiting the patient, from the patient's perspective.

The truth of each of these claims is subject to empirical evaluation in actual decision-making situations. Very little evaluation of this kind has been done, and what has been reported often raises concerns as to the validity of these key contentions.

Are Patients Willing to Make Health Care Decisions in Advance?

Despite widespread media attention and the mandatory educational intervention of the PSDA, the majority of seriously ill patients do not have a written advance directive (Teno et al. 1997a; Emanuel et al. 1994). For these patients, decisions are usually made by informal mechanisms such as family collaborating with a physician or other health care provider to make decisions, generally reflective of a substituted judgment or best interests principle. An intervention that relied on physician counseling (Schneiderman et al. 1992) resulted in two of every three patients completing a directive, whereas a mass mailing of an educational booklet resulted in less than one in five patients creating a written directive (Rubin et al. 1994). Few health care decisions are likely to be guided by clearly written advance directives, leaving many decisions to a surrogate applying either the substituted judgment principle or best interests principle.

To date, limited research has examined patients' desires to discuss advance care planning. Most persons note that they want to be involved in medical decisions (Emanuel et al. 1991; Teno et al. 1990; Gamble, McDonald, and Lichstein 1991). Yet, in the case of hospitalized patients surveyed about whether they wanted to discuss resuscitation with their physicians, researchers found that only one in two wanted to discuss CPR (Frankl, Oye, and Bellamy 1989). Perceived barriers to discussion about advance care planning include physicians not initiating the conversation, the belief that directives are only relevant for the old and sick, patients not wanting to discuss the topic, and a desire that decision making be based on the guidance of family members rather than on a written directive (High 1993a; Emanuel et al. 1991; Elder et al. 1992). Based on his surveys of the decision-making preferences of older subjects in Kentucky, High proposed that policy should be changed to endorse automatic delegation of surrogate health decision-making authority to family members (High 1993a). However, there is no authoritative answer to the question of whether patients could be moved to make important health care decisions in advance.

Do Directives Provide Clearly Stated Instructions?

In order to be effective, directives must be written with an understanding of what the decision entails, take into account the impact of alternative choices on the patient, and be communicated effectively. What counsel do patients receive about their advance care planning? Do persons discuss their directives with their named proxy or their health care providers? Studies to date raise concerns regarding whether the process of completing a written directive is based on adequate communication between the person completing the directive and surrogates or health care providers, both before crafting the directive, in order to shape it adequately, and after completing the directive, in order to ensure that it is interpreted correctly (Teno et al. 1990; Yellen, Burton, and Elpern 1992).

Similar concerns are noted about the degree to which written directives provide additional information that actually shapes medical decision making. In a review of 638 written directives placed in the medical record since the PSDA became law, we have found that only 13 percent of documents provided additional specific information beyond naming a surrogate or stating the preferences noted in a standard living will (Teno et al. 1997c). Thirty-six directives (less than 1 percent) continued specific instructions about the use of life-sustaining treatments, and only 22 voiced a preference to forgo life-sustaining treatments in the patient's current situation.

Are Preferences Stated in Directives Valid and Enduring?

Everyone is familiar with preferences changing as situations change. Reasonably, one might be concerned that preferences of relatively healthy patients anticipating illness may not be the same as those patients have when actually ill. Thus, one must be concerned as to whether preferences or instructions noted by competent patients in advance directives are applicable during a period of incompetence that is also marked by much more serious illness. Beyond conflicting anecdotes, there is very little evidence on this issue.

An important limitation of the validity of preferences about care is to what extent health care providers and patients discuss the patients' preferences and values noted in the directive and the degree to which future medical decisions can be anticipated. Brett (1991) has pointed out that checklists of "intervention-focused directives" may lead to inconsistent responses. In a pilot survey of persons attending a workshop on advance directives, Forrow and colleagues (1991) found that 10 of 29 respondents stated both that they "never want to be on a respirator in an intensive care unit" and "If a short period of extremely intensive medical care could return me to near normal condition, I would want it." The creators of the medical directive note that inconsistencies occur about 1 percent of the time (Emanuel and Emanuel 1993). Of course, a health care provider can probably reconcile these inconsistencies with an informative discussion. How often such discussion occurs and how successful it is have not been examined.

A preference may be valid at time of counseling; however, whether it represents an enduring and deeply held conviction bears important relevance to theory and policy regarding decision making for incompetents. Preferences may be insubstantial, transitory, or both. Some patients may hold their treatment preference with deepest conviction and little leeway, whereas others desire that family have great latitude in decision making (Sehgal et al. 1992; Lynn 1991). Research that examines endurance of preferences shows only moderate stability, with change occurring in both directions (Emanuel et al. 1994; Everhart and Pearlman 1990; Silverstein et al. 1991). These studies have not examined the degree to which preferences are stable when appropriately counseled by a health care provider. If a previously voiced preference remains only moderately stable or a person's intent is that surrogates should have discretion in interpreting the directive, the implied lexical ordering of the advance directive guidance principle over the substituted judgment and best interests principle should be reconsidered.

Do Advance Directives Affect Decision Making or Outcomes?

Advance directives will be of limited value unless they improve both the process of decision making and patient outcomes. Research that has examined the impact of written advance directives suggests a rather limited impact on end-of-life decision making. Schneiderman et al. (1992) conducted a randomized trial of physician counseling about advance directives and the placing of that directive on the medical record for each hospital admission. They found virtually no impact on decision making (e.g., the medical treatments provided at the end of life), patient outcomes (e.g., satisfaction, well-being, health related quality of life), and societal outcomes (e.g., cost of care). However, in this study, most of the patients retained decision-making capacity up until the time of death. In only three patients' cases was implementation of advance directives really appropriate.

In an observational study of decision making in seriously ill patients in the two years before and the two years after the PSDA became law (the Study to Understand Prognoses and Preferences for Outcomes and Risks of Treatments, or SUPPORT), we have examined the impact of written advance directives on the process of decision making (e.g., documentation of preferences for resuscitation or information about the directive in the permanent medical record, interview report of discussion about CPR), actual decisions made (e.g., timing and whether there is decision to forgo resuscitation), patient outcomes (e.g., survival to hospital discharge, having a DNR order, intensity of treatment), and societal outcomes (e.g., hospital charges and hospital length of stay) (Teno et al. 1997b). Similar to Schneiderman et al. (1992), we found that advance directives did not have clinically relevant impact on treatments. After enactment of the PSDA, fewer than one of every three subjects who reported having a written advance directive ordinarily had documentation about that directive in the medical record. Unlike Schneiderman's study, about one-third of our patients were comatose or intubated in their first week of hospitalization, and nearly one in four subjects died on that hospital admission. Despite SUPPORT patients' being very ill and often incompetent, advance directives had no discernible effect.

Chambers and colleagues (1994) found that among 474 Medicare beneficiaries who died at a university hospital, 132 subjects had documentation of discussion about advance directives in the first three days. These patients who had early discussion of advance directives noted in the medical record had one-third of the hospital costs of those without such documentation (see also Weeks et al. 1994). SUPPORT yielded a marked contrast to this. Advanced directives in SUPPORT had no correlation with costs, once virtually all advance directives were documented (Teno et al. 1997b).

These preliminary results highlight the need for further understanding of current practices about written directives (e.g., whether directives are ignored, whether preferences shape decision making, whether communication occurs) and the degree that written directives impact other outcomes (e.g., the sharing of power in decision making and decisions to forgo hospitalization). Decision making that relies solely on surrogate input without any specific instructions needs to be compared with decision making that relies upon patient-stated instructions in advance.

Review of the Literature: Surrogate Decision Making

Conditions for Effective Surrogate Decision Making

Because most Americans will not have made a decision, much less have written an advance directive, that applies to the situation they face when sick and incompetent, decision making for previously competent patients will often rely on decisions made in conjunction with kith and kin. Judicial rulings and clinical practice have generally turned to family members to collaborate in medical decisions for the incompetent patient. Indeed, when the PSDA required states to articulate their state law, 35 states addressed the role of family in decision making (Teno et al. 1997a). Almost all states favored the informal practice of turning to families, often even when there was no clear state law or judicial rulings. Justifications for reliance on family in decision making include (1) that families are most concerned for the patient's welfare, (2) that they are most likely to be knowledgeable about the patient's preferences and values, and (3) that the family is an important social unit that intrinsically merits a sphere of privacy and autonomy into which states should be reluctant to intrude (President's Commission 1983). Of course, some patients do not have a family or any other potential surrogate. Decision making for this group follows no assured guidelines and has not been studied. The sections below summarize research concerning decision making with a previously competent patient, now incompetent, who has a natural surrogate decision maker.

The reliance on surrogates for decision making has come under close scrutiny. Emanuel and Emanuel (1992) recommend that policy should not trust informal surrogates. Instead, patients should complete comprehensive instruction directives and name a proxy. Otherwise, population-based databases about preferences should be developed to guide decision making for incompetent persons without advance directives. Those who question the role of proxy decision makers note that the following conditions need to be met before one can rely upon surrogates:

1. A surrogate has to be willing to participate in decision making.

2. The surrogate has to be able to reflect on knowledge about the patient so that decisions reflect the patient's preferences.

3. Decisions must be made without undue influence of financial impact, pressure from the emotional burdens of caregiving, or pressure from the victimizing behavior of dysfunctional families.

4. Reliance on surrogates must result in better outcomes for the patient as the patient would reasonably be thought to evaluate them (in comparison with alternate public policies, such as uniform decisions based on a given condition or assigning public guardians as decision makers).

Are Proxies Willing to Participate in Decision Making?

Some contend that asking a loved one to participate in end-of-life decision making is too much of a burden to impose on an individual and that health care providers should protect the surrogate from this burden. Others have felt that this sort of "burden" is what defines a family. The overwhelming empirical evidence is that families do participate in decisions to forgo resuscitation as well as other life-sustaining treatments (Bedell et al. 1986; Evans and Brody 1985; Jonsson, McNamee, and Campion 1988; Smedira et al. 1990). Whether doing so is a benefit or burden and whether the responsibility could be adapted appropriately to match the surrogate's capabilities have not been studied.

Are Surrogates Able to Present Patient Preferences?

With or without written directives, people do not often discuss their preferences and values with their families, even about end-of-life care (Harvey and Shubat 1989; Gamble et al. 1991). Responses to survey questions about hypothetical situations have shown that surrogates often are unable to replicate their patients' responses. The answers are usually not much better than random guesses based on the population's prior probabilities would be. Some feel that this provides strong evidence to question the moral authority of surrogates (Hare and Nelson 1992; Ouslander et al. 1989; Seckler et al. 1991; Uhlmann, Pearlman, and Cain 1988). Before endorsing this interpretation, one must recognize that these studies involve patients who do not actually face the decision in question and have not had discussion and counseling about end-of-life decision making. Furthermore, the moral authority of surrogates might not lie in their ability to predict the patients' choices but in the patients' preferences for contemporaneous decision making by family members, rather than reliance on advance directives. Lynn et al. (1994), High (1993b), and Seghal (1992) have shown that many older persons would want their family to make decisions (rather than adhering to advance directives) and that individuals ordinarily want leeway to be given to a surrogate in interpreting preferences.

Do Surrogate Biases Influence Decision Making?

The case of the nefarious family member is often used as the textbook example of patients being harmed by a surrogate's conflict of interest. Yet there are little empirical data examining how often such cases arise or how serious a risk the conflict of interest presents. Ethics committees do encounter these cases of surrogates with questionable intent (LaPuma 1988). However, the rate is not clear and would seem to be quite low. These cases may well be the exception to the rule that most families will take on tremendous burden to themselves in order to help a loved one. Given that decisions are made jointly between health care provider and surrogate, clinicians are responsible for ensuring that (1) there is no serious conflict of interest or history of abuse, (2) decisions are consistent with what is known about the patient's values and preferences, and (3) choices are made within medically sound alternatives (Buchanan and Brock 1989). It may well be the case that these protections and the risks of retrospective prosecution for decisions made abusively are sufficient.

Does Surrogate Decision Making Result in Good Outcomes?

No studies of the decision-making process and patient outcomes specifically address the role of participation by informal surrogates, which would especially need to be contrasted with decision making in cases with advance directives and in cases with court authority. Schneiderman et al. (1992) found no discernible merit in relying upon physician counseling on advance directives, as compared with customary decision making which is usually based on the guidance of surrogates. Reliance on the courts can result in great delays in decision making, but no comparison among the merits of courts, advance directives, and informal family decision making has been made.

Resolving the Case: Persistent Vegetative State with a Conflict between the Advance Directive and the Surrogate

Should it be disconcerting that bioethics consultants differ on the management of the patient in a persistent vegetative state who has written a directive that articulates a preference to forgo life-sustaining treatment and has a family who desires that "everything be done?" Existing guidelines tend to endorse following a written directive but do not strongly proscribe attending to the family's preferences (President's Commission 1983; Council on Scientific Affairs 1990; Hastings Center 1987; Institute of Medical Ethics 1991; Coordinating Council 1991). The Appleton International Conference on guidelines for forgoing life-sustaining treatment notes that "where a patient has lost capacity to make decisions but has given a valid advance directive to refuse treatment and/or has appointed a representative to make decisions about refusal of treatment, such directives and decisions should be respected by doctors and other health-care workers" (Stanley 1992, 6). "Respect" might be a word used to indicate that the directive should be followed. However, it might also mean that the directive should usually be followed but that family and other considerations might make the proper course more difficult to discern and might justify the consideration of other factors.

For example, a written directive should have substantial moral weight only if stated preferences are based on effective communication between health care provider and patient about the nature of possible treatments and outcomes and if the situation envisioned in the written directive is reasonably similar to the one that the patient now faces. Guidelines must give due consideration to the process of decision making. The clinician would have to be blind to human realities to view the patient as an "island to himself" without acknowledging the important role of families. Families shape the possibilities for outcomes and the context of their interpretation. The clinician faced with a conflict between a patient's advance directive and the surrogate's preferences should have an obligation to undertake a process of communication with family members to understand their interpretation of the directive and their concerns and to provide the necessary emotional support. The family's interests might be sufficient to take precedence over the stated preferences of the patient. For example, a patient who asked to be allowed to die unattended might have a family whose self-respect entails attending to the dying person. None of these issues has benefited from descriptive research or ethical commentary.

A clinician might be inclined to comply with a family request rather than an advance directive because the family is more likely to litigate (in order to enforce their preference or to punish those whose actions were contrary). Although such litigation seems both rare and rarely successful and compliance with an advance directive gains a certain degree of immunity from litigation under law, it remains the case that the surviving family has some authority to interpret or question an advance directive that may overcome the advocacy of clinicians caring for a dying patient.

Surrogate Decision Making at the Crossroads

Tremendous strides have been made in the past several decades in improving decision making for incompetent adults. Only twenty years ago, hospitalized patients did not often merely die, but they died after a failed resuscitation attempt, with full efforts to rectify all physiological abnormalities and to forestall death. In contrast, now the majority of deaths involve no attempt at resuscitation, and honoring patient preferences to forgo artificial hydration and nutrition has become acceptable. This progress has been the result of judicial decisions, distinguished professional organizations writing guidelines, media attention to these issues, and consumer organizations who have advocated individual rights. We are now at an important crossroads on how best to define appropriate safeguards and structure legal guidance in decision making for incompetent adults. We are unlikely to accord all cases individual due process through the courts. Doing so would be too costly, too slow, and not clearly useful for most situations. As safeguards, we may need some supervision of clinicians and appropriate referral to institutional ethics committees and the courts. Most importantly, good policy might require overt authorization of automatic family decision making in the absence of instruction from the patient.

Wise policy formulation requires both sound theory and empirical research. To date, the empirical information has been especially weak. Formulation of further policy without consideration of the realities of effective implementation places patients at considerable risk. The complexity of decision making, and how little we understand it, should receive substantial attention (Brock 1994).

Specific Questions

How Are Advance Directives and Durable Powers of Attorney Assessed within Your Profession in Your Country?

The question of how advance directives and durable powers of attorney are assessed can be answered from both a theoretical and an empirical perspective. From a theoretical perspective, a valid advance directive is assumed to carry more moral authority than a surrogate's substituted judgment. The physician's role in defining the validity of an advance directive needs much more clarification.

Physicians in Arkansas were surveyed from an empirical perspective regarding their attitudes toward advance directives. Davidson et al. (1989) found that 83.5 percent of those respondents experienced with advance directives stated that experience had made their attitudes more positive. These results were in conflict with Zinberg (1988), who conducted a qualitative survey regarding advance directives with physicians in Vermont and California. Using physician responses to hypothetical scenarios, physicians who initially opposed a feeding tube changed their decisions if the families "pushed" for it (Ely et al. 1992). Physicians were more likely to follow therapy-specific advance directives than a directive that employed a general statement (Mower and Baraff 1993).

As noted earlier, however, the generally positive attitude of health care professionals toward advance directives does not translate into many being completed, counseling about them being common, or their having an impact upon treatment.

How Could or Should Advance Directives and Durable Powers of Attorney Be Used?

1. Advance directives and durable powers of attorney should be written evidence of comprehensive advance care planning that reflects a thoughtful anticipation of the likely futures facing the patient and the preferences of the patient from among the alternatives.

2. Clinicians should focus efforts to use advance directives (instructional or proxy-naming) in these situations when patients have no natural surrogate or multiple contenders for surrogacy who would not be expected to cooperate, when they have unusual preferences, when their natural surrogates or designated proxies are not likely to follow the patient's preferences without the added guidance of written direction, or when the patient is anxious and gains peace of mind by having attended to these matters.

3. Advance directives can also be used to relieve families of the feeling of being burdened by decision making, or to push surrogates and caregivers to consider elements beyond the patient's health, such as family financial burden or religious obligations in the management of the dying process.

4. It should be possible to accomplish most aims with oral communication and documentation in the medical record without formal documentation or statutory protection.

5. There are multiple types of advance directives. The type that is employed probably should be targeted to the patient's needs, the law of the state, and the practice in the region.

What Influence Does Law and Regulation Have on the Conduct of Your Profession and on Patient Attitudes and Goals?

The PSDA represents an excellent opportunity to examine the impact of laws and regulation on patient attitudes and decision making. SUPPORT collected data at a time prior to and in the two years after the passage of the PSDA. In seriously ill patients, there has been only a small increase in the writing of formal directives from 20 to 24 percent. There has been a sixfold increase in documentation about directives. As noted earlier, this increased documentation has not altered the absence of an impact by advance directives on decision making about, and outcomes of, resuscitation (Teno et al. 1997a). Teno et al. (1994) examined the impact of the PSDA in a 10-state survey of nursing home residents and found that the rate of DNR orders increased from 30 to 51 percent. However, this increase in DNR orders began prior to the implementation of the PSDA. Although this seems to be an improvement, the newly more prevalent DNR orders were not examined as to their appropriateness and may represent a trend that would have occurred without the PSDA.

Law and regulation on the centrally important issue of the determination of incompetence are determinative of the course of decision making in many cases but are rarely examined. A few states have a method of deciding incompetence for health care matters that requires no involvement of the courts. Each state has a formal method for declaring incompetence in court, a process that is probably applied to very few patients. Yet, the decision that the patient is incompetent can determine the patient and family role in receiving information, participating in discussions, and making decisions. There are no population studies of the rate of incompetence, its sensitivity to various potential standards, or the modes of determination now in use. In addition, important theoretical issues about the responsiveness of the standard to the seriousness of the issue and to focal or fluctuating cognitive or emotional deficits persist.

What Role Could or Should Law Play in Supporting Important Professional Goals or Cultural and Moral Values in Caring for Those Who Are Terminally Ill and Incompetent?

Persons who are seriously and progressively ill and likely to die face a series of important questions that will shape their life possibilities. When the patient is incompetent, decisions have to be made by others. Although law and social convention shape these decision-making processes and their outcomes, good reasons abound for decision making to allow informal processes and reliance upon family when they are present and show concern for the well-being of the patient. How to do this while still defending the state's interest and obligation to protect the lives of its citizens (under the Fourteenth Amendment to the Constitution) is the challenge for policy.

In addition, treatment options are shaped by funding and resource-allocation decisions. Although we often take these constraints as part of the unchanging forces that shape possibilities, in fact, they constitute the most significant role played by the law—the laws that do or do not provide financial support for certain kinds of care.

Law and regulation also shape the availability of courses of care that end life. As we have written elsewhere, there are good reasons for the law to continue to prohibit outright killing. To do otherwise risks acceptance of inadequate care systems for the severely ill and disabled as well as the erroneous killing of individual persons whose needs would be misunderstood or unaddressed (Teno and Lynn 1991).

What Are the Major Areas and Matters of Conflict between Law and Actual Behavior?

Law conflicts with clinical practice in many aspects of decision making:

1. Informed consent is an ethical goal and a legal requirement but is often missing from clinical medicine.

2. The ethical and legal mandates exist for effective communication about options and outcomes. Yet such communication is absent.

3. Which standards of evidence should be used in adjudication about advance direction? Should it be "clear and convincing" or a lesser standard such as "preponderance of the evidence"? The former is allowed but not required by the *Cruzan* opinion of the U.S. Supreme Court.

4. Many elements of the "real" case cannot be presented in court (e.g., the suffering of the family, the costs of care, the other patients turned away).

5. The law cannot enforce living wills that have no enforceable direction but only poetic statements of general proclivities. Because the vast majority of living wills are not specific, the enforcement provisions seem to promise more than can be accomplished.

6. The boundary between good care and murder is often difficult to state precisely.

7. The law requires forms and witnesses, which are poorly understood.

Which Areas and Matters Require Further Transdisciplinary and Transcultural Study; How Should Those Studies Be Conducted?

Future research needs to be conducted on thantoepidemiology (population studies of the process of dying) in order to assure further refinement of the process of advance care planning. For example, what should be the communication process and content of advance care planning? What is the proper balance of specificity and flexibility? In addition, the role of surrogates in decision making for incompetent adults requires further study, and evaluation of the role of institutional and federal policy in end-of-life decision making should be undertaken. Very little such research is available about the dominant American cultures; even less has been done in ethnic minorities or in transcultural designs.

We recommend that research on advance directives ordinarily be conducted by interdisciplinary teams composed of social scientists, health care providers, philosophers, and attorneys, using both qualitative and quantitative research methods.

Where Do You See Areas or Subjects That Need Resolution of Conflict between Law and Actual Behavior, or between Patients' Interests, Professional Conduct, and Legal Parameters?

The most pressing areas for reflection are the following:

1. Circumstances when clinicians, ethics committees, or the courts should "trump" advance directives or decision making that relies on surrogates need to be articulated.

2. A regular decision-making process needs to be designed with safeguards that are flexible and efficient. Decision-making processes must incorporate reliance on family members and other informal surrogates.

3. The pluralism in the United States suggests the need to design flexible systems of care and decision making that accommodate the cultural and

religious beliefs of a diverse population.

4. Consensus is needed about the weight that the interests of others (e.g., family or society) should have in decision making. Perhaps patient autonomy should not always take precedence.

What Do You Expect to Be Prime Future Questions in This Area? How Would You Go About Resolving Them? Which Principles Should Govern Surrogate Decision Making and Advance Directives?

The primary issues are the following:

1. ethnic issues in framing decision making,
2. suspicion of withholding treatment to save money,
3. patients without surrogates (the unbefriended patient),
4. how to target advance care planning so it is desired and helpful,
5. integration of the emergency care system, and
6. how to fund adequate care of the chronically ill and dying and how to organize health care systems to provide such care effectively.

Suggestions for how to resolve these issues are the following:

1. more thoughtful literature,
2. more broadly available advance directive information,
3. more adequate descriptive research,
4. more definitive intervention trials, and
5. involvement of multiple disciplines.

Principles that should guide surrogate decision making and advance directives are as follows:

1. Decisions for incompetent adults should be guided by advance directives when doing so serves the needs of the patient.
2. Decisions for incompetent adults, when made by the courts or other strangers, should not generally be dramatically different from those chosen by competent adults with similar medical problems.
3. Systems for medical decision making should be evaluated by better outcomes in terms of health and satisfaction, not just in terms of having adhered to a justifiable process.

4. The decision-making process must involve the consideration of an adequate array of potential care plans and characterization of their likely outcomes.

References

Bedell, Susanna E., Denise Pelle, Patricia L. Maher, and Paul Cleary. 1986. "Do-Not-Resuscitate Orders for Critically Ill Patients in the Hospital." *Journal of the American Medical Association* 256:233–37.

Brett, Alan S. 1991. "Limitations of Listing Specific Medical Interventions in Advance Directives." *Journal of the American Medical Association* 266:825–28.

Buchanan, Allan E., and Dan W. Brock. 1989. *Deciding for Others: The Ethics of Surrogate Decision Making.* Cambridge: Cambridge University Press.

Chambers, Christopher V., James J. Diamond, Robert L. Perkel, and Lori A. Lasch. 1994. "Relationship of Advance Directives to Hospital Charges in a Medicare Population." *Archives of Internal Medicine* 154:541–47.

Coordinating Council on Life-Sustaining Medical Treatment Decision Making by the Courts. 1991. *Guidelines for State Court Decision Making in Authorizing or Withholding Life-Sustaining Medical Treatment.* Williamsburg, Va.: National Center for State Courts.

Council on Scientific Affairs and Council on Ethical and Judicial Affairs. 1990. "Persistent Vegetative State and the Decision to Withdraw or Withhold Life Support." *Journal of the American Medical Association* 263:426–30.

Cruzan v. Director, Missouri Department of Health. 1990. 110 S. Ct. 2841.

Davidson, Kent W., Chris Hackler, Debra R. Caradine, and Ronald S. McCord. 1989. "Physicians' Attitudes on Advance Directives." *Journal of the American Medical Association* 262:2415–19.

Elder, Nancy C., F. David Schneider, Steven C. Zweig, Philip G. Peters, and John W. Ely. 1992. "Community Attitudes and Knowledge about Advance Care Directives." *Journal of the American Board of Family Practice* 5:565–72.

Ely, John W., Philip G. Peters, Steven Zweig, Nancy Elder, and F. David Schneider. 1992. "The Physician's Decision to Use Tube Feedings: The Role of the Family, the Living Will, and the Cruzan Decision." *Journal of the American Geriatrics Society* 40:471–75.

Emanuel, Ezekiel J., and Linda L. Emanuel. 1992. "Proxy Decision Making for Incompetent Patients: An Ethical and Empirical Analysis." *Journal of the American Medical Association* 267:2067–71.

———. 1993. "Decisions at the End of Life: Guided by Communities of Patients." *Hastings Center Report* 23:6–14.

Emanuel, Linda L., Michael J. Barry, John D. Stoeckle, Lucy M. Ettelson, and Ezekiel J. Emanuel. 1991. "Advance Directives for Medical Care: A Case for Greater Use." *New England Journal of Medicine* 324:889–95.

Emanuel, Linda L., and Ezekiel J. Emanuel. 1989. "The Medical Directive: A New Comprehensive Document." *Journal of the American Medical Association* 261: 3288–93.

Emanuel, Linda L., Ezekiel J. Emanuel, John D. Stoeckle, Lacinda R. Hummel, and Michael J. Barry. 1994. "Advance Directives: Stability of Patients' Treatment Choices." *Archives of Internal Medicine* 154:209–17.

Evans, Andrew L., and Baruch A. Brody. 1985. "The Do-Not-Resuscitate Order in Teaching Hospitals." *Journal of the American Medical Association* 253:2236–39.

Everhart, Maria A., and Robert A. Pearlman. 1990. "Stability of Patient Preferences Regarding Life-Sustaining Treatments." *Chest* 97:159–64.

Forrow, Lachlan, Edward Gogel, and Elizabeth Thomas. 1991. "Advance Directives for Medical Care [Letter]." *New England Journal of Medicine* 325:1255.

Fox, Ellen, and Carol Stocking. 1993. "Ethics Consultants' Recommendations for Life-Prolonging Treatment of Patients in a Persistent Vegetative State." *Journal of the American Medical Association* 270:2578–82.

Frankl, David, Robert K. Oye, and Paul E. Bellamy. 1989. "Attitudes of Hospitalized Patients toward Life Support: A Survey of 200 Medical Inpatients." *American Journal of Medicine* 86:645–48.

Gamble, Elizabeth R., Penelope J. McDonald, and Peter R. Lichstein. 1991. "Knowledge, Attitudes, and Behavior of Elderly Persons Regarding Living Wills." *Archives of Internal Medicine* 151:277–80.

Gibson, Joan. 1990. "National Values History Project." *Generations* 14 (Supplement): 51–63.

Hare, Jan, Clara Pratt, and Carrie Nelson. 1992. "Agreement between Patients and Their Self-selected Surrogates on Difficult Medical Decisions." *Archives of Internal Medicine* 152:1049–54.

Harvey, Lynn K., and Stephanie C. Shubat. 1989. *Physician and Public Attitudes on Health Care Issues.* Chicago: American Medical Association.

Hastings Center. 1987. *Guidelines on the Termination of Life-Sustaining Treatment and the Care of the Dying.* Bloomington: Indiana University Press.

High, Dallas M. 1993a. "Advance Directives and the Elderly: A Study of Intervention Strategies to Increase Use." *Gerontologist* 33:342–49.

———. 1993b. "Why Are Elderly People Not Using Advance Directives?" *Journal of Aging and Health* 5:497–515.

Institute of Medical Ethics Working Party on the Ethics of Prolonging Life and Assisting Death. 1991. "Withdrawal of Life-Support from Patients in a Persistent Vegetative State." *Lancet* 337:96–98.

Jonsson, Palmi V., Michael McNamee, and Edward W. Campion. 1988. "The 'Do Not Resuscitate' Order: A Profile of Its Changing Use." *Archives of Internal Medicine* 148:2373–75.

Kutner, Luis. 1969. "COMMENTS: Due Process of Euthanasia: The Living Will, a Proposal." *Indiana Law Journal* 44:539–54.

LaPuma, John, Carol B. Stocking, Marc D. Silverstein, Andrea DiMartini, and Mark Siegler. 1988. "An Ethics Consultation Service in a Teaching Hospital." *Journal of the American Medical Association* 260:808–11.

Lynn, Joanne. 1991. "Why I Don't Have a Living Will." *Law, Medicine & Health Care* 19:101–4.

Lynn, Joanne, F. Cohn, J. H. Pickering, J. Smith, and A. M. Stoeppelwerth. 1997. "American Geriatrics Society on Physician-Assisted Suicide: Brief to the United States Supreme Court." *Journal of American Geriatircs Society* 45:1–11.

Lynn, Joanne, and David DeGrazia. 1991. "An Outcomes Model of Medical Decision Making." *Journal of Theoretical Medicine* 12:325–43.

Lynn, Joanne, and Joan Teno. 1993. "After the Patient Self-determination Act: The Need for Empirical Research on Formal Advance Directives." *Hastings Center Report* 23 (1): 20–24.

Lynn, Joanne, J. Teno, R. S. Phillips, R. E. Phillips, N. Wenger, B. Virnig, A. Connors, A. Galanos, for the Help Investigators. 1994. "Preferences for Instructional Directives or Family Decision-making among Older Patients [Abstract]." American Geriatrics Society, May 21, Los Angeles.

Molloy, David W., Roger M. Clarnette, E. Ann Braun, Martin R. Eisemann, and B. Schneiderman. 1991. "Decision Making in the Incompetent Elderly: 'The Daughter from California Syndrome.'" *Journal of the American Geriatric Society* 39:396–99.

Mower, William R., and Larry J. Baraff. 1993. "Advance Directives: Effect of Type of Directive on Physicians' Therapeutic Decisions." *Archives of Internal Medicine* 153:375–81.

Ouslander, Joseph G., Alexander J. Tymchuk, and Bita Rahbar. 1989. "Health Care Decisions among Elderly Long-Term Care Residents and Their Potential Proxies." *Archives of Internal Medicine* 149:1367–72.

President's Commission for the Study of Ethical Problems in Medicine and Biomedical and Behavioral Research. 1983, *Deciding to Forego Life-Sustaining Treatment.* Washington, D.C.: Government Printing Office.

Rubin, Susan M., William M. Strull, Michael F. Fialkow, Sarah J. Weiss, and Bernard Lo. 1994. "Increasing the Completion of the Durable Power of Attorney for Health Care: A Randomized, Controlled Trial." *Journal of the American Medical Association* 271:209–12.

Schloendorff v. Society of New York Hospital. 1914. J. Cardozo, dissenting, 211 NY 125, 105 NE 92.

Schneiderman, Lawrence J., and John D. Arras. 1985. "Counseling Patients to Counsel Physicians on Future Care in the Event of Patient Incompetence." *Annals of Internal Medicine* 102:693–98.

Schneiderman, Lawrence J., Richard Kronick, Robert M. Kaplan, J. P. Anderson, and R. D. Langer. 1992. "Effects of Offering Advance Directives on Medical Treatments and Costs." *Annals of Internal Medicine* 117:599–606.

Seckler, Allison B., Diane E. Meier, Michael Mulvihill, and Barbara E. Cammer. 1991. "Substituted Judgement: How Accurate Are Proxy Predictions?" *Annals of Internal Medicine* 115:92–98.

Sehgal, Ashwini, Allison Galbraith, Margaret Chesney, Patricia Schoenfeld, Gerald Charles, and Bernard Lo. 1992. "How Strictly Do Dialysis Patients Want Their Advance Directives Followed?" *Journal of the American Medical Association* 267: 59–63.

Silverstein, Marc D., Carol B. Stocking, Jack P. Antel, Janese Beckwith, Raymond P. Roos, and Mark Siegler. 1991. "Amyotrophic Lateral Sclerosis and Life-Sustaining Therapy: Patients' Desires for Information, Participation in Decision Making, and Life-Sustaining Therapy." *Mayo Clinical Proceedings* 66:906–13.

Smedira, Nicholas G., Bradley H. Evans, Linda S. Grais, Neal H. Cohen, Bernard Lo, Molly Cooke, William P. Schecter, Carol Fink, Eve Epstein-Jaffe, Christine May, and John M. Luce. 1990. "Withholding and Withdrawal of Life Support from the Critically Ill." *New England Journal of Medicine* 322:309–15.

Stanley, John M, ed. 1992. "The Appleton International Conference: Developing Guidelines for Decisions to Forgo Life-Prolonging Medical Treatment. Part 1: Decisions Involving Patients Who Have Decision-Making Capacity or Patients Who Have Executed an Advance Directive before Losing This Capacity." *Journal of Medical Ethics* 18 (Supplement): 6–9.

Strong, Carson. 1993. "Patients Should Not Always Come First in Treatment Decisions." *Journal of Clinical Ethics* 4:63–65.

Teno, Joan. 1994. "Lack of Concern from Bioethics Consultants: Is It Time for a New Cook or a New Cookbook?" *Geriatric Research Application Digest* xx:yy–zz.

Teno, J. M., K. J. Branco, V. Mor, C. D. Phillips, C. Howes, J. Morris, and B. E. Fries. 1997a. "Changes in Advance Care Planning in Nursing Homes before and after the Patient Self-determination Act: Report of a 10-State Survey." *Journal of the American Geriatrics Society* 45:939–44.

Teno, Joan, John Fleishman, Dan Brock, and Vincent Mor. 1990. "The Use of Formal Prior Directives among Patients with HIV-Related Diseases." *Journal of General Internal Medicine* 5:490–94.

Teno, J., and J. Lynn. 1991. "Voluntary Active Euthanasia: The Individual Case and Public Policy." *Journal of the American Geriatrics Society* 41:827–30.

Teno, J. M., J. Lynn, A. F. Connors Jr., N. Wenger, R. S. Phillips, C. Alzola, D. P. Murphy, N. Desbiens, and W. A. Knaus. 1997b. "The Illusion of End-of-Life Resource Savings with Advance Directives." *Journal of the American Geriatrics Society* 45: 513–18.

Teno, J., J. Lynn, R. S. Phillips, D. Murphy, S. J. Youngner, D. Bellamy, A. F. Connors Jr., N. A. Desbiens, W. Fulkerson, and W. A. Knause. 1994. "Do Formal Advance Directives Impact on Resuscitation Decisions and Resource Utilization among Seriously Ill Patients?" *Journal of Clinical Ethics* 5 (1): 23–30.

Teno, Joan M., Charles Sabatino, Lauren Parisier, Fenella Rouse, and Joanne Lynn.

1993a. "The Impact of the Patient Self-determination Act's Requirement That States Describe Law Concerning Patients' Rights." *Journal of Law, Medicine, & Ethics* 21:102–8.

Teno, Joan, et al. 1993b. "Do Advance Directives Provide Personal Instructions Which Direct Care? [Abstract]." *Gerontologist* 33:143–44.

Teno, Joan M., et al. 1997c. "Do Advance Directives Provide Instructions That Direct Care?" *Journal of the American Geriatric Society* 45:508–12.

Teno, Joan M., et al. 1997d. "Advance Directives for Seriously-Ill Hospitalized Patients: Effectiveness with the Patient Self-determination Act and the Support Intervention." *Journal of the American Geriatrics Society* 45:500–507.

Uhlmann, Richard F., Robert A. Pearlman, and Kevin C. Cain. 1988. "Physicians' and Spouses' Predictions of Elderly Patients' Resuscitation Preferences." *Journal of Gerontology* 43:M115–M121.

Weeks, W. B., L. L. Kofoed, A. E. Wallace, and H. G. Welch. 1994. "Advance Directives and the Cost of Terminal Hospitalization." *Archives of Internal Medicine* 154:2077–83.

Yellen, Suzanne B., Lauren A. Burton, and Ellen Elpern. 1992. "Communication about Advance Directives: Are Patients Sharing Information with Physicians?" *Cambridge Quarterly of Healthcare Ethics* 4:377–87.

Zinberg, Joel M. 1989. "Decisions for the Dying: An Empirical Study of Physicians' Responses to Advance Directives." *Vermont Law Review* 13 (winter): 445–91.

2

Legal Issues in Decision Making for Incompetent Patients

Advance Directives and Surrogate Decision Making

ALAN MEISEL, J.D.

Introduction

Twenty years ago the term *advance directive* did not exist, the term *living will* was not a household word, and a durable power of attorney was used to avoid guardianship proceedings for the management of financial affairs. Today, every state has recognized the validity of advance directives through statute, case law, or both. All states but three (Massachusetts, Michigan, New York) have adopted living will legislation, and all have enacted durable health care power of attorney legislation. Close to three-quarters have enacted statutes intended to clarify the status of family members as surrogate decision makers, and the number of these statutes is growing so quickly that it is difficult to get an accurate count (much as it was with living will and health care power of attorney statutes in the late 1980s and early 1990s).

A legal consensus has emerged over the last two decades about how decisions are to be made about the initiation, continuation, and termination of life-sustaining medical treatment for patients who no longer possess the capacity to decide these matters for themselves (Meisel 1992a). However, consensus is not unanimity, and the consensus often consists of broad generalities—for example, close family members have the legal authority to make decisions for incompetent patients without advance directives—that raise more questions than they answer. Who is a close family member? How should we resolve conflicts between family members? What kinds of conflicts of interest are serious enough to warrant the dishonoring of a close family member's decision? Even the statutes, which the courts have repeatedly implored the legislatures to enact, do not always answer all the important questions. For instance, a surrogate decision-making statute may provide that an incompetent patient's adult children are to serve as surrogates if the patient's spouse is deceased but fail to explain how differences of opinion among the children are to be resolved.

This chapter discusses some of the more prominent legal issues that arise in the process of making decisions about forgoing life-sustaining treatment for incompetent persons.[1] It is primarily written from the perspective of the law and secondarily from the perspective of the kinds of concerns that lawyers have about advance directives.

Case Discussion

The following cases provide examples of the kinds of dilemmas that can arise in making decisions about forgoing life-sustaining treatment for patients who have advance directives.

Case 1: Statement of the Case

Mr. Jones is a 32-year-old man who was diagnosed five years ago as having AIDS. Despite several hospitalizations in the last two years, he continues to work normal hours in his career as an editor at a publishing house, he continues to be an avid skier and runner, and, on balance, he tries to and mostly succeeds in living life as he did before he became infected. There are periods of time when he is seriously fatigued and restricts most of his activities except work, but as of late work has begun to be affected too. He has begun to cut out working many evenings and weekends, which previously had been a normal part of his life.

He is committed to maintaining as active a life as possible for as long as possible, but he is also resigned to the inevitability of death at an early age. Having witnessed the prolonged deaths of countless friends and acquaintances from AIDS, he is also committed to not prolonging his own death merely for the sake of staying alive.

In order to ensure that this wish will be carried out, he has had his lawyer draw up an advance directive. The state in which he lives has no living will statute. The attorney drafts a living will using as a guide a living will form produced by a nonprofit organization whose purpose is to provide advice to those who need assistance in exercising their right to refuse medical treatment. The living will says in relevant part: "If I should be in an incurable or irreversible mental or physical condition with no reasonable expectation of recovery, I direct my attending physician to withhold or withdraw treatment that merely prolongs my dying." The form also contains a provision stating "I especially do not want the following treatments," followed by a list of treatments in which one can check those that one does not want. These treatments are CPR, dialysis, a feeding tube, ventilator, or antibiotics; Mr. Jones checked them all as treatments he would not want.

Mr. Jones was hospitalized three days ago complaining of persistent fever, a bad cough, and increasing difficulty breathing. X-rays confirm his doctor's initial diagnosis of pneumonia, and lab tests further confirm that it is pneumocystic carinii. At this time, although very fatigued, Mr. Jones is still in possession of decision-making capacity. His doctor tells him that he is putting him on heavy doses of antibiotics and that if his breathing gets any worse, he will be transferred to the ICU where he can be placed on a ventilator. Mr. Jones does not object to either of these statements. His difficulty breathing does worsen, and he is now delirious. His doctor orders transfer to the ICU and intubation. Mr. Jones appears only vaguely aware of what is going on. Because of the intubation and his mental status, it is no longer possible to communicate with him.

Two days after admission to the ICU, which is his fifth day in the hospital, his parents arrive from out of town to visit him. After they are briefed by his physician about his medical status, they remind the doctor of the advance directive that Mr. Jones had executed. The doctor consults his office record and finds it. Two days pass in which Mr. Jones's condition shows neither any worsening nor any improvement, and his parents ask the doctor to remove him from the ventilator and to discontinue antibiotics because they violate his wishes as expressed in his advance directive and because he frequently pulls on the ventilator tube.

His doctor hesitates and after some consideration declines to do so because he believes that the advance directive was written to prevent a prolonged and possibly painful process of dying, and he believes that it is likely that, with an adequate course of antibiotics and ventilation, Mr. Jones will recover from this current episode of pneumonia.

Case 2: Statement of the Case

Suppose that, in addition to the facts in case 1, Mr. Jones's lawyer also explained proxy directives to him. After listening to his lawyer explain the difference between the instruction and proxy directives and the pros and cons of each, he concluded that he would rather leave his fate in the hands of those who knew him best, loved him, and would do only what they thought was best for him—his parents. Thus, the substance of his advance directive states: "In the event that I lose decision-making capacity, I direct my doctor(s) to rely on my parents as my agents for decision making and to be bound by their decisions in the same manner and to the same extent as they would be bound by my own decisions if I had not lost decision-making capacity. However, I do not want my parents to authorize any treatment that would merely prolong the process of my dying."

His parents have been present since the time of Mr. Jones's admission to the hospital. It is now two weeks after his admission to the ICU. The doctor now believes that there is very little chance that Mr. Jones can ever be weaned from the ventilator or leave the hospital alive. He has been comatose for the last ten days and seems to experience no pain or suffering. The doctor believes that it is now time to turn off the ventilator and allow Mr. Jones to die if he cannot breathe on his own.

The doctor is aware of Mr. Jones's proxy directive appointing his parents to make decisions for him. In this case, Mr. Jones's parents vehemently disagree with this proposal. They believe that the termination of treatment is not the proper course because Mr. Jones consented to treatment before losing decision-making capacity and because they believe that Mr. Jones would want to be treated, leave the hospital, and resume leading life in much the same way as he did prior to hospitalization. They do not believe the doctor's prognosis, although it is supported by pulmonary and neurological consultants.

The doctor believes that the parents' instructions are inconsistent with Mr. Jones's own wishes and that the parents are motivated primarily by their inability to come to terms with the fact that their son has AIDS, that he is homosexual, that he is dying, and that little can be done to prevent it.

Case 3: Statement of the Case

Mrs. Smith is an 87-year-old woman who has lived in Pleasant Manor Nursing Home for the last five years. She originally moved into the nursing home's intermediate care unit after she suffered a mild stroke that left her right arm paralyzed because she felt that she could no longer adequately care for her house. At the time she sold the house before moving into the nursing home, she also had her lawyer write an instruction directive, without a proxy provision, for her. Because Mrs. Smith had witnessed the prolonged deterioration of many friends and relatives in nursing homes, who lingered for years after losing their mental faculties, she did not want this to happen to her, and she especially wanted to avoid being kept alive by artificial nutrition and hydration. Mrs. Smith's lawyer advised her that her state's living will statute applied only to patients who were terminally ill or permanently unconscious, but he agreed to add the following provision because she was so adamant about it: "I do not wish to have the process of dying prolonged even if I am not terminally ill or not permanently unconscious. If I am suffering from an incurable disease—for example, serious dementia—and treatment will only prolong dying—for example, a feeding tube—I want treatment to be forgone."

Two years after she moved into the nursing home, Mrs. Smith began to experience a variety of other medical problems. She was intermittently incontinent—which caused her great embarrassment—she began to lose her eyesight and hearing, and she increasingly lost the ability to feed herself and had to be spoon-fed by an attendant. At this time, four years after moving into the nursing home, Mrs. Smith is no longer able to walk, to obtain adequate nutrition and hydration by being fed by others, or to recognize her children and grandchildren who come to visit her once a week. Although she can talk, it usually consists of ramblings about events that happened long ago and that are disconnected from the current context. She often does not answer direct and simple questions, and when she does, her answers are seldom responsive.

Nursing home personnel are worried about her debilitated state because of her inability to obtain adequate nutrition and hydration. They ask the nursing home physician to evaluate her, and he says that she needs to have a feeding tube inserted. Her family reminds the doctor and the nursing home personnel of her advance directive, which is in her nursing home record.

The doctor does not want to follow the advance directive because the state living will statute requires that a patient be terminally ill or permanently unconscious for the advance directive to become operative. He believes that Mrs. Smith is not terminally ill (and she is surely not permanently unconscious), because with a feeding tube she is likely to live for a substantial period of time.

Review of the Legal Literature

American lawyers and lawmakers have a tendency, frequently shared by health care professionals and the public, to think of advance directives as a magic bullet that will solve the dilemma posed by decision making about life-sustaining treatment for patients who no longer possess decision-making capacity. In the wake of the Supreme Court's *Cruzan* decision (*Cruzan* 1990), many feared, based on a misreading of that decision, that across the nation the termination of life support would become increasingly difficult, if not impossible. Others feared, more realistically—but, as it has turned out, incorrectly (Meisel 1992b)—that other states would follow Missouri's lead and legislatively or judicially adopt more stringent standards for the termination of life support. Certainly this was the thinking behind the passage of the Patient Self-determination Act, a monumental effort that has borne meager fruit.

Since the *Quinlan* case (*Quinlan* 1976) and in many subsequent ones, state courts have called for the promulgation of legislative rules to aid doctors, patients, and families in making decisions about forgoing life-sustaining treatment so that they will not feel it necessary to bring these cases to the courts for resolution. The legislative response has been half-hearted at best. Although every state has enacted some legislation—living will statutes, health care power of attorney statutes, surrogate decision making statutes, Do Not Resuscitate (DNR) statutes, or some combination—no state has enacted a truly comprehensive statute for guiding decision making about life-sustaining treatment.

Advance directive (and related) legislation has not been unhelpful in resolving some of the dilemmas that arise in decision making for incompetent patients, but we should be careful not to equate legislation with progress. Probably the most significant benefit of such legislation has been to eliminate or reduce health care professionals' anxiety about whether or not the forgoing of life-sustaining treatment is "legal" and whether advance directives are a legitimate basis for making such decisions.

However, advance directive legislation reflects a very formalistic approach to decision making. Too often, people who execute advance directives and lawyers who counsel them expend extraordinary amounts of energy obsessively trying to "get the form right," as if the "right" word formula will somehow assure that people get the kind of medical care they want at some future date. We know—or at least we ought to—that disease, medical treatment, and individual preferences cannot be reduced to a recipe.

That is a problem endemic to advance directives whether statutorily based or not, but advance directives drafted in conformance with state statutes suffer from another problem. Advance directive statutes contain a maze of technical and substantive requirements and sometimes seem to require physicians to provide treatments they believe are not medically indicated. This maze of requirements can also be easily used to evade compliance with an advance directive that a physician would prefer to ignore.

The Legal Basis for Advance Directives and the Problem of Generally "Nonconforming" Advance Directives

One of the most fundamental legal questions about advance directives is whether they are valid in the absence of a statute (case 1 raises this issue). Although most states now have advance directive statutes, not all do, and not too long ago there were many states that did not.

There were advance directives long before there were advance directive statutes (Kutner 1969). Were they valid? The answer is plainly yes, so much so that these advance directives have generated very little litigation.[2] I refer to these prestatutory advance directives as "nonstatutory" advance directives because the courts that have recognized their validity have done so on the basis of the common-law and/or constitutional right of competent individuals to make decisions about their medical care. Included, by extension, is the right to make these decisions anticipatorily as well as contemporaneously, that is, in advance of their losing decision-making capacity (hence the term *advance* directive).

The widespread enactment of advance directive statutes, rather than mooting the question of the validity of nonstatutory advance directives, has led to its reformulation: Are advance directives that deviate from statutory requirements legally valid and effective? The answer to this question is central in responding to the issue raised by case 3 as to whether, in a jurisdiction that does have an advance directive statute, an advance directive that does not conform—and may conflict—with the statute is legally effective. An advance directive may deviate from an advance directive statute's requirements in two general ways. First, the advance directive may simply ignore the statutory requirements or explicitly disavow them. Second, an advance directive may appear to or purport to comply with statutory requirements but in fact contain a provision that conflicts with the statute.

This is a very important issue. Many advance directive statutes contain serious limitations on what kinds of decisions can be made. People will, and probably already do, attempt to write advance directives that circumvent these restrictions, and courts will consequently be faced with the prospect of attempting to reconcile these "nonconforming" advance directives and the advance directive statutes that they appear to violate. This is exemplified by case 3, in which the advance directive contains an instruction—to terminate artificial nutrition and hydration—that the statute appears not to permit.

In most instances, the answer again is that nonconforming advance directives should be presumed to be valid even in a jurisdiction that has enacted advance directive legislation. There are several reasons for this conclusion that might seem odd at first glance. First, many advance directive statutes contain provisions stating that they are intended to preserve, rather than limit, common-law rights (Meisel 1995, § 10.12). Second, the purpose of advance directive statutes is generally acknowledged to be the conferral of legal immunity through a set of procedures, rather than the preemption of substantive rights or even the prescription of a particular method for executing an advance directive. Third, although most living will statutes contain an advance directive form, there is usually an accompanying statutory provision stating that use of the form is optional or may be modified (ibid., §§ 11.3, 12.11).

Judicial decisions have also provided grounds for the conclusion that nonconforming advance directives are valid. The Florida Supreme Court's *Browning* decision permitted the enforcement of an advance directive, a provision of which—a request not to be kept alive by artificial nutrition and hydration—directly violated the state's advance directive statute (which, at that time, prohibited the enforcement of a request for the forgoing of artificial nutrition and hydration). The court did not hold the statute unconstitutional nor did it look to other provisions of the statute that might have allowed for the enforcement of a nonconforming advance directive. It merely held that the patient's state constitutional right of privacy guaranteed her the right to forgo any form of medical treatment, including artificial nutrition and hydration, and that the nonstatutory advance directive that she had written was the means by which she sought, and was entitled, to implement this right (*Browning* 1990). Finally, in a number of cases, the argument has been made that treatment could not be forgone under the circumstances of the cases because the advance directive statute did not permit it. When the patient in question did not have an advance directive, courts have rejected these arguments on the basis that the advance directive statute does not apply to patients who do not have advance directives (*Rasmussen* 1987; *Degrella* 1993; *Myers* 1993).

On the other side of the ledger, there are no statutory provisions or appellate cases specifically requiring that advance directives comply with the provisions of advance directive statutes. However, one state appellate court has looked to its advance directive statute as source of law to restrict patients' decisional rights even in the absence of advance directives (*Cruzan* 1988). Furthermore, there are at least some provisions of advance directive statutes that are worded in such a way as to suggest that they apply to patients without advance directives as well as to those with advance directives.

On balance, however, the better view and the one likely to prevail is that advance directive statutes were not enacted to *create* the right to make treatment decisions anticipatorily, for the existence of that right predated the enactment of the statute. Rather, they were enacted to provide assurance to health care professionals seeking to honor such choices that they would not incur legal liability if they did so, and to provide them with a specific statutory grant of immunity if the manner in which the advance directive was executed conformed to statutory requirements.

All of this is something of a tempest in a teapot because the courts have held that health care professionals who comply with the decisions of surrogates in the absence of *any* advance directive are also presumed to be immune from liability. The Kentucky Supreme Court has specifically addressed this issue, stating that "[f]uture criminal sanctions or civil liability turn not on the existence or absence of a court order, but on the facts of the case. . . . No liability attaches to a decision to refuse or withdraw treatment in a case of this nature once the necessary facts are established and carefully documented by the parties involved" (*Degrella* 1993, 710). Almost ten years earlier, the Florida Supreme Court had issued a similar ruling that "court approval to terminate extraordinary life support systems was not necessary in this type of case in order to relieve the consenting family members, the attending physicians, and the hospital and its administrators of civil and criminal liability (*Bludworth* 1984, 922). "To be relieved of potential civil and criminal liability," the court held, "guardians, consenting family members, physicians, hospitals, or their administrators need only act in good faith (ibid., 926).

A fortiori, compliance with a decision made by the patient before losing decision-making capacity (e.g., a nonstatutory directive) should carry with it at least the same immunity, though it is true that the presumption of immunity flowing from an advance directive is probably more difficult to overcome than is nonstatutory immunity. Further, since advance directive statutes generally provide that an advance directive in the statutory form complies "substantially" with the act and thereby acquires immunity, there is the question of how much an advance directive may deviate from the statutory form and still be considered a statutory advance directive, adherence to which clothes the physician with immunity.

Specific Types of Nonconforming Advance Directives

In addition to the problem of general noncompliance with advance directive statutes, there are three important ways in which individuals might seek to implement advance directives that specifically conflict with advance directive statutes. These are the frequently encountered provisions in advance directive statutes (1) requiring that the patient be suffering from a terminal illness or be in a state of permanent unconsciousness for the advance directive to become effective, (2) limiting the forgoing of artificial nutrition and hydration on the basis of an advance directive, and (3) limiting the forgoing of treatment on the basis of an advance directive if the patient is pregnant. A closely related fourth issue is whether some of the requirements of advance directive statutes apply to individuals who have not executed an advance directive.

THE "TERMINAL ILLNESS/PERMANENT UNCONSCIOUSNESS" REQUIREMENT. The most significant restriction imposed by most living will, and by a smaller number of health care power of attorney, statutes is that statutory advance directives become effective only for patients who are *terminally ill* or *permanently unconscious*. These terms are frequently defined in such a manner that patients with dementing illnesses who are not in the final stages of these illnesses, yet who are quite incapable of making their own health care decisions, are not covered by the statute. This is the situation in case 3. This limitation is a result that is probably neither intended by nor known to most people who execute a statutory advance directive, and it may not even be something of which many lawyers are aware.[3]

For the most part, the case law—based on the common law, state constitutions, and the federal constitution—contains no such restrictions. There is certainly no requirement that a *competent* patient be terminally ill for medical treatment to be forgone. For example, the appellate courts of various states have affirmed the right of a nonterminally ill patient suffering from cerebral palsy to be free from an unwanted feeding tube (*Bouvia* 1986) and of nonterminally ill quadriplegic accident victims to have ventilatory support terminated (*McAfee* 1989; *McKay* 1990; *Thor* 1993). There are now a significant number of cases affirming the right of competent people who are not even suffering from any chronic illness or injury to refuse treatment for an acute condition, the refusal of which is said to be likely to lead to their death and the acceptance of which is said to be virtually certain to save their lives. The most notable of these cases involve the refusal of blood transfusions by members of the Jehovah's Witness faith (*Wons* 1989; *Ramsey* 1985; *Fosmire* 1990; *Munoz* 1991; *Dubreuil* 1993; *Jackson* 1985; *Stamford Hospital* 1996; *Harrell* 1996).

THE "ARTIFICIAL NUTRITION AND HYDRATION" RESTRICTION. Another restriction contained in some advance directive statutes involves the forgoing of artificial nutrition and hydration. This restriction is far less common today than it was just a few years ago. Yet, despite the repeal of some of these restrictions in the wake of the *Cruzan* case, such restrictions still exist in some advance directive statutes. Rather than absolutely prohibiting the forgoing of artificial nutrition and hydration as they formerly did, most statutes now merely require that such measures be provided if it is necessary for the patient's comfort even if the patient had expressed no such limitation in the advance directive (Meisel 1995, §§ 11.12, 12.26).

Statutory restrictions on the forgoing of artificial nutrition and hydration in general represent a serious limitation of common-law and constitutional rights. Of the 21 jurisdictions with state appellate or federal trial court decisions involving the forgoing of artificial nutrition and hydration,[4] only two have shown any inclination to treat this matter as substantially different from the forgoing of other kinds of life-sustaining medical treatment (*Cruzan* 1988; *Grant* 1988).[5] Thus, with the possible exception of these two states, all other courts who have ruled on this issue consider artificial nutrition and hydration to be a form of medical treatment and permit it to be forgone under the same conditions as any other life-sustaining medical treatment. Consequently, the advance directive statutes that limit or prohibit the forgoing of artificial nutrition and hydration appear to restrict preexisting rights.

These restrictions are probably not constitutionally defensible. As previously discussed, the Florida Supreme Court in the *Browning* case, while skirting the issue of the constitutionality of the prohibition in the advance directive statute on forgoing artificial nutrition and hydration, evaded its impact by finding that the construction of an advance directive containing such an instruction was authorized by the state constitutional right of privacy. In her concurring opinion in the *Cruzan* case, Justice O'Connor chose not to enter the fray about whether artificial nutrition and hydration is a medical treatment because such a procedure is a serious invasion of bodily integrity, and thus its nonconsensual administration would violate a constitutionally protected liberty interest (*Cruzan* 1990, 288).

THE "PREGNANCY" RESTRICTION. Some advance directive statutes contain stringent limitations on the forgoing of life-sustaining treatment if the patient is pregnant (Meisel 1995, §§ 11.11, 12.27). Unlike the restrictions imposed on the forgoing of artificial nutrition and hydration and the restrictions imposed by the requirements of "terminal illness" or "permanent unconsciousness," there is only very sparse precedential case law on this topic (ibid., §§ 5.39, 9.55). What does exist, however, suggests that a woman's decision-making rights under the advance directive statutes are restricted to a greater extent than by the common-law (and possibly constitutional) requirements.

As is the case with artificial nutrition and hydration, these restrictions are constitutionally suspect, though not *as* suspect. Certainly until her fetus is viable, a woman has the right to terminate a pregnancy for any reason (*Roe* 1973), and a critical illness is probably among the better reasons for doing so (*A.C.* 1990). To do so anticipatorily might prove to be no weaker a right than to do so contemporaneously. However, after the fetus has reached viability, the state's interest in potential human life is sufficient to prevent termination of the pregnancy at least insofar as doing so would not threaten the mother's life (*Roe* 1973). Furthermore, states may impose other restrictions at different points in the pregnancy (*Casey* 1992). Thus, states that choose to impose limitations on forgoing life-sustaining treatment under such circumstances might be within their constitutional prerogatives to do so. Nonetheless, a state that chooses to impose such a limitation through an advance directive statute that is applicable only to women who have executed advance directives—and probably applicable only to women who have executed a statutorily based advance directive—runs the risk that such a prohibition will constitute a denial of equal protection.

CONCLUSION. If a statutory advance directive is the sole legally enforceable means for executing an advance directive, then the substantive rights of incompetent individuals to forgo life-sustaining treatment have been seriously restricted by these statutes. Probably the most restrictive of the provisions is the one that permits a statutory advance directive to take effect only if the patient is "terminally ill" or "permanently unconscious." If that is the case, people who wish to forgo or limit treatment in the event of a long, debilitating illness such as Alzheimer's disease or other dementiform conditions such as stroke will have those wishes thwarted. Ironically, although this particular restriction is the most sweeping, it is also the least visible. That this is so becomes clear merely from reading an advance directive statute with limitations on forgoing artificial nutrition and hydration or on forgoing any treatment from a pregnant patient. The limitation imposed by the requirement that the patient be terminally ill or permanently unconscious, however, is phrased in such a way that it might not be at all apparent to nonmedically trained people—and especially to people who execute advance directives and even to the lawyers who might draft them—that a statutory advance directive will not become effective in the situation that they most fear: dying a slow, debilitating, possibly painful, and probably expensive death.

Applicability of Advance Directive Statutes to Nondeclarants

Because advance directive statutes tend to restrict the scope of common-law rights to refuse medical treatment, it is important to know not only whether these restrictions can be avoided by individuals who wish to have broader advance directives but also whether they restrict the rights of people who become incompetent but have not executed an advance directive.

The theory of advance directives strongly, if not unquestioningly, suggests that the provisions of advance directive statutes should not apply to people who have not executed a directive. Again, the purpose of advance directive statutes is not to create legal rights—specifically, the right to make anticipatory medical decisions—but to provide a nonexclusive mechanism by which these rights may be implemented.

This question has been the subject of some, though not extensive, attention by a number of courts, and there seems to be a split of authority. For instance, the Kentucky Supreme Court found in the living will statute

> a reaffirmation of the common-law right, a legislative finding "that all adults have the fundamental right to control the decisions relating to their own medical care, including the decision to have medical or surgical means or procedures calculated to prolong their lives provided, withheld, or withdrawn." KRS 311.622(1). The statute goes on from there to specify one method by which a competent adult, through a "living will" as detailed in the Act, can "make a written declaration . . . instructing the adult's physician to withhold or withdraw life-prolonging treatment in the event such person is diagnosed as having a terminal condition." KRS 311.622(2). (*Degrella* 1993)

According to this court, the statute "does not purport to be exclusive, or to supersede common law rights" (ibid., 706). It therefore concluded that the provisions of the living will statute were of no effect in the case of a patient who had not executed a living will. By contrast, the Pennsylvania Superior Court (in an opinion that it subsequently vacated) took its general direction from the state's advance directive statute. The court applied a substantial number of the statute's requirements in the case of a patient who had never made his wishes about treatment known, orally or in writing, pursuant to the advance directive statute or otherwise. However, it also concluded that "the Act creates no presumption concerning the intent of any person who has not executed" an advance directive (*Fiori* 1993, *9).

An intermediate position was adopted by the Missouri Supreme Court in the *Cruzan* case. The court agreed that the living will statute did not apply because the patient had made no living will (and could not have pursuant to the statute because the statute was not enacted until long after the patient became incompetent) but nonetheless relied on it "as an expression of the policy of this State with regard to the sanctity of life" (*Cruzan* 1988, 420).

Advance Directives and Competent Patients

When does an advance directive become operative? There are actually two parts to this question, as suggested by case 1. The more frequently occurring of the two is the question of when a patient is to be considered incompetent such that his or her advance directive applies. This question arises only with patients, such as those with moderate dementia, who are not *unquestionably* incapable of making decisions (e.g., *Lane* 1978). The second and less frequently occurring aspect of this question is whether an advance directive has any relevance to decision making (and, if so, what kind and how much) when a patient is unquestionably competent. An example of this occurs when a doctor writes a DNR order for a hospitalized competent patient on the basis of the fact that the patient has an advance directive that states that he or she does not want CPR.

Although courts have not had occasion to address these questions, some guidance can be intuited from the fundamental purpose of advance directives and from the probable intent of those who make them. The purpose of advance directives is to provide people with a means for influencing, if not directing, decisions about their medical treatment after they have lost the capacity to do so contemporaneously. As a general rule, doctors should assume that as long as patients remain competent, their contemporaneous *decisions* govern rather than their advance directives. The only exception should be when the patient has expressly stated in a health care power of attorney that it is his or her intent to transfer decision-making authority to a proxy upon execution rather than upon the patient's loss of decision-making capacity.[6] Even in that case, however, it is probably better practice for doctors to specifically ask patients whether they should deal with the patient or with the proxy. In addition, physicians most certainly must observe competent patients' objections to any decision made by a proxy.

Closely related to this issue is the question of whether the patient's conduct and decisions about treatment while competent should be taken to modify or even revoke the provisions of an advance directive if the patient subsequently becomes incompetent. For example, in case 1, Mr. Jones contemporaneously consents—or at least his lack of objection is taken by the doctor as consent—to ventilation and antibiotic therapy. There is nothing inherently inconsistent between that consent and the advance directive, even though it specifically says that he does not want these treatments. The advance directive should only be interpreted as meaning that Mr. Jones, when he contemplated some future time at which he might not be able to decide for himself, decided that under such circumstances he did not want a variety of treatments, including ventilation and antibiotics. When Mr. Jones does, in fact, lose decision-making capacity, his prior refusal of such treatment, through his advance directive, comes into conflict with his prior contemporaneous consent to such treatment before losing decision-making capacity. Which should govern?

There is no specific legal guidance in judicial opinions or in legislation about this issue. I suggest the following way of analyzing the problem. At the outset, Mr. Jones's contemporaneous consent to these treatments must govern because he is competent. When he loses decision-making capacity, the treatments to which he has consented should continue if they are still medically indicated. The mere fact that a patient loses the ability to make decisions—one of the conditions necessary for an advance directive to go into effect—does not, in itself, mean that treatments already in progress should be stopped or even reevaluated, even if the advance directive directs that he does not want the treatment in question. It is reasonable to assume in Mr. Jones's case, given our knowledge of how he wanted to live and die, that he was not opposed to ventilators and antibiotics per se, but rather he was opposed to medical treatment that would only prolong the process of dying and would provide no reasonable probability of restoring his health. If that were the case, then the treatments in question could be—and should be—stopped, not simply because Mr. Jones now lacks decision-making capacity but because further treatment will not effectuate his goals. It is pretty safe to say that if Mr. Jones could recover, he would want to, but if treatment is only postponing death, he does not want it. However, the doctor is uncertain about whether the treatment will accomplish Mr. Jones's goal of restoring his health or whether it will undermine his goal of avoiding a lingering death.

The "Checklist" Approach to Advance Directives

Most living will statutes contain forms that, as previously discussed, may be, but are not required to be, used to make an advance directive. Many of these forms contain a list of treatments that the patient can check that he or she wants or does not want. These forms and lists have been included in the statutes, first, to encourage the execution of advance directives by providing people with a simple way to make an advance directive without either having to consult a lawyer to have one written or having to design one by oneself. Second, by providing physicians and health care administrators with a familiar-looking form, these lists are intended to decrease the chance that an advance directive will be ignored because it is viewed by a physician as "illegal."

Despite these admirable objectives, this approach to writing advance directive legislation and to writing advance directives puts form over substance. Case 1 illustrates that reliance on this approach can be unwise. Worse than unwise, reliance on forms can be dangerous. Suppose that in case 1, Mr. Jones recovers and leaves the hospital. While crossing the street in front of the hospital, he is struck by a bus. His advance directive is in his shirt pocket. The emergency medical technicians provide stabilizing care and take him to the hospital's emergency room, where his advance directive is discovered. The professional staff there know that Mr. Jones is terminally ill with AIDS, they see that he does not want CPR or ventilation, so they halt all resuscitative efforts. Given that Mr. Jones had just completed a successful hospitalization, it is fairly certain that he *does* want to be resuscitated even though he has a terminal illness. What this example illustrates is that most people probably mean to imply a causal link between the terminal illness and the treatment in question, a link that is absent when Mr. Jones's need for treatment is brought about not by the terminal illness but by some other infelicitous event.

Although reliance on forms is likely to be both the patient's and the lawyer's approach, it should not be the physician's. For a superior approach to work, however, physicians must take the initiative to discuss advance medical planning with patients, to achieve an understanding of the patient's goals and values, and to acquire an understanding of the *patient.* Otherwise, patients who want to plan for medical decision making when they can no longer decide for themselves are forced to fall back on lawyers, legal forms, and self-help advance directive forms, all of which are inherently mechanistic.

My chief concern with reflexive reliance on forms for executing advance directives is that the form will substitute for substance. This is not a hypothetical concern. We have enough experience with the use of so-called informed consent forms in medical therapy and research to know that physicians become obsessively concerned with getting patients to sign forms at the expense of explaining to patients the information that they need to know to make intelligent decisions and instead of undertaking efforts, through a discussion, to determine if patients understand what they have been told (Katz 1984). The same is true of institutional review boards (IRBs), which not uncommonly seem far more concerned with making sure that the consent forms for clinical research contain all necessary information—sometimes so much information that it makes it difficult for potential subjects to determine what is relevant and what is not—than with ensuring that subjects understand what they need to know to make intelligent decisions and that the research, as designed, should be undertaken at all. Ethics committees and courts, if they were to review advance directives, could easily fall prey to the same kind of thinking.

Another concern, as previously discussed and as illustrated by case 3, is that statutory advance directive forms, like the statutes that they are intended to implement, place some serious restrictions on what treatment may be forgone, restrictions that some (and perhaps many) people wish to avoid. Because these restrictions probably do not apply to nonstatutory directives, one might avoid them by refraining from using the statutory form. However, the sense of security provided by statutory forms is frequently too hard for patients, their lawyers, and their doctors to resist.

Fine-Tuning Instructions through the Use of Health Care Agents

One of the reasons that living wills often prove to be less useful in making actual decisions than their proponents would like them to be is that they run the dual opposing risks of either being too general or too specific. As to the former, for example, there are probably very few people who object in principle to a particular kind of treatment—who really mean that they would *never* want to be kept alive by a ventilator—but many whose living wills actually say that. What they really object to is the administration of any medical treatment other than palliative and hygienic care when there is no reasonable hope for recovery in a state of existence and a quality of life that they would find acceptable.

Gradually, legislatures have come to realize what many physicians have long known: that it is far more useful in making decisions about life-sustaining treatment for doctors to know *who* has authority to speak for the patient than what the patient's wishes are (or, more likely, are purported to be). Legislatures have done this by the enactment of health care power of attorney statutes. Even before these statutes were as widespread as they are today, the use of an ordinary durable power of attorney for health care decision making received the imprimatur of the few courts that had occasion to consider them (*Peter* 1987; *Rasmussen* 1987; *O'Connor* 1988; *Crabtree* 1990; *Cruzan* 1990, O'Connor, J., concurring).

Appointing an agent for medical decision making provides a great deal more flexibility than can ever be incorporated in any meaningful, simple, and sensible way into an instruction directive because it is simply not possible to anticipate in advance all the different medical decisions that might need to be made and the circumstances under which they might arise. Nor is it possible to anticipate all the subtleties of medical decision making even for a patient who is clearly dying from a particular disease.

Rather than attempting to decide all things in advance, one who executes a proxy directive implicitly acknowledges that such detailed advance planning is either not possible or, if possible, not desirable because it is too inflexible. The proxy directive is, in effect, interstitial decision making in the form of a statement by the person who executes it that he or she entrusts decision making to a representative about his or her future medical care, should the person be unable personally to participate in decision making.

Case 1 illustrates the need for fine-tuning an advance directive. Under these kinds of conditions of uncertainty, what role should doctors, families and close friends, and proxies have in this fine-tuning and applying of an advance directive? How certain must the doctor be that the patient will recover in order to treat him despite the advance directive and the parents' invocation of it?

Proxy directives can be combined with instruction directives so that one can both invest an agent with decision-making authority and provide evidence of one's wishes. When this is done, it is probably best for patients to express their wishes in precatory, rather than binding, terms, lest they undercut the very flexibility that is the hallmark of a proxy directive. The essence of the proxy directive is the avoidance of categorical decisions, such as "I never want to be on a ventilator," because the fact is that the declarant would *want* to be on a ventilator if it were necessary to sustain his or her breathing until he or she recovered enough from an illness or injury to breathe without mechanical assistance, as illustrated by case 1.

Fine-tuning an advance directive can also be enhanced by the patients' stating their treatment goals, what quality of life they find acceptable, as well as indicating that they do not want treatment that is not likely to achieve those goals and that quality of life.

Surrogate Decision Making without Advance Directives

Advance directives are helpful only if people have them, and most people do not (Emanuel and Emanuel 1989). Although unlikely, perhaps someday everyone will have an advance directive, but even if they did, the foregoing discussion elucidates the fact that advance directives rarely answer all questions about decision making, and sometimes they create new ones. Thus, other devices also need to be employed for making medical treatment decisions for incompetent patients.

Because most people do not have advance directives, we have a great deal of experience in facilitating decision making for incompetent patients without these documents. Decision making without advance directives raises procedural questions about who is to serve as a surrogate for a patient lacking in decision-making capacity, how that person is to acquire the authority to act, and how to make decisions in the face of irresolvable disagreements among surrogates, family members (and possibly close friends of the patient), and health care professionals. Decision making without advance directives also raises the central substantive issue of surrogate decision making: by what standards are surrogates to make decisions for incompetent patients?

PROCEDURAL ISSUES: SURROGATE DECISION-MAKING STATUTES. When a patient has failed to designate a surrogate prior to losing decision-making capacity, the courts have made it abundantly clear that the patient's family has legal authority to make decisions for the patient, and to do so without one of them being judicially appointed to serve as the patient's guardian (Meisel 1995, § 5.14). This is consistent both with clinical practice, which traditionally has relied upon family members to make decisions for patients unable to do so for themselves (Smedira et al. 1990), and with the wishes of many patients (Cohen-Mansfield et al. 1991; Gamble, McDonald, and Lichstein 1991).

This general rule of law is frequently far easier to state than to implement in the clinical setting. A handful of questions immediately arise: Who is the patient's "family"? How are decisions to be made by a group of people? What if the patient has no family? What if the patient has family members, but has a close friend who may seem at least as appropriate as family to act as surrogate (such as a domestic partner to whom he is not married)?

Although judicial decisions exhibit a strong general preference for having these issues resolved without recourse to the courts, they have provided little specific guidance. This has served as an impetus for many state legislatures, in the wake of the *Cruzan* decision, to enact statutes recognizing who possesses the legal authority to make medical decisions on behalf of patients who are unable to do so for themselves and who have not themselves designated another to do so. These are usually referred to as "surrogate decision-making" statutes, but sometimes as "family decision-making" statutes (Orentlicher 1994).

The main feature of these statutes is a list, in order of priority, of persons who are legally authorized to act as surrogate decision makers (Meisel 1995,

§ 14.4). The person usually heading the list is the patient's spouse. Also high on the lists are the patient's adult offspring, parents, and adult siblings. Beyond that the statutes vary widely, listing (in descending order of frequency) a guardian of the person, nearest living relative or competent relative, grandchild, grandparent, friend, and attending physician. Some also include a guardian of the patient's estate, heirs at law, clergy, domestic partner, religious superior if a member of a religious order, or other person to whom one's wishes were made known.

Although the intent of such priority lists is a good one—to eliminate possible uncertainty about who, if anyone, has the legal authority to make decisions for incompetent patients—the result of surrogate designation pursuant to such a list is not only mechanical but can be contrary or even inimical to the patient's wishes or best interests (Loewy 1992). This would occur, for example, if the patient were estranged from his or her spouse or parents. However, it is not clear that the result would be much different in the absence of a statute since the ordinary custom of physicians is to look to incompetent patients' close family members to make decisions for them. In the absence of a statute, the physician might ignore a spouse whom he or she knows to be estranged from the patient in favor of other close family members as surrogates. Because there is nothing in most statutes to prohibit an estranged spouse from acting as surrogate, the result could be worse under a statute than in its absence if the statute is mechanically applied.

Most statutes do not specifically anticipate that there may be disagreement among the persons in a particular class who are designated to serve as surrogate (e.g., the patient's adult offspring or the patient's siblings), or that there may be disagreement between the person who is authorized to act as a surrogate by virtue of a high priority on the list (e.g., the patient's spouse) and someone lower on the priority list (e.g., a sibling of the patient) who would be authorized to act as surrogate if a higher priority individual were not available. In practice, disagreements of these kinds may not be at all infrequent, and therefore the failure of most statutes to address them could easily lead to precisely the kind of uncertainty (and potentially lead to litigation) that surrogate decision-making statutes were enacted to avoid. Although some statutes do recognize that there may be disagreement, the manner in which this disagreement is to be resolved varies considerably.

SUBSTANTIVE ISSUES: STANDARDS FOR SURROGATE DECISION MAKING. The most fundamental problem of decision making for incompetent patients is the standard by which such decisions are to be made. This issue has received voluminous attention from courts and commentators—and increasingly from legislatures (Meisel 1995, § 14.8)—that have overwhelmingly concluded that, in order to promote individual autonomy, decision making should be guided by the now-incompetent patient's *wishes.*[7] Others have felt that this conclusion is ultimately a fiction (Harmon 1990; Robertson 1991; Dresser 1986)—and the *clinical experience* with the difficulties arising from the use of advance directives possibly bears out their objections[8]—and therefore have urged the use of some variation on a best interests standard. Some courts permit the use of a best interests standard when a patient's wishes cannot be ascertained (Meisel 1995, § 7.12), but only one judicial decision has suggested that this standard should always be used, even if the patient's wishes are known (*Drabick* 1988).

One way to avoid the difficulties associated with determining the wishes of a person who can no longer express them is to attempt to devise objective standards for forgoing life-sustaining treatment. These principles may be used either when we do not know a patient's wishes with a sufficient degree of confidence, or instead of relying on a patient's wishes altogether. A variation on this proposal is to create a presumption that when these objective criteria are met, life support will be terminated unless the patient has previously "opted out" through an advance directive. This is essentially the approach that is used in the transmission of decedents' estates. If an individual does not execute a will directing how his or her property is to be transmitted to the heirs, there are rules of state law that govern how the estate is to be distributed.

One aspect of the standards issue that has received little attention is the question of what standard for decision making is to apply when a patient *has* executed an advance directive. At first, this seems like an absurd question because an advance directive—or at least an instruction directive—is intended to address this issue by providing clear and convincing evidence of the patient's own wishes about treatment, thereby precluding any further need for attention to the standard for surrogate decision making.[9]

However, advance directives do not always hit the nail squarely on the head. There are two kinds of situations in which the standard for surrogate decision making might *not* be satisfied by the existence of an advance directive. First, the advance directive might be an instruction directive that is too general or of uncertain applicability to the current situation. A generic advance directive stating that the patient does not want any "extraordinary or heroic" treatment is an example of an overly general advance directive. The advance directive in case 1 stating "If I should be in an incurable or irreversible mental or physical condition with no reasonable expectation of recovery, I direct my attending physician to withhold or withdraw treatment that merely prolongs my dying" is an another example of a directive that might or might not have anticipated the current set of circumstances. Such an advance directive would probably not satisfy the "specific-subjective-intent" standard required in New York (*O'Connor* 1988) and might not even satisfy the widely accepted substituted judgment standard.

Second, the advance directive might be a proxy directive—that is, it might appoint an agent for making decisions rather than providing any instructions. Such a directive does not *in fact* satisfy any standard for surrogate decision making; nonetheless, it might be *legally* satisfactory. A proxy directive could be thought of as a waiver by the patient of the application of the prevailing standard for surrogate decision making; in effect, it is an instruction from the patient to the proxy for the proxy to use his or her own judgment in determining what treatment decisions to make, rather than an injunction to use good faith in making a decision that best reflects what the proxy believes are the patient's wishes or best interests (*Cruzan* 1990, 289; *Mack* 1993, 757–58; *O'Connor* 1988, 612 n.2).

Suppose that the patient seeks to modify the prevailing standard for decision making for incompetent patients through his advance directive. For example, in New York, a surrogate may forgo life-sustaining treatment for an incompetent patient only if the surrogate has clear and convincing evidence of the patient's wishes. If an advance directive appoints a proxy and gives him or her explicit authorization to make such medical decisions "that the proxy believes are in my best interests," is New York law satisfied if the proxy does not know what the patient's wishes are but in good faith makes a decision that he or she believes to be best for the patient? Or suppose that the patient has appointed his spouse as proxy and then given the direction that the proxy "is to make whatever decision she wishes, taking into account the impact of my condition and its treatment on her and on my children"—in effect, a direction to make decisions in the best interests of the patient's family, a standard not currently accepted in law. It is not certain whether such directives are legally enforceable.

What is to happen when the proxy makes decisions that are thought to be inconsistent with the patient's wishes or with the patient's best interests? If the patient attempts to control the proxy's discretion in specific ways, then the dangers of an instruction directive (inflexibility and excessive specificity) once again arise. If the patient attempts to control the proxy's discretion by some more general standard—such as "make decisions that are in my best interests"—then the directive may be so general as to be unhelpful.

Nonetheless, there will be situations in which the patient's doctor will be concerned that the proxy is choosing a course of action that either goes against the patient's wishes or is not in the patient's best interests, or both. For example, in case 1, the doctor believes that treatment should continue because it was Mr. Jones's own goal to get out of the hospital to resume life as it was before he developed pneumonia. Furthermore, his consent (or, at least, his lack of objection) to ventilation and antibiotics demonstrates that he sought to pursue this goal in these particular circumstances, and these treatments stand a reasonably good chance of achieving his goal. The doctor therefore believes that the agent's decision to terminate treatment, if implemented, would not effectuate the patient's own wishes.

A more graphic example of this same general problem of what standards should apply to decision making by a patient-appointed agent is exemplified by case 2. Here, the physician believes that continued treatment will not accomplish the patient's goals and seeks to withdraw it but is confronted with a proxy who wants "everything possible" done for the patient. The proxy's instruction may be based on a different understanding of what the patient's goals were or a different interpretation as to whether those goals can be achieved. Alternately, the proxy may be considering his own interests—such as assuaging the proxy's guilt about his prior relationship with the patient or a financial interest in keeping the patient alive (e.g., retirement benefits, trust beneficiary)—rather than the patient's.

These problems also arise in decision making for incompetent patients who have not made any kind of advance directive and who thus have a common-law or statutory surrogate. Do the standards set forth in the judicial precedents or in the surrogate decision-making statutes in which surrogates are charged with making decisions for incompetent patients apply when the patient appoints the surrogate through a proxy directive? Does the patient have the authority to vary these standards?

Conflict of Interest

Another problem that exists in decision making for incompetent patients and that advance directives do not, and probably cannot, avoid is conflicts of interest between surrogates and patients. To some extent, conflicts of interest are built into the decision-making process for incompetent patients because the application of any of the accepted standards for surrogate decision making is substantially enhanced by the surrogate's familiarity with the patient and knowledge of his or her preferences, goals, and values. We need and want someone who knows the patient well to act as the surrogate, but someone who knows the patient well is also likely to be someone who will be personally affected in some way by the decision he or she makes for the patient. Thus, if the existence of a conflict of interest alone were to disqualify an individual from serving as a surrogate, precisely the people we want to make decisions for incompetent patients would be barred from doing so.

Conflicts of interest will almost always exist in decision making about life-sustaining treatment (*Cruzan* 1990, 286). The standards for making such decisions for incompetent patients demand that, if at all possible, the surrogate be someone who knows the patient's wishes and interests well. Such a person is likely to be one who personally stands to lose or gain in some way from the patient's death. The only way to avoid conflicts of interest is either to insist that patients make such decisions for themselves before losing decision-making capacity or to utilize as surrogates individuals who have no personal stake in the outcome of the decision. Most courts have rejected both approaches as impractical and not consistent with what most patients would want. Consequently, what is essential is not whether there is a conflict of interest but how extensive it is. Only when a surrogate decision is motivated primarily by something other than concern for what is best for the *patient* should recourse to the courts be sought (*Drabick* 1988, 861 n.38; *Conroy* 1985, 1218–19; Pa. Cons. Stat. Ann. 1993, § 5511[F]).

The law about conflicts of interest is woefully underdeveloped. Judicial decisions have only given cursory attention to the threshold issue—namely, that the existence of a conflict of interest is one of the reasons for seeking recourse to the courts in decision making about life-sustaining treatment (Meisel 1995, § 5.35). However, a conflict of interest should not prima facie disqualify a surrogate or require judicial supervision of the decision-making process, for this would effectively cripple this process in most cases.

Neither courts nor legislatures have provided any significant guidance about what constitutes a conflict of interest serious enough to disqualify the surrogate or to require recourse to the courts. Probably the clearest kind of potential conflict of interest exists when the surrogate is an heir of the patient or is financially responsible for the patient's health care costs and stands to gain financially by the patient's death.[10] In addition to financial conflicts of interest, there may be an "emotional conflict of interest" between the surrogate and the patient. A surrogate might be motivated, perhaps unconsciously, by a wish to put an end to a tremendous emotional strain on his or her own life caused by the patient's illness (*Cruzan* 1990, 2855–56; *A.C.* 1990, 1250). Not all conflicts of interest will incline the surrogate to terminate life-sustaining treatment; some may create an incentive to *continue* treatment, either for financial or emotional reasons.

Not all conflicts of interest should bar a surrogate from acting or should require a surrogate to act only under judicial supervision. Only when a surrogate's decision is motivated *primarily* by something other than concern for what is best for the patient should recourse to the courts be sought (*Drabick* 1988, 861 n.38; *Conroy* 1985, 1218–19). There are difficulties with this test, and indeed with any test. First, there is the problem of determining what motivates any person in any circumstance, let alone what *primarily* motivates someone. Second, it is unclear what the role of health care professionals should be in ascertaining the existence, nature, and depth of a conflict of interest in any particular case. Health care professionals should attempt to verify that surrogates are making decisions motivated primarily by the patient's wishes and interests. Special attention must be paid to possible "economic considerations, family pressures, or other factors of undue influence [that] could cloud a surrogate's judgment" (*Browning* 1989, 274), but just how this is to happen will require a great deal of work by courts, commentators, and clinicians.

Futility

Case 2 illustrates a problem that has been lurking in the shadows of decision making for incompetent patients for quite some time and has only recently begun to emerge. This problem—usually referred to as "futility"—concerns the authority of family members to compel the provision of treatment that physicians believe no longer serves the patient's interests—for example, patients for whom treatment is thought to be futile. It is a problem common to both patients with and without advance directives, and it is a problem that advance directive legislation does not expressly address.[11] Advance directive legislation can, however, exacerbate this problem. Some statutory checklists are accompanied by a section in which declarants are invited to signify whether they do not or *do* want a particular treatment. If they signify that they do want a treatment, this could easily trigger a battle between a physician who believes that such treatment is not warranted and the patient's family who contend, on the basis of the advance directive, that the patient wanted it to be provided.

There is little case law on the topic, though it is beginning to be the subject of litigation. The well-known *Wanglie* case (1991) was the first to raise the issue in court, though in a very oblique manner, and the result of this case was entirely inconclusive. The second case, *In re Doe* (1992), was a definitive ruling holding that physicians could not refuse to administer cardiopulmonary resuscitation that they believed was not medically indicated in the face of the surrogate's insistence that it be administered if needed. However, the ruling was based on a fairly narrow Georgia statutory ground and might not be persuasive to other courts faced with similar problems but not bound by the statute. In a later case, one judge of the Georgia Court of Appeals suggested that there might be a constitutional basis for patients to claim an entitlement to treatment (*Velez* 1995, Beasley, S.J., concurring), but it is doubtful that there is any such right under the federal constitution (Meisel 1995, § 19.10).

The third futility case, the *Baby K* case (1994), also held that treatment could not be forgone in the face of the refusal of the surrogate to consent to its termination. The basis for this holding—the federal Emergency Medical Treatment and Active Labor Act (EMTALA 1992)—is of much broader applicability than the statute on which the *Doe* decision is based and seemed to create the possibility that physicians would legally not be able to resist demands for medically futile treatment.

However, the scope of the *Baby K* decision has been significantly narrowed by a later decision of the same court (*Bryan* 1996). More recent litigation has also been inconclusive. The notorious *Gilgunn* case (1995), in which a patient in a persistent vegetative state was removed from a ventilator over the express wishes of her daughter, resulted in a jury verdict for the doctor and hospital, but because this was not appealed, it does not constitute a legal precedent. A similar case is making its way through the Pennsylvania courts, and it is possible that it will yield a more definitive precedent than any of the other cases (*Rideout* 1996).

Conclusion

Judges, legislators, health care professionals, academic commentators, and the public have all put their money on advance directives (and the closely related surrogate decision-making statutes) to solve the inherent dilemma of making a decision about forgoing or administering life-sustaining treatment to people who are no longer able to make their own decisions. Although these advocates should not be faulted for trying, the truth is that the solutions are halfway at best and may create as many new dilemmas as they resolve. If advance directives do not work well in the United States with its substantial emphasis on individualism and rationality, it is not likely that they will work much better in more paternalistic societies.

Advance directives are not the only problem, nor are they the only solution, in decision making for incompetent patients. There are other, and possibly better, ways to ease the burden of decision making for incompetent patients, involving a clarification of substantive standards, procedural changes (e.g., surrogate decision-making statutes), or both. Lawyers—whether acting as legislators, judges, counselors to individual patients, or counselors to health care professionals and institutions—need to redirect their energies from emphasizing legislation and drafting solutions that rely on formalities to addressing the truly fundamental problem of decision making for patients who have lost their decision-making capacity, namely, the standard by which such decisions should be made.

Notes

1. I use the term *incompetent persons* as a shorthand expression for patients who lack decision-making capacity in fact but who have not necessarily been adjudicated incompetent. If a patient has been adjudicated incompetent, a guardian will have been appointed and probably clothed with the authority to make medical decisions, so that questions about advance directives and surrogate decision making are either nonexistent or very attenuated.

2. The question has not received a great deal of attention from the courts. Two Florida courts have ruled on the validity of nonstatutory living wills (*Corbett* 1986; *Browning* 1990), both finding them valid. A small number of courts (*Peter* 1987; *Rasmussen* 1987; *O'Connor* 1988; *Crabtree* 1990) have considered the validity of using an ordinary durable power of attorney for the purpose of medical decision making, finding it permissible to do so (see Meisel 1995, § 10.11).

3. Any lawyer who recommends the use of a statutory advance directive to a client who is not aware of this limitation (and others) and of the possible ways of evading it might be a subject to liability for professional negligence.

4. Arizona, California, Connecticut, Delaware, Florida, Illinois, Indiana, Kentucky, Maine, Maryland, Massachusetts, Michigan, Missouri, New Jersey, New York, North Carolina, Ohio, Pennsylvania, Rhode Island, Washington, Wisconsin.

5. The Missouri Supreme Court treats artificial nutrition and hydration differently from other forms of treatment. In fact, it does not consider artificial nutrition and hydration to be a form of medical treatment. In the court's words, "This is not a case in which we are asked to let someone die. . . . This is a case in which we are asked to allow the medical profession to make Nancy die by starvation and dehydration. . . . And common sense tells us that food and water do not treat an illness, they maintain a life" (*Cruzan* 1988, 412, 423). Consequently the Missouri court will permit artificial nutrition and hydration to be forgone from an incompetent patient only if there is "clear and convincing evidence" that the patient herself decided upon their termination prior to losing decision-making capacity—for example, through an advance di-

rective. The fact that the applicability of this high standard is limited to artificial nutrition and hydration is demonstrated by the Missouri Court of Appeals' *Warren* (1993) decision in which it permitted a cardiopulmonary resuscitation to be withheld on the basis of a best interests standard.

The state of Washington might preclude the forgoing of artificial nutrition and hydration altogether, unlike Missouri, which permits it to be forgone pursuant to an advance directive. It is difficult to know just where the Washington Supreme Court stands on this issue. In the *Colyer* (1983) and *Hamlin* (1984) cases, the court permitted the termination of "life support systems" from patients who were in a persistent vegetative state. Presumably, this included artificial nutrition and hydration, but the court's opinions do not say this specifically. In the next right-to-die case to come before that court (*Grant* 1987), by a 5 to 4 vote the court specifically permitted the withholding of artificial nutrition and hydration. Seven months later, the court issued a new, two-sentence opinion, which stated that the name Justice Durham, who had voted with the 5 to 4 majority, "is removed" from the majority opinion and "is appended at the end of the [dissenting] opinion" (*Grant* 1988).

Illinois requires judicial review for forgoing artificial nutrition and hydration (*Longeway* 1989; *Greenspan* 1990). An Ohio appellate case appeared to prohibit the forgoing of artificial nutrition and hydration (*Couture* 1989), but according to a subsequent case (*Crum* 1991), new advance directive legislation now permits the forgoing of artificial nutrition and hydration.

6. A durable power of attorney can be drafted so as to take effect upon execution or on the happening of some condition, generally the "incapacity" (or similar language) of the principal. The latter is referred to as a *springing* durable power of attorney. The disadvantage of the former is that the agent is empowered to act for the principal immediately even though the principal may have no need or wish to delegate authority at present. In practice, however, should the agent seek to assert authority when the principal is competent and does not wish the agent to act, the principal may revoke the power of attorney (Uniform Durable Power of Attorney Act 1983, § 5). The Uniform Health Care Decisions Act (1993, § 2[c]) presumes that a health care power of attorney is springing unless the document states otherwise.

7. Determining the wishes of one who can no longer express them is necessarily a hypothetical exercise. The primary point of divergence among courts subscribing to the consensus is *how* hypothetical an exercise they will permit it to be. The New York courts require that there be "clear and convincing evidence" that the patient made a solemn declaration of his wishes (*Eichner* 1980; *O'Connor* 1988), which is sometimes referred to as a "subjective standard"; perhaps Missouri (*Cruzan* 1988; *Warren* 1993) and Maine (*Gardner* 1987; *Swan* 1990) do also, and Michigan (*Martin* 1995) and Wisconsin (*Edna F.* 1997) do under limited circumstances. All other courts that have considered this issue permit the use of the "substituted judgment standard," which in effect permits surrogates to make their best approximation of what patients

would want were they able to express their wishes. Some, but not all, of the courts subscribing to the substituted judgment standard permit a best interests standard to be used if there is inadequate evidence or no evidence of the patient's wishes (Meisel 1995, § 7.2).

8. The evidence about whether family members accurately reflect patients' views is mixed. Tomlinson et al. (1990, 59) report that "close family members performed slightly better than physicians in reflecting patients' wishes. But . . . the use of family members does not in itself improve protection of the elderly patient's interests unless they are also required to act on the basis of a substituted judgment standard." Danis et al. (1988, 799) report that "families' preferences were similar to those of surviving patients." However, Zweibel and Cassel (1989, 620) report that "middle-generation family proxies" of widowed elderly patients underestimated patients' preferences for resuscitation and "often choose care . . . that goes against what the patients would choose for themselves"; and Uhlmann, Pearlman, and Cain (1988) report that spouses overestimate patients' preferences for CPR.

9. Although most surrogate decision-making statutes provide some guidance about the standard that the surrogate is to apply in decision making, these standards tend to follow the common-law pattern of a preference for implementing the patient's wishes and thus have not seized the opportunity to attempt to provide a more detailed account of an objective best interests standard than the courts have provided (Meisel 1995, § 14.8).

10. A classic example of this is illustrated by an unreported Florida case (*Stone* 1991), in which the patient's wife claimed that the patient's son was trying to terminate life support to inherit his father's estate and to deprive her of an expectancy under an antenuptial agreement. The patient's son claimed (and the trial court found) that he was merely trying to enforce his father's wishes, and that the patient's wife was "only trying to prolong Mr. Stone's life so that she can gain more monies" (*Stone* 1991, 3).

11. It is also a problem that can arise with competent patients. However, when patients are competent, their medical condition is presumably such that treatment should be provided if that is what they request. There are, however, limits to which treatments should be provided to competent patients, too. Terminally ill people will sometimes grasp at straws if a treatment holds out a possibility, however remote, of providing a permanent or temporary cure.

Cases

A.C. 1990. In re A.C., 573 A.2d 1235 (D.C. 1990).

Baby K 1994. In re Baby "K," 16 F.3d 590 (4th Cir. 1994).

Bludworth 1984. John F. Kennedy Memorial Hosp. v. Bludworth, 452 So. 2d 921 (Fla. 1984).

Bouvia 1986. Bouvia v. Superior Court (Glenchur), 225 Cal. Rptr. 297 (Ct. App. 1986).

Browning 1989. In re Browning, 543 So. 2d 258 (Fla. Dist. Ct. App. 1989).
Browning 1990. In re Browning, 568 So. 2d 4 (Fla. 1990).
Bryan 1996. Bryan v. Rectors & Visitors of the University of Virginia, 95 F.3d 349 (4th Cir. 1996).
Casey 1992. Planned Parenthood of Southeastern Pa. v. Casey, 112 S. Ct. 2791 (1992).
Colyer 1983. In re Colyer, 660 P.2d 738 (Wash. 1983).
Conroy 1985. In re Conroy: 1985, 98 N.J. 321, 486 A. 2d 1209.
Corbett 1986. Corbett v. D'Alessandro, 487 So. 2d 368 (Fla. Dist. Ct. App.), *review denied,* 492 So. 2d 1331 (Fla. 1986).
Couture 1989. Couture v. Couture, 549 N.E.2d 571 (Ohio Ct. App. 1989).
Crabtree 1990. In re Crabtree, No. 86-0031 (Haw. Fam. Ct. 1st Cir., Apr. 26, 1990).
Crum 1991. In re Crum, 580 N.E.2d 876 (Probate Ct. Franklin County, Ohio 1991).
Cruzan 1988. Cruzan v. Harmon, 760 S.W.2d 408 (Mo. 1988).
Cruzan 1990. Cruzan v. Director, 497 U.S. 261 (1990).
Degrella 1993. Degrella v. Elston, 858 S.W.2d 698 (Ky. 1993).
Doe 1992. In re Doe, 418 S.E.2d 3 (Ga. 1992).
Drabick 1988. In re Drabick, 245 Cal. Rptr. 840 (Ct. App. 1988).
Dubreuil 1993. In re Dubreuil, 629 So. 2d 819 (Fla. 1993).
Edna F. 1997. In re Edna M.F. v. Eisenberg, 563 N.W.2d 485 (Wis. 1997).
Eichner 1980. In re Eichner, 426 NYS 2d 517.
Fiori 1993. In re Fiori, 1993 Westlaw 471460 (Pa. Super. Ct. Nov. 16, 1993), *opinion vacated,* 652 A.2d 1350 (Pa. Super. 1995), *aff'd,* 673 A.2d 905 (Pa. 1996).
Fosmire 1990. In re Fosmire, 551 N.E.2d 77 (N.Y. 1990).
Gardner 1987. In re Gardner, 534 A.2d 947 (Me. 1987).
Gilgunn 1995. Gilgunn v. Massachusetts General Hospital, No. SUCV92-4820 (Superior Court, Suffolk County, Mass., verdict April 21, 1995).
Grant 1987. In re Grant, 747 P.2d 445 (Wash. 1987).
Grant 1988. In re Grant, 757 P.2d 534 (Wash. 1988).
Greenspan 1990. In re Estate of Greenspan, 558 N.E.2d 1194 (Ill. 1990).
Hamlin 1984. In re Hamlin, 689 P.2d 1372 (Wash. 1984).
Harrell 1996. Harrell v. St. Mary's Hosp., Inc. 678 So. 2d 455 (Fla. Dist. Ct. App. 1996).
Jackson 1985. Mercy Hosp. Inc. v. Jackson, 489 A.2d 1130 (Md. Ct. App. 1985).
Lane 1978. Lane v. Candura, 376 N.E.2d 1232 (Mass. App. Ct. 1978).
Longeway 1989. In re Longeway, 549 N.E.2d 292 (Ill. 1989).
Mack 1993. Mack v. Mack, 618 A.2d 744 (Md. 1993).
Martin 1995. Martin v. Martin, 538 N.W.2d 399 (Mich. 1995).
McAfee 1989. State v. McAfee, 385 S.E.2d 651 (Ga. 1989).
McKay 1990. McKay v. Bergstedt, 801 P.2d 617 (Nev. 1990).
Munoz 1991. Norwood Hosp. v. Munoz, 564 N.E.2d 1017 (Mass. 1991).
Myers 1993. In re Myers, 610 N.E.2d 663 (Probate Ct., Summit County, Ohio 1993).

O'Connor 1988. In re O'Connor, 531 N.E.2d 607 (N.Y. 1988).

Peter 1987. In re Peter, 529 A.2d 419 (N.J. 1987).

Quinlan 1976. In re Quinlan 1976, 70 N.J. 10, 355 A. 2d 647, *cert. denied sub nom. Garger v. New Jersey*: 1976, 429 U.S. 922, overruled in part, In re Conroy: 1985, 98 N.J. 321, 486 A. 2d 1209.

Ramsey 1985. St. Mary's Hosp. v. Ramsey, 465 So. 2d 666 (Fla. Dist. Ct. App. 1985).

Rasmussen 1987. Rasmussen v. Fleming, 741 P.2d 674 (Ariz. 1987).

Rideout 1996. Rideout v. Hershey Medical Center, 16 Fiduc. Rep. 2d 181 (C.P. Dauphin County, Pa. 1996).

Roe 1973. Roe v. Wade, 410 U.S. 13 (1973).

Stamford Hosp. 1996. Stamford Hosp. v. Vega, 674 A.2d 821 (Conn. 1996).

Stone 1991. In re Stone (1991), No. 90-5867 (Cir. Ct. 17th Dist. Broward County, Fla., June 24, 1991).

Swan 1990. In re Swan, 569 A.2d 1202 (Me. 1990).

Thor 1993. Thor v. Superior Court, 855 P.2d 375 (Cal. 1993).

Velez 1995. Velez v. Bethune, 466 S.E.2d 627 (Ga. Ct. App. 1995).

Wanglie 1991. In re Wanglie, No. PX-91-283 (4th Dist. Ct. Hennepin County, Minn., July 1, 1991).

Warren 1993. In re Warren, 858 S.W.2d 263 (Mo. Ct. App. 1993).

Wons 1989. Wons v. Pub. Health Trust, 541 So. 2d 96 (Fla. 1989).

Legislation

EMTALA 1992. 42 U.S.C.A. 1395dd (West 1992).

Uniform Durable Power of Attorney Act, § 5, 8A U.L.A. 275 (1983).

Uniform Health Care Decisions Act (1993).

References

Cohen-Mansfield, Jiska, et al. 1991. "The Decision to Execute a Durable Power of Attorney for Health Care and Preferences Regarding the Utilization of Life-Sustaining Treatments in Nursing Home Residents." *Archives of Internal Medicine* 151: 289–94.

Danis, Marion, et al. 1988. "Patients and Families' Preferences for Medical Intensive Care." *Journal of the American Medical Association* 260: 797–802.

Dresser, Rebecca. 1986. "Life, Death, and Incompetent Patients: Conceptual Infirmities and Hidden Values in the Law." *Arizona Law Review* 28: 373–405.

Emanuel, Linda L., and Ezekiel J. Emanuel. 1989. "The Medical Directive: A New Comprehensive Advance Care Document." *Journal of the American Medical Association* 261: 3288–93.

Gamble, Elizabeth R., Penelope J. McDonald, and Peter R. Lichstein. 1991. "Knowledge, Attitudes, and Behavior of Elderly Persons Regarding Living Wills." *Archives of Internal Medicine* 151: 277–80.

Harmon, Louise. 1990. "Falling off the Vine: Legal Fictions and the Doctrine of Substituted Judgment." *Yale Law Journal* 100: 1–71.

Katz, Jay. 1984. *The Silent World of Doctor and Patient.* New York: Free Press.

Kutner, Luis. 1969. "Due Process and Euthanasia: The Living Will, A Proposal." *Indiana Law Journal* 44:539–54.

Loewy, Erich H. 1992. "Advance Directives and Surrogate Laws: Ethical Instruments or Moral Cop-out?" *Archives of Internal Medicine* 152: 1973–76.

Meisel, Alan. 1992a. "The Legal Consensus about Forgoing Life-Sustaining Treatment: Its Status and Its Prospects." *Kennedy Institute of Ethics Journal* 2: 309–45.

———. 1992b. "A Retrospective on Cruzan." *Law, Medicine, and Health Care* 20: 340–53.

———. 1995. *The Right to Die.* 2d ed. New York: John Wiley.

Orentlicher, David. 1994. "The Limits of Legislation." *Maryland Law Review* 53: 1255–1305.

Robertson, John. 1991. "Second Thoughts on Living Wills." *Hastings Center Report* 21 (Nov-Dec): 6–9.

Smedira, Nicholas G., et al. 1990. "Withholding and Withdrawal of Life Support from the Critically Ill." *New England Journal of Medicine* 322: 309–14.

Tomlinson, Tom, Kenneth Howe, and Mark Notman. 1990. "An Empirical Study of Proxy Consent for Elderly Persons." *Gerontologist* 30: 54–64.

Uhlmann, Richard F., Robert A. Pearlman, and Kevin C. Cain. 1988. "Physicians' and Spouses' Predictions of Elderly Patients' Resuscitation Preferences." *Journal of Gerontology* 43: M115–21.

Zweibel, Nancy R., and Christine K. Cassel. 1989. "Treatment Choices at the End of Life: A Comparison of Decisions by Older Patients and Their Physician-Selected Proxies." *Gerontologist* 29: 615–21.

3

Ethical Dimensions of Advance Directives and Surrogate Decision Making in the United States

ROBERT M. VEATCH, PH.D.

Overview

Advance directives in the United States emerged in the late 1960s and early 1970s as a major social and medical phenomenon as a result of the confrontation of two major social ethics that had, until the middle of the twentieth century, coexisted without confronting one another. One, which dominated professional physician ethics, has its roots in the Hippocratic ethic. The norm of the practice of medicine in the United States (and much of the rest of Western and non-Western cultures as well) until the confrontation began about 1970 was that the physician's duty was to benefit the patient according to the physician's own ability and judgment. In classical Hippocratic writings it was clear that the physician was expected to recognize the limits of the physician's skill. There came a time when disease could not be mastered. The physician was to discontinue the struggle. In modern medicine, especially in the twentieth century, however, the revival of the Hippocratic commitment to strive to benefit the patient was combined with a new belief that death should be fought to the very end. When combined with a belief in the goodness of preserving life regardless of its condition, this Hippocratic mandate led physicians to believe that they had the right and the obligation to preserve life, regardless of the wishes of the patient. Of course, ancient Hippocratic ethics would not be expected to include notions of patient autonomy and informed consent. Those concepts are much more modern. But what is more striking is that even twentieth-century ethics in the Hippocratic tradition still omits or at least de-emphasizes such notions. This was an ethic that had no place for the autonomous self-determination of patients. The notion of patient consent, or refusal of consent, was totally alien to this modern version of the Hippocratic ethic. American professional medicine of this period renewed its paternalistic Hippocratic commitment grounded in a predemocratic elitist ideal while abandoning its traditional acknowledgment of its limits.

Coexisting in American culture, but seemingly oblivious to it, was a dominant nonmedical social-political philosophy of liberalism. It has its roots in the political philosophy of Locke, Hobbes, Rousseau, and Kant and in the affirmation of the individual as decision maker of the Judeo-Christian tradition, especially that of the Protestant Reformation. Outside of medicine, this affirmation of the individual as a rights-bearing, decision-making being dominated American culture from its beginnings. It permeates the key documents of American public culture: the Declaration of Independence, the Bill of Rights of the Constitution, and Lincoln's Gettysburg Address. It is identified as central to American culture in de Tocqueville's *Democracy in America.* It provided the foundations for the two most important moral principles of American culture: autonomy and justice. Together they provide the moral norms that challenge consequentialist devotion to benefiting patients and protecting them from harm.

The benevolent paternalism of the medical profession existed as an illiberal island in a sea of democratic egalitarian individualism. But the turmoil of the 1960s in the United States with its all-encompassing civil rights movement and its militant antiwar movement generated a focus on the rights of the underdog: the racial minority, the student, the woman, and the young. A patients' rights movement followed on the heels of racial rights, women's rights, students' rights, and children's rights. American liberalism finally penetrated into American medicine. The results have been hundreds of court cases, every one of which has affirmed the legal as well as the moral right of competent American adults to refuse any medical treatment whatsoever provided that treatment is offered for the patient's own good, literally millions of copies of advance directives (originally called "living wills"), and laws in every state authorizing both substantive and proxy instructions, that is, those that specify which treatments are desired or rejected and those that specify who should serve as a proxy in case individuals are unable to speak for themselves.

Key Cases

Even before the famous public cases of the 1970s, there were hints of the clash between medical paternalism and the affirmation of the patient as self-determining decision maker. The American interest in advance directives has its roots in this clash between the Hippocratic and liberal worldviews that were first manifest in the emergence of the doctrine of informed consent beginning early in the twentieth century (Faden and Beauchamp 1986; Pernick 1982; Katz 1984; Veatch 1976). In the 1914 case of Schloendorff v. Society of New York Hospitals, a patient was subjected to an operation for a fibroid tumor after consenting to an abdominal examination under anesthesia but explicitly refusing an operation. Justice Benjamin Cardozo's finding is often cited as the definitive statement of the American commitment to patient self-determination: "Every human being of adult years and sound mind has a right to determine what shall be done with his own body; and a surgeon who performs an operation without his patient's consent commits an assault, for which he is liable in damages" (*Schloendorff*).

By the 1960s, the consent doctrine was taking shape as an expression of the American commitment to self-determination in medical decision making (*Salgo; Natanson*). Liberal political philosophy was beginning to challenge the hegemony of the Hippocratic ethic in medical ethics. This notion of patient self-determination was applied to cases involving life-or-death decisions to forgo life-sustaining medical treatments.

Often these cases reflected the deep-seated American commitment to freedom of religion. Central to the American founding ideology is an affirmation of freedom of religious belief. Although the right to act on that belief is not absolute when such action impinges on the rights of others, the right to act based on one's religious convictions is given very high status. Hence, early cases involving the freedom of patients to refuse life-prolonging medical treatment often were motivated by religious convictions.

In 1964 Mrs. Bernice Brooks suffered from a peptic ulcer for which she required a blood transfusion that was deemed by her physician to be necessary to save her life. She had repeatedly informed her physician that she was a Jehovah's Witness and had refused all blood transfusions. The physician successfully sought to have a conservator appointed who authorized the transfusion, but that decision was later overturned, giving priority to the patient's own convictions (*Brooks*). Similar results have occurred in other cases involving adult religious objectors to medical treatment (*Erickson; Phelps; Holmes; Fox*).

It is important to realize, however, that the patient's refusal of life-prolonging treatment need not be religiously based. A number of patients have refused interventions such as life-prolonging amputations simply on the grounds of self-determination; they exercised their autonomy to choose a life plan that foreclosed the medical treatment even though it was expected to prolong life (*Raasch*). The moral principle of autonomy that is manifest in the legal notion of self-determination emerges as paramount in its conflict with traditional paternalistic professional physician ethics in the Hippocratic school.

By the mid-1970s this ethical position was so firmly established that it was rare that there would be any public controversy over treatment refusals by patients who were clearly competent. The one major exception involved adults with minor children.[1] The parent's obligation to the child was recognized as a legitimate ethical obligation that could take precedence over the notion of self-determination (*Wallace; Georgetown; Jones; Raleigh*). Nevertheless, limits on one's duty to one's children were also recognized. In one case, a father was permitted to refuse a blood transfusion believed to be lifesaving in spite of the fact that he had two small children. The family claimed that adequate arrangements had been made to care for the children if their father should die. (His brothers would provide a father figure and help in the family business.) The father was permitted to refuse the blood (*Osborne*). Only compelling social responsibilities involving matters of public health or family obligation justify overriding the fundamental notion of self-determination by competent adults.

By the mid-1970s the American people were ready for a prolonged public debate over a series of issues related to terminal illness treatment decisions, advance directives, and surrogate decision making. The following four cases illustrate the most public and most controversial issues.

Karen Quinlan and the Legitimacy of Surrogate Decisions

In 1975, 21-year-old Karen Ann Quinlan was left in a permanently unconscious, persistently vegetative state on a ventilator, having been rendered unconscious after what was probably an overdose of a combination of alcohol and a tranquilizing medication (*Quinlan*). Her father, Joseph Quinlan, sought to be appointed her guardian with the express power of authorizing the discontinuance of all extraordinary procedures for sustaining his daughter's vital processes. The attending physician, Dr. Robert Morse, had objected to removal of the respirator, claiming that doing so "would not conform to medical practices, standards, and traditions" (*Quinlan,* 655).

It is doubtful that, by 1975, removal of a ventilator from such a patient in these circumstances would actually have failed to conform to medical practice. However, one of the important issues in this case was whether such matters should be resolved by appeal to the standard medical practice of the time or should, instead, be resolved by appeal to the wishes of the patient or her appropriate surrogate. The New Jersey court concluded that the standard of practice of the physician's colleagues was not definitive. They held that "the question is whether there is such internal consistency and rationality in the application of such standards as should warrant their constituting an ineluctable bar to the effectuation of substantive relief for plaintiff at the hands of the court. We have concluded not" (45–46).

In lay language, the court rejected the claim that the standard of practice of Dr. Morse's colleagues was definitive, appealing instead to such criteria as "consistency" and "rationality." Substantively, the court affirmed the acceptability of a nontreatment decision as long as there was no reasonable possibility of the patient's recovering to what was called a "cognitive, sapient state," a notion that would eventually prove controversial, as we shall see below.

The Quinlan case consolidated the normative cultural consensus that had been emerging in professional and legal circles for over a decade. It is not unethical to decide to forgo life-sustaining medical treatment. The final decision is not one that is to be made unilaterally by the medical professional; it is one to be left to the patient or appropriate surrogate.[2] The era of Hippocratic paternalism in the United States was over (even if individual clinicians to this day were to retain some residual resistance to the liberal alternative).

Karen Quinlan, of course, never had a written advance directive. One of the implications of grounding the right of refusal in the moral principle of autonomy and the correlated legal notion of self-determination is that a physical, written advance directive or living will is not essential. What is important is knowing what the patient actually would choose given the patient's beliefs and values. The written document, whether it be an advance directive refusing medical treatment or a form consenting to treatment, is necessary only to help make the patient's wishes clear.

To this day, it is not clear exactly on what grounds the New Jersey Court authorized Mr. Quinlan to decide for his daughter. One view is that he was designated because, as her parent, he would best know her wishes. In fact, the court makes an ambiguous reference to the notion of "substituted judgment," the term usually used in American discussion to refer to judgments based on what the patient would have wanted. That would be an approach completely consistent with the primacy of the patient's wishes in medical treatment decisions.

It is also possible, however, that Mr. Quinlan was given the authority to make the choice that he thought was best for her under the circumstances. That could be a decision not necessarily based on the patient's beliefs and values. It is what is now usually referred to as the "best interests" standard.

It could be argued that by 1976 in the United States, if the patient's wishes were known, that would clearly be sufficient to stop the treatment regardless of the involvement of the parent. The social impact of Quinlan was to condone significant parental involvement in decisions to forgo treatment even in cases in which the patient's own views are not clear.[3] This thus not only solidified the primacy of patient self-determination when the patient's wishes are known, but also opened the door to familial surrogate decision making, a matter that would become more significant in the next decade.

Claire Conroy and the Legitimacy of Forgoing Nutrition, Hydration, and Other Simple Treatments

A second case that embodies the American controversy over terminal illness treatment decisions, advance directives, and surrogate decision making is that of Claire Conroy (*Conroy*). Also decided in New Jersey, it involved an 84-year-old woman who in 1983 had long suffered from organic brain syndrome. She had been legally incompetent since 1979. Her nephew was her only living relative, and he was appointed her guardian.

In July 1982 she entered a hospital for treatment of a gangrenous left foot. Her nephew claimed that Miss Conroy had always resisted medical involvement and refused amputation of her foot on those grounds. The fact that he was not challenged for basing his decision on his understanding of her wishes shows how quickly the doctrine of substituted judgment was accepted among clinicians and the public.

While she was hospitalized, a nasogastric tube was inserted. Her nephew now insisted that she would not want the tube even though forgoing it would certainly mean her death. This case led to a major public ethical discussion over whether patients or their surrogates could exercise their right of self-determination by refusing routine, simple medical procedures such as nasogastric feeding, gastrostomies, medical hydration, antibiotics, and cardiopulmonary resuscitation.

The philosophical and ethical discussion focused first on whether the complexity of the technology was a morally relevant consideration in deciding to forgo a treatment. Earlier discussion, particularly within the tradition of Catholic moral theology, had led to the conclusion that when a treatment is labeled "extraordinary," the word *extraordinary* is to be taken in a normative sense. It is not the technical complexity of the treatment that makes it morally expendable, but rather whether the benefits of the treatment exceed the burdens. Clinicians and lawyers often do not grasp this normative use of the term *extraordinary,* but religious and philosophical ethicists as well as the key participants in the public policy discussion now clearly accept the notion that a treatment may be morally expendable if it does not offer proportional benefit regardless of how simple or basic it is (President's Commission 1983). This means that nutrition or hydration medically supplied as well as antibiotics and cardiopulmonary resuscitation will be assessed by the same criteria as any more complex medical treatment. Simple as well as complex treatments will be deemed expendable when they do not offer benefits that exceed burdens. Moreover, in the liberal tradition of the American culture, these are judgments that, whenever possible, are to be made by the patient drawing on his or her own beliefs and values.

Although Claire Conroy died before the final decision was rendered, that decision clearly confirmed the legitimacy of surrogate decisions to forgo nutrition and hydration when there is clear evidence that the patient would not have wanted them. The decision also opens the door further to surrogate use of the best interests standard, authorizing surrogates to forgo treatment when the "burdens clearly and markedly outweigh the benefits" (even if the patient's wishes are not known at all). It also suggests the existence of a hybrid basis for decision making when there is some indication the patient would have refused and the treatment would only prolong suffering. What is clearly emerging is a liberal hierarchy of authority relying first on the patient's own life choices and, to the extent they are not known, on the judgment of the appropriate surrogate about the best interests of the patient.

Philip Becker and the Legitimation of Surrogacy

By the mid-1980s the victory of liberal political philosophy in its conflict with Hippocratic physician paternalism was just about settled, at least in the minds of the theorists who attempted to articulate the moral foundations for making terminal illness treatment decisions, even if individual clinicians may not have been fully converted and individual practicing attorneys might not have grasped the full impact of the change. The emerging liberal consensus (Meisel 1992, 1996) was that the free choice of the competent adult was the first priority insofar as the individual has indicated his or her preferences. There is some emerging controversy over whether those preferences expressed while competent should continue to prevail when a person's mental status has left him or her with no continuity of personal identity with the individual who expressed those wishes. Some are suggesting that if a patient with advanced dementia has no remaining mental continuity with the individual who expressed a life plan in an advance directive, then a "new person" has been created, and the advance directive may be superseded by the wishes or interests of this new person (Buchanan and Brock 1989, 184–89; Dresser and Robertson 1989), while others warn of the dangers of overturning advance directives and undermining the hard-won victory for patient autonomy (Veatch 1993, 16–17).

The most controversial aspect of advance directives and surrogate decision making, however, involves the role of surrogates. One of the cases that best illustrate the issue is that of a youngster named Phillip Becker. Phillip had Down's syndrome and a congenital heart defect that is sometimes associated with it. This disorder involved a cardiac septal defect and elevated pulmonary blood pressure. In 1978, at age 12, he had not yet had the heart condition evaluated. He would suffer progressive loss of energy and vitality until he was forced to lead a bed-to-chair existence. A pediatric cardiologist recommended catheterization to determine if surgery was appropriate. The boy's parents resisted the test, pointing to a surgical mortality risk of 5 to 10 percent if the operation were to be performed. Without the surgery he would face severe incapacitation, whereas with the surgery he might live 20 more years. The court supported the parental refusal, mentioning specifically that "it is fundamental that parental autonomy is constitutionally protected. The United States Supreme Court has articulated the concept of personal liberty found in the Fourteenth Amendment as a right of privacy which extends to certain aspects of a family relationship" (*Becker*).

Phillip was transferred to an institutional facility in 1972. A volunteer, Mrs. Patsy Heath, became involved and soon after began to bond with Phillip. Eventually Mrs. Heath and her husband, Herbert, asked for and were awarded custody of Phillip, making clear that it was their intention to authorize the diagnosis and, if appropriate, the surgery.

Does this imply that the Heaths made a more rational choice and were given custody on that basis? Probably not. Although little was made of it at the time, the Beckers had been advised to institutionalize Phillip and minimize contact with him. Although that would not be the advice given today, it was considered acceptable at the time. When the Heaths established a close relationship with Phillip they became his de facto parents. The second court case resembled an unusual custody fight characterized by the attempt to establish which pair should be Phillip's parents. The courts ruled in favor of the Heaths, but there is no evidence that they did so based on the substance of the clinical decision to proceed. The court opinion makes it difficult to interpret this issue, but it could be that the judge reached the conclusion that the Heaths, having a much closer relationship with Phillip than his natural parents, were the appropriate ones to function as parents. The court called them his "psychosocial parents."

This case is crucial for understanding American views about the role of parents as surrogate decision makers. It is often claimed that in such cases the parents must do what is in the best interests of the child. (The substituted judgment standard is meaningless for small children or those with severe retardation.) Even though we often talk about doing what is *best,* it is clear that the courts and the American public do not really believe that such a high standard is necessary or even appropriate.

It seems quite possible that in the original decision that granted the Beckers authority to refuse the treatment, the judge believed that having the treatment would be *best,* but that refusal was sufficiently within reason that it was a tolerable choice. Given the commitment to familial autonomy in matters of child raising, the judge may have accepted their decision even though he did not think it was best.

Interestingly, by the time the Heaths' claim was heard, the procedures previously contemplated were considered more risky. It might even be argued that by that time, refusing the surgery was best. Nevertheless, once the Heaths were considered to be most appropriately in the parenting role, the same tolerance for parental autonomy that originally led to supporting the less plausible choice of the Beckers could now support the now less plausible choice of the Heaths. In neither case would the *best* choice have been made, but in each case one that was arguably within reason. Several American commentators are now questioning whether surrogate decision makers, either family members or other surrogates with a previously existing social bond with the incompetent one, need to be held literally to the standard of doing what is best. If there are several decisions that are within reason, then a society that extends liberal principles so that there is some range of limited autonomy for the family as well as the individual will support discretion by familial surrogates as long as the choice is within the range of reasonableness (Veatch 1984). There is widespread de facto support for such familial discretion not only among theorists, but also among clinicians and among members of the legal community (Areen 1987). There remains, however, among American bioethicists, considerable dispute over both the grounding and the range of such familial discretion. When one realizes that surrogate authority for discretion in deciding either what the patient wants or what is in the patient's best interests cannot itself be grounded in liberal individualism, one begins to see the reason for the uncertainty. Nevertheless, there is substantial support in practice for giving legitimate familial surrogates a range of discretion in fulfilling their duties of surrogacy.

Baby K and the Limits of Familial Discretion to Demand Care Deemed Futile

Most recently, the victory for liberal individualism in American terminal illness treatment policy has been challenged from a new front. In the early days of the clash between liberal political philosophy and Hippocratic paternalism, the medical profession was governed by the primacy of the value of preserving human life in any form. This meant that whenever there was a disagreement between physician and patient, the physician was pressing for preserving life, and the patient was pressing for ceasing treatment.

As the right of the patient or surrogate to refuse consent has become more established, many physicians have acknowledged the wisdom of forgoing life support in cases in which the envisioned benefits do not exceed the envisioned risks. In turn some patients, particularly those in the minority religious communities of Orthodox Judaism and fundamentalist Christianity, and those associated with the right-to-life movement, have held to the view that biological life is sacred and to be preserved whenever possible.

Baby K was born October 13, 1992, with a diagnosis of anencephaly. She had a brain stem, but the cerebral cortex was rudimentary or absent. All parties agreed that she was permanently unconscious and could not hear or see. She did not feel pain. She manifested only rudimentary reflexive actions. Baby K's mother, who had previously been advised by physicians to terminate the pregnancy, understood the severity of his child's condition but nevertheless insisted that she wanted life support, including maintenance of respiration by a ventilator if necessary to prolong life.

The hospital at which the baby was being cared for sought the legal authority to withhold ventilatory support. The hospital stipulated that it was not proposing to deny ventilator support to Baby K because of any lack of adequate resources or inability of the mother to pay for the treatment. A lower court refused to grant the hospital the right to unilaterally withhold the ventilator (*Baby K I*). The decision was sustained on appeal to the Fourth Circuit of the United States Court of Appeals (*Baby K II*).

Although the court decided the matter on technical grounds having to do with the law regarding the duty of the hospital to provide emergency treatment, many debating the case assume that the moral foundation of the mother's claim for a right of access is the principle of autonomy and the authority of the surrogate to make medical treatment choices that has been outlined in the previous cases.

There is a philosophical complexity here, however. Autonomy, especially within the tradition of liberal Western political philosophy, has been seen as creating what is called a liberty right—a right to be left alone. As long as physicians were demanding the right to treat and patients or their surrogates were demanding nontreatment, autonomy functioned well to support the right of patients to withdraw from the medical enterprise. But in the case of Baby K, the mother was demanding a right of access—what is usually called an entitlement right, not a liberty right.

Entitlement rights are grounded in moral principles other than autonomy. They may stem from a principle of justice or a principle of beneficence, either of which might create a claim to an entitlement. But autonomy, as it is normally interpreted by American ethicists, simply gives one the right to be self-determining in the sense of having a right of noninterference in living one's life according to one's own life plan. It does not give one a right of access to the resources needed to live that life; it only provides noninterference.

In fact, if autonomy is at stake at all in so-called futile care cases, it is the provider's autonomy that is at stake. Physicians, like other citizens, have a right to self-determination in choosing which patients they will see. This libertarian notion is long-affirmed by organized professional medicine in the United States.

This does not imply that physicians never have a moral or legal duty to treat. It merely implies that if there is such a duty it cannot come from the moral principle of autonomy. There are many reasons why the autonomy of health professionals might be constrained in such a way that physicians would have a duty to treat against their consciences. They might have executed legally binding contracts providing a right of access. Morally this could be seen as a duty of promise-keeping. They might have moral obligations grounded in beneficence or justice. It seems likely, for example, that it would be immoral and perhaps even illegal for physicians to refuse to treat a patient solely on the grounds of race (even if the physician sincerely held some strange conscientious position requiring him or her to discriminate).

There are several similar cases involving claims by providers that the care being demanded is what the provider believes to be "futile" (Miles 1991; Angell 1991; *Jane Doe*). The implications of Baby K and similar so-called futile care cases for advance directives are immense. Traditionally, advance directives have focused on specifying the nature of the treatment being refused and spelling out the implications of the principle of autonomy for such a right of refusal. Now, however, people who desire certain kinds of care that are usually not provided will have a burden of executing advance directives specifying their desires. Furthermore, the moral and legal grounds for their requests will no longer be simply autonomy and self-determination. They will have to be spelled out in terms of contractual obligations or entitlement claims grounded in beneficence or justice.

Review of the Literature

It is striking that the cases that have just been described generally do not involve formally written advance directives. Some involve advance expressions of wishes about terminal care communicated orally in more or less formal ways. I have suggested that, from the point of view of the principle of respect for patient autonomy, these oral communications are perfectly adequate (although there may be considerable risk of disagreement about the exact meaning of the individual expression of preference). It is not surprising that there are relatively few clinical cases involving formally prepared advance directives. Written directives have been available for only about 25 years, and, to date, only a relatively small percentage of the American population (probably no more than 20 percent) has prepared a written directive (Emanuel et al. 1991; Harvey and Shubat 1989; Hughes and Singer 1992).

Although many of the cases of importance involve oral communication of a patient's wishes, almost all involve surrogate decision making. It is strange that although most of the clinical decisions involve surrogates and most of the complex ethical controversy surrounds surrogacy, still most of the literature has addressed the preparation of formal written advance directives. Perhaps this is because decisions by competent adults themselves fit so much more neatly into the framework of autonomy and self-determination that provides the moral underpinnings of the advance directive movement.

American Advance Directive Literature

THE ORIGINAL "LIVING WILL." Luis Kutner, a Chicago attorney, is usually credited with developing the first American advance directive in the 1930s (Kutner 1969). He called it a *living will.* In the 1960s he provided a copy to the Euthanasia Educational Council, a large, public, educational organization. In 1968, it began circulating the living will. By now, millions of copies have been distributed. Although some of its features are now considered controversial and anachronistic, it has served as the prototype for advance directives. To distinguish it from other, later forms, I will use the term *living will* to refer only to Kutner's document and the one circulated by the Euthanasia Educational Council and its successor organizations.[4] The term *advance directive* will be used more generically, referring to any of a wide range of documents designed to convey wishes about terminal care. It will be used to refer to both substantive directives (those specifying which treatments are desired or refused) and proxy directives (those specifying a person to function as surrogate in case the individual is not capable of speaking for him- or herself).

The original living will is a modest document. It explicitly states that it is not legally binding. When this document emerged, defenders of patient choice were too timid to challenge the authority of the Hippocratic regime directly. Instead, it pleads with physicians, saying "I hope [you will] feel morally bound to follow" the request. It also assumes that all parties interested in refusing treatment will fit the terms of the document, which asks that the signer "be allowed to die and not be kept alive by artificial means or heroic measures," terms that are both vague and potentially restricting. Such a document, thus, is not necessarily consistent with the goal of furthering autonomous choice based on the patient's own life plan, as would be more in keeping with a full-blown shift to the liberal ethic.

THE CHRISTIAN AFFIRMATION OF LIFE. That this advance directive approach was compatible with the mainstream of American Catholicism is made clear by the distribution in 1974 of the "Christian Affirmation of Life" by the Catholic Hospital Association (1974). It is, in fact, an advance directive endorsed by American Catholicism with key operative language nearly identical to that of the living will. That the Catholic Church was facilitating decisions to forgo "extraordinary means" of life support is not surprising; this has long been the position of the Catholic Church. The uniquely American emphasis is on encouraging the patient to take an active role as the decision maker. The major European Catholic documents accept decisions to forgo disproportionally burdensome treatment, but they tend to see the clinician rather than the patient as the one with the authority to make such decisions (Sacred Congregation for the Doctrine of the Faith 1980). Still, this early model of an advance directive puts the communication in the form of a request rather than an instruction, as would be more in keeping with a view of the patient as an autonomous decision maker. It states, "I request that, if possible, I be consulted concerning the medical procedures," hardly an aggressive affirmation of patient autonomy.

Developments in Advance Directives in the 1970s

Beginning in the early to mid-1970s, efforts were made to bring the advance directive more in line with what would be appropriate for an ethic grounded in liberal political philosophy and the doctrine of informed consent that derives from it. In 1973, as part of a project for the Hastings Center's Research Group on Death and Dying, I drafted an advance directive intended for my own use, but also as a model for others. It was eventually published in 1976 (Veatch 1976, 184–85). It was explicitly intended to be a legally binding expression of the signer's beliefs and values. It asks anyone signing it to spell out more specifically the point at which treatment is refused, and it encourages a signer to preface the document with a statement of the individual's religious, moral, and philosophical convictions relevant to forgoing treatment. My personal advance directive was revised extensively for the second edition of *Death, Dying, and the Biological Revolution* (Veatch 1989, 154–55) but holds to the same general principles. The second edition adds a specific designation of physicians, lawyers, and moral counselors to assist the signer's proxy and specifies the state where he or she would want to receive critical medical care, a device necessary in the United States to help assure that care will be provided in a state with laws supportive of advance directive decision making. It also makes clear that the signer would want to refuse nutrition and hydration that was not, in the eyes of my proxy, offering benefit that exceeds the burdens of treatment based on the criterion of substituted judgment.

As far as I know, this was the first advance directive that specifically incorporated the appointment of a proxy to act for the signer in the event that the one signing the directive was unable to speak for him- or herself. Sissela Bok soon thereafter published a similar set of "personal directions" that includes the appointment of a proxy decision maker (Bok 1976). Both of these publications make clear that the appointment of a proxy is for the purpose of making a substituted judgment, that is, to have the proxy make the choice based on the signer's own personal beliefs and values. Thus, the one designated as proxy should not necessarily be one competent in medicine (such as the physician), but one who knows the signer's worldview.

Enriching the Possibilities for Autonomous Choice

A number of others have published model advance directives incorporating their personal views about terminal illness care and their own variations to make them more consistent with their own personal values (Weir 1989,

191–93; Cantor 1990; Cantor 1993, 149–58). Cantor's directive provides separate mechanisms for substantive and proxy directives.

Several other commentators, recognizing the importance of the individual's personal values in crafting an individual and nuanced statement of which treatments should be provided and which ones should be refused, have set out to help patients inventory their own beliefs. Cantor (1993, 166–71) provides several pages of a "value profile" that can be completed by a patient to assist in formulating a personal advance directive. The document can be completed in the company of one's physician or family to help them understand the patient's concept of good medical care. The radical implication of this new view of medical decision making is that it is literally impossible for the physician to know what counts as good medical care for a particular patient without asking the patient or having the patient instruct the physician about what care is appropriate.[5] The value profile is a very useful device for accomplishing this.

Kielstein and Sass (1993) summarize four types of efforts to survey patient values. They include taking a "value history" (Doukas and McCullough 1991), creating a "value inventory list" (Gibson 1990), establishing a "value preference list" (Emanuel and Emanuel 1990), and creating a "value journal" (Grundstein-Amato 1992). To these methods, Kielstein and Sass add the approach of using stories or case scenarios to establish patient values. All of these methods share the insight important to the American approach to advance directives: the patient's own beliefs and values are the basis upon which key medical choices must be made.

Books

In addition to Cantor's volume (1993), three other books deserve special mention because of their contribution to an understanding of the American approach to advance directives, its dependence on liberal political values, and the priority that has been placed on patient self-determination. Nancy M. P. King's *Making Sense of Advance Directives* (1991) was the first full-length monograph devoted specifically to the American approach to advance directives. The report of the President's Commission for the Study of Ethical Problems in Medicine and Biomedical and Behavioral Research, *Deciding to Forego Life-Sustaining Medical Treatment* (1983), set the basic moral framework and established some of the vocabulary used in the discussion about advance directives. The Hastings Center's *Guidelines on the Termination of Life-Sustaining Treatment and the Care of the Dying* (1987) provides specific applications to specific treatments and disease entities as well as an extensive general framework for making treatment decisions and a briefer analysis of the ethics involved. That analysis relies on four values (or what are often called principles): patient well-being, autonomy or self-determination, the integrity of the health care professional, and justice. Both the President's Commission report and the Hastings Center document, as political projects authored by committees, make occasional openings to the more traditional Hippocratic concern with patient well-being, but both make clear that when patient autonomy conflicts with well-being, autonomy takes priority. Moreover, they both emphasize that when the patient's own beliefs and values cannot be determined, a familial surrogate is next in priority as the decision maker, subject only to the limits of reasonable discretion discussed above. These documents, together with the individually authored books on death and dying, provide the basis for an understanding of the ethical framework brought to bear on advance directives in the United States.

More Theoretical Medical, Ethical, and Bioethical Literature

The vast literature dealing with advance directives in the American context should be seen as a playing out of a crucially important social change in the underlying medical ethical and bioethical theory of the American culture in the past twenty years. The emergence of patient autonomy and surrogate decision making as the foundations for advance directives is a symptom of a much more fundamental philosophical and ethical change. Although Hippocratic ethics in medicine has coexisted with a broader liberal political philosophy in American culture since its origins, only in the past 20–25 years has their incompatibility been recognized vividly.

A broad consensus on an ethical framework has dominated much of this period. The dominant approach has been one relying on a set of general ethical principles from which more specific ethical conclusions on specific clinical and policy questions can be derived.[6] Only recently have important differences among the advocates of this approach been emphasized. All draw on several basic principles, but they sometimes include different numbers of principles, define the principles differently, or give them different priorities. Beauchamp and Childress (1994) balance the principles of beneficence, nonmaleficence, autonomy, and justice, refusing to give any one absolute priority. The National Commission for the Protection of Human Subjects' Belmont Report (1978) works with three principles: beneficence (under which is subsumed nonmaleficence), justice, and respect for persons (under which is subsumed autonomy). That report also balances competing principles. By contrast, my own theory (Veatch 1981) includes these four plus additional principles of fidelity to promises, veracity, and avoidance of killing. In my theory, the consequence-oriented principles (beneficence and nonmaleficence) are always subordinated to those principles not oriented to maximizing consequences. H. Tristram Engelhardt (1986), a libertarian philosopher, gives first priority to the principle of autonomy, or what he now prefers to call the "principle of permission," reducing beneficence to a subordinate role. Edmund D. Pellegrino (1988) gives first priority to beneficence but interprets beneficence (doing good) more broadly to include several elements of good. Respecting patient autonomy is one of those elements, and it is given priority over the production of medical goods, such as preserving life.

The net effect of these apparently different theories is that all agree that the autonomous patient always (or virtually always) has the right to refuse life-sustaining medical treatment when that treatment is offered for the patient's own good. There is room for greater disagreement over matters of resource allocation and conflicts between maximizing justice and maximizing social utility, but it is the nature of most advance directive cases that the central moral conflict is between autonomy and paternalistically doing what the clinician believes is good for the patient, even if the patient does not want the purported benefit. One way or another, virtually all American theorists now accept the priority of autonomy in such conflicts.

Special Issues

Assessment of Advance Directives and Durable Powers of Attorney

As suggested above, the general concepts of advance directives and durable powers of attorney have been very well received by American bioethicists. There is, in theory, almost universal acceptance of the legitimacy of these devices as ways of furthering the autonomy of individuals, but two types of doubts arise.

First, there remains considerable skepticism over whether advance directives really achieve their purpose of facilitating decisions based on the patient's actual beliefs and values. It is pointed out that most people still do not have written advance directives, and, when they do, often they are not made available to care providers. When they are made available, there is doubt about whether they are followed (Perkins, Bauer, and Hazuda 1990; Zinberg 1989). Recall that the medical profession, at least until recently, felt a sense of moral duty to act paternalistically. Clinicians have been heard to say with pride that they can persuade patients to consent to anything. Other clinicians persist in believing that patients cannot possibly know what they want—that they either cannot understand the implications of specific treatments or cannot know what their actual preferences will be in a moment of crisis. At the level of practical application, there remains considerable doubt about the use of advance directives. Evidence supporting this skepticism is seen in the chapter by Joan Teno and Joanne Lynn in this volume (see also Teno et al. 1994).

Second, there remains doubt at the margins where the moral consensus supporting autonomous decisions of patients is inapplicable because the patient is marginally competent or clearly incompetent. Controversies exist over whether all conceivable decisions should be included within the range of tolerable free choice—whether active euthanasia or the forgoing of nutrition and hydration should be included, for instance.

How Could or Should Advance Directives Be Used?

American culture is intrigued with the technical fix. That a written piece of paper, especially one enforceable by a court, could solve profound moral and existential problems appeals to the American psyche. No doubt great benefit can come from using advance directives. In a culture that is so radically pluralistic, fragmented, and mobile, it is beyond reason to hold to the old myth of the physician who can know his or her patient well enough to know when to stop life-sustaining treatment. Every adult should go through the exercise of formulating a set of goals for terminal medical treatment. Those conclusions normally should be reduced to writing and shared with family, friends, clergy, lawyer, and physician. But it would be a serious mistake to assume that the successful completion of that exercise would ensure that the delivery of medical care remain under the control of the terminally ill patient. The advance directive would still have to be seen as one component of a newly structured health care delivery system if the patient is to receive medical interventions consistent with his or her beliefs, values, and life plan.

The Influence of Law and Regulation

Bioethicists are remarkably free from the control of law and regulation. There has been some interest in controlling entry into the ethicist profession due to concern about incompetent or inadequately trained practitioners. Some have no formal training in ethics at all. There is something odd about the ease with which those trained in other professions begin using the appellation "ethicist" while militantly resisting letting uncertified practitioners call themselves lawyer or physician. Nevertheless, there is a substantial consensus in the United States that doing ethics should be an art that all may try without fear of retribution from a professional disciplinary and licensure body.

The Role of Law

The United States probably provides the most visible role for law pertaining to advance directives of any nation in the world. Literally hundreds of judicial actions have educated the public and provided the framework for most decisions involving advance directives and surrogate decision making. Moreover, statutory law provides the framework for preparing and acting on advance directives.

Many clinicians protest this aggressive involvement of the law, but I would speculate that, especially in a pluralistic, liberal society, there would chaos if the statutory and judicial system failed to provide a mechanism for public resolution of dispute and clarification of public policy at the margins. There are enormous and dramatic disputes over the care of the terminally ill. Clinicians would probably protest as loudly if the public system of rational and systematic problem solving were absent. Many of the policy questions require decisions, however arbitrary.

Conflict between Law and Actual Behavior

Perhaps the most dramatic tension between law and actual behavior arises between clinical practice and legal structure. There is something about the nature of clinical practice that attracts personalities that are repulsed by bureaucratic rationality and disciplined rule following. Clinicians in the United States (and probably elsewhere) possess a certain sense of being above the law, of feeling morally obliged to bear the burden of doing whatever it takes to benefit patients even if it means circumventing the law. Hence, physicians such as Timothy Quill, Jack Kevorkian, and any clinician who has failed to get an adequately informed consent feel authorized to place themselves above the law. Physicians are on record lying to patients about diagnoses (Oken 1961), lying about the cause of death on death certificates (Quill 1991; Belkin 1993), and refusing to follow legally binding advance directives (Zinberg 1989; Danis et al. 1991; Hughes and Singer 1992; Perkins et al. 1990). In the Netherlands, the best data indicate that over a thousand patients a year are actively killed without the mandated persistent and voluntary request. That constitutes more than one deviant death for every three patients actively killed under the agreed procedures for voluntary euthanasia (Van der Maas et al. 1991). Similar willingness to violate the law in order to make patients dead is reported in the United States (Quill 1991; "Its Over Debbie" 1988; Kevorkian 1991). At the same time, clinicians are willing to refuse to follow valid advance directives when they believe patients would be better off if these documents were ignored. If this society is to rely on advance directives to assure its deeply held commitment to liberal values, some method will have to be found to see that valid advanced directives are followed.

Areas for Further Transdisciplinary and Transcultural Study

One reason advance directives have such potential importance in the United States is that our culture is so pluralistic. No health care provider can possibly be expected to understand the beliefs and values that motivate patients coming from significantly different religious and cultural systems. Still, the extent and range of those variations in beliefs and values is not well documented. Many providers, especially those with little transcultural experience, fail to grasp the enormous differences among peoples of different traditions. Documenting the range of variation within and among Germany, Japan, and the United States will help to begin establishing the necessary database, but it would be more helpful if a broader range of cultures could be studied to show their range of views about terminal care and the use of advance directives.

Areas of Conflict and Future Questions

Although in the United States a substantial consensus has emerged, especially on matters involving the rights of substantially autonomous patients, a new set of "second-generation" problems is emerging that will require attention in the future. These problems generally involve situations in which patients cannot be said for certain to have the power to exercise autonomous choices to refuse treatment. Among the issues that have yet to be resolved are the following:[7]

1. Refusals that go beyond those authorized by state statute (such as refusals by patients who are neither terminally ill nor permanently vegetative, those who are refusing oral nutrition and hydration, those who suffer cardiac arrest in the operating room, and those who suffer arrest outside of medical settings).

2. Damages and compensation for patients who are treated against their will in violation of an advance directive.

3. Refusals in cases in which third parties have an interest in keeping the patient alive either because the third party is a dependent of the one attempting to refuse treatment or because of the social consequences of letting the individual die.

4. Refusals that are said to violate the ethical integrity of the medical profession or the individual professional.

5. Refusals by patients who are borderline competent.

6. The forgoing of treatment for surrogateless incompetent patients without advance directives.

7. The forgoing of treatment when there is conflict among plausible surrogates.

8. The forgoing of treatment based on bonded surrogate decisions that appear to be in pursuit of something less than the literal best interests of the patient.

9. The forgoing of treatment for patients who have so lost continuity of identity with the one who executed an advance directive that they can be said to be "new persons."

10. The possibility of extending the authority of patients to the point that they might make life-ending decisions that encompass physician-assisted suicide and active killing for mercy as well as merely forgoing treatment (*Washington et al.;* Quill 1991).

Notes

1. For a fuller discussion of the limits on the right of competent adults to exercise self-determination in refusing life-prolonging medical treatment see Veatch (1976, 155–61). For example, society acknowledges special cases of people "willing to be coerced." Some religious objectors insist they cannot consent to medical treatment such as blood transfusions, but would not object to being ordered by a court to undergo such treatments (*Powell; George*). Prisoners present another special case. Sometimes treatment is ordered against the wishes of prisoners never declared incompetent because it is deemed necessary to protect other prisoners or guards (such as in a political protest involving a hunger strike). In other cases, prisoners who are clearly mentally deranged are never formally declared incompetent as they would have to be in civilian legal proceedings.

2. This was the clear impact of the Quinlan case even though the actual opinion uses the language of having the physician make the choice to stop the ventilator. The court said that the responsible attending physicians may conclude that "there is no reasonable possibility of Karen's ever emerging from her present comatose condition to a cognitive, sapient state and that the life-support apparatus now being administered to Karen should be discontinued" (*Quinlan,* 671–72).

Technically, this makes both the technical prognostic decision and the normative decision to forgo life support rest with the physician. The court in 1976 apparently did not grasp that the first decision was essentially neurological, for which the physician may claim some expertise, while the second was entirely nontechnical, for which in the liberal tradition physicians can claim no expertise. This problem was pointed out immediately in commentaries of the day and was subsequently corrected in the New Jersey State Department of Health's "Guidelines for Health Care Facilities to Implement Procedures Concerning the Care of Comatose Non-Cognitive Patients" (1977). Because Mr. Quinlan was clearly given the authority by the court to hire and fire the physician, presumably if he found a physician who determined that his daughter was in a vegetative state but who was nevertheless unwilling to conclude the life-support apparatus should be withdrawn, he could dismiss the physician and keep appointing new ones until he got the normative answer he sought. It would have been more consistent with the values of the court's decision to ask the physician to determine prognosis and the family to determine whether to stop the treatment.

3. Ten years later, the New Jersey courts clarified their position with regard to the basis of the parental choice in *Quinlan.* They point out that they had originally ruled out the use of reports of statements Karen Quinlan made to friends as a basis for the court's determining Karen's wishes. (That, of course, does not establish that Mr. Quinlan, who knew his daughter much more intimately, could not still have had a basis for estimating her views.) Now, while ruling on the case of another patient, they say regarding statements made to friends, "Such evidence is certainly relevant to shed light on whether the patient would have consented to the treatment if competent to make the decision." This seems to suggest that the court would by the mid-1980s be more willing to authorize forgoing treatment based on its understanding of the patient's wishes—a position that would be consistent with the evolving dominance of self-determination and the tradition of liberal political philosophy. It is also consistent with the case of Nancy Cruzan, which would become one of the most celebrated public cases by the end of the decade—a case finally decided on the basis of the understanding of the patient's wishes as expressed by friends of the patient reconstructing their conversations with her.

4. The Euthanasia Educational Council eventually separated into two organizations, Concern for Dying and the Society for the Right to Die. The former focused more on education, while the latter devoted its attention to legislative and other legal concerns. They have now merged back together into the organization Choice in Dying.

5. For a fuller discussion of the notion that deciding what constitutes good medical care is something that can only be known by the patient see Veatch (1991), especially chapter 27.

6. This general approach of basing bioethics on a set of ethical principles is sometimes referred to as the "Georgetown mantra" because many of its advocates have at one time or another been associated with the Kennedy Institute.

7. This list is based on Veatch (1993).

Cases

Baby K I: In the Matter of Baby K, 1993, WL 343557 (E.D. Va., Civ. A. No. 93-68-A).

Baby K II: In the Matter of Baby "K," 1994, United States Court of Appeals for the Fourth Circuit, February 10, No. 93-1899.

Becker: In the Matter of Phillip Becker, 1979, 92 Cal. App. 3d 796, 156 Cal. Rptr. 48, *cert. denied sub nom. Bothman v. Warren B.,* 1980, 445 U.S. 949.

Brooks: In re Brooks Estate, 1965, 32 Ill. 2d 361, 205 N.E. 2d 435.

Erickson: Erickson v. Dilgard, 1962, 44 Misc 2d 27, 252 N.Y. S. 2d, 705 (Sup. Ct.).

Fox: In the Matter of Father Philip K. Eichner, S.M. on behalf of Brother Joseph Charles Fox v. Denis Dillon, 1981, N.Y. Court of Appeals, 426 N.Y.S. 2d 517.

George: United States v. George, 1965, 33 U.S.L.W. 2518 (D.C., Conn., March 24).

Georgetown: In re President and Directors of Georgetown College, Inc., 1964, 331 F. 2d 1000 (D.C. Cir.), *cert denied sub nom.*

Holmes: Holmes v. Silver Cross Hospital of Joliet, 1972, Illinois 340 F. Supp. 125.

Jane Doe: In re Jane Doe, a minor, 1991, Civil Action File No. D-93064, Superior Court of Fulton County, State of Georgia, October. *In re Doe,* 1992, 418 S.E. 2d 3 (Ga.).

Jones: Jones v. President and Directors of Georgetown College, Inc., 1964, 377 U.S. 978.

Natanson: Natanson v. Kline, 1960, 186 Kan. 393, 350 P. 2d 1093.

Osborne: In the Matter of Charles P. Osborne, 1972, 2942 A. 2d 372 (D.C. Cir.).

Phelps: In re Phelps, 1972, No. 459-207, Milwaukee County Co., filed July 11.

Powell: Powell v. Columbian [sic] Presbyterian Medical Center et al., 1965, 49 Misc. 2d 215, 267. N.Y.S. 2d, 450 (Sup. Ct.).

Quinlan: In re Quinlan, 1976, 70 N.J. 10, 355 A. 2d 647, *cert. denied sub nom,* Garger v. New Jersey, 1976, 429 U.S. 922, overruled in part, In re Conroy, 1985, 98 N.J. 321, 486 A. 2d 1209.

Raasch: Guardianship of Gertrude Raasch, 1972, County Co. for Milwaukee, Probate Div., No. 455-996, decided Jan. 25.

Raleigh: Raleigh Fitkin-Paul Morgan Memorial Hospital v. Anderson, 1964, 42 N.J. 421, 201 A. 2d 537; *cert. denied,* 337 U.S. 985.

Salgo: Salgo v. Leland Stanford Jr. University Board of Trustees, 1957, 317 P. 2d 170.

Schloendorff: Schloendorff v. Society of New York Hospitals, 1914, 211 N.Y. 128, 105 N.E. 92.

Wallace: People ex. rel. Wallace v. Labrenz, 1952, 411 Ill. 613, 104 N.E. 2d 769.

Washington et al.: Washington et al. v. Blucksberg et al., Supreme Court of the United States No. 96-110, June 27, 1997.

References

Angell, Marcia. 1991. "The Case of Helga Wanglie: A New Kind of 'Right to Die' Case." *New England Journal of Medicine* 325 (7): 511–12.

Areen, Judith. 1987. "The Legal Status of Consent Obtained from Families of Adult Patients to Withhold or Withdraw Treatment." *Journal of the American Medical Association* 258 (2): 229–35.

Beauchamp, Tom L., and James F. Childress. 1994. *Principles of Biomedical Ethics.* 4th edition. New York: Oxford University Press.

Belkin, Lisa. 1993. "There's No Such Thing as a Simple Suicide." *New York Times Magazine,* November 14, 48–56, 74–75.

Bok, Sissela. 1976. "Personal Directions for Care at the End of Life." *New England Journal of Medicine* 295:367–69.

Buchanan, Allen E., and Dan W. Brock. 1989. *Deciding for Others: The Ethics of Surrogate Decision Making.* Cambridge: Cambridge University Press.

Cantor, Norman L. 1990. "My Annotated Living Will." *Law, Medicine & Health Care* 18 (1–2): 114–22.

———. 1993. *Advance Directives and the Pursuit of Death with Dignity.* Bloomington: Indiana University Press.

Catholic Hospital Association. 1974. "Christian Affirmation of Life." St. Louis: Catholic Hospital Association.

Danis, Marion, Leslie I. Southerland, Joanne M. Garrett, Janet L. Smith, et al. 1991. "A Prospective Study of Advance Directives for Life-Sustaining Care." *New England Journal of Medicine* 324 (13): 882–88.

Doukas, David J., and Laurence B. McCullough. 1991. "The Values History: The Evaluation of the Patient's Values and Advance Directives." *Journal of Family Practice* 32 (2): 145–53.

Dresser, Rebecca S., and John A. Robertson. 1989. "Quality of Life and Non-treatment Decisions for Incompetent Patients: A Critique of the Orthodox Approach." *Law, Medicine, & Health Care* 17 (3): 234–44.

Emanuel, Ezekiel J., and Linda L. Emanuel. 1990. "Living Wills: Past, Present, and Future." *Journal of Clinical Ethics* 1 (1): 9–19.

Emanuel, Linda L., Michael J. Barry, John D. Stoeckle, et al. 1991. "Advance Directives for Medical Care: A Case for Great Use." *New England Journal of Medicine* 324 (13): 889–95.

Engelhardt, H. Tristram. 1986. *The Foundations of Bioethics.* New York: Oxford University Press.

Faden, Ruth, and Tom L. Beauchamp, in collaboration with Nancy M. P. King. 1986. *A History and Theory of Informed Consent.* New York: Oxford University Press.

Gibson, Joan McIver. 1990. "Reflecting on Values." *Ohio State Law Journal* 51 (2): 451–71.

Grundstein-Amato, Rivka. 1992. "Narrative Inquiry: A Method for Eliciting Advance Health Care Directives." *Humane Medicine* 8 (1): 31–39.

Harvey, Lynn K., and Stephanie C. Shubat. 1989. *Physician and Public Attitudes on Health Care Issues*. Chicago: American Medical Association.

Hastings Center. 1987. *Guidelines on the Termination of Life-Sustaining Treatment and the Care of the Dying*. Briarcliff Manor, N.Y.: Hastings Center.

Hughes, David L., and Peter A. Singer. 1992. "Family Physicians' Attitudes toward Advance Directives." *Canadian Medical Association Journal* 146 (11): 1937–44.

"It's Over Debbie." 1988. *Journal of the American Medical Association* 259 (2): 272.

Katz, Jay. 1984. *The Silent World of Doctor and Patient*. New York: Free Press.

Kevorkian, Jack. 1991. *The Goodness of Planned Death*. Buffalo, N.Y.: Prometheus Books.

Kielstein, Rita, and Hans-Martin Sass. 1993. "Using Stories to Assess Values and Establish Medical Directives." *Kennedy Institute of Ethics Journal* 3 (3): 303–25.

King, Nancy M. P. 1991. *Making Sense of Advance Directives*. Boston: Kluwer.

Kutner, Luis. 1969. "Due Process of Euthanasia: The Living Will, a Proposal." *Indiana Law Journal* 44 (4): 539–54.

Meisel, Alan. 1992. "The Legal Consensus About Forgoing Life-Sustaining Treatment: Its Status and Its Prospects." *Kennedy Institute of Ethics Journal* 2 (4): 309–45.

———. 1996. "The Right to Die: A Case Study in American Lawmaking." *European Journal of Health Law* 3:49–74.

Miles, Steven H. 1991. "Informed Demand For "Non-beneficial" Medical Treatment." *New England Journal of Medicine* 325 (7): 512–15.

National Commission for the Protection of Human Subjects of Biomedical and Behavioral Research. 1978. *The Belmont Report: Ethical Principles and Guidelines for the Protection of Human Subjects of Research*. Washington, D.C.: Government Printing Office.

New Jersey State Department of Health. 1977. *Guidelines for Health Care Facilities to Implement Procedures Concerning the Care of Comatose Non-cognitive Patients*.

Oken, Donald. 1961. "What to Tell Cancer Patients: A Study of Medical Attitudes." *Journal of the American Medical Association* 175:1120–28.

Pellegrino, Edmund D., and David C. Thomasma. 1988. *For the Patient's Good: The Restoration of Beneficence in Health Care*. New York: Oxford University Press.

Perkins, Henry S., Richard L. Bauer, and Helen P. Hazuda. 1990. "Impact of Legal Liability, Family Wishes, and Other "External Factors" on Physicians' Life Support Decisions." *American Journal of Medicine* 89 (2): 185–94.

Pernick, Martin S. 1982. "The Patient's Role in Medical Decisionmaking: A Social History of Informed Consent in Medical Therapy." In *Making Health Care Decisions: A Report on the Ethical and Legal Implications of Informed Consent in the Patient-Practitioner Relationship*, 3:1–35. President's Commission for the Study of

Ethical Problems in Medicine and Biomedical and Behavioral Research. Washington, D.C.: Government Printing Office.

Pope Pius XII. 1958. "The Prolongation of Life: An Address of Pope Pius XII to an International Congress of Anesthesiologists." *The Pope Speaks* 4:393–98.

President's Commission for the Study of Ethical Problems in Medicine and Biomedical and Behavioral Research. 1983. *Deciding to Forego Life-Sustaining Treatment: Ethical, Medical, and Legal Issues in Treatment Decisions.* Washington, D.C.: Government Printing Office.

Quill, Timothy E. 1991. "Death and Dignity: A Case of Individualized Decision Making." *New England Journal of Medicine* 324 (10): 691–94.

Sacred Congregation for the Doctrine of The Faith. 1980. *Declaration On Euthanasia.* Rome: Sacred Congregation for the Doctrine of the Faith.

Teno, Joan M., Joanne Lynn, Russell S. Phillips, Donald Murphy, Stuart J. Youngner, Paul Bellamy, Alfred F. Connors Jr., Norman A. Desbiens, William Fulkerson, and William A. Knaus. 1994. "Do Formal Advance Directives Affect Resuscitation Decisions and the Use of Resources for Seriously Ill Patients?' *Journal of Clinical Ethics* 5 (1): 23–30.

Van der Maas, Paul J., Johannes J. M. Van Delden, Loes Pijnenborg, and Casper W. N. Looman. 1991. "Euthanasia and Other Medical Decisions Concerning the End of Life." *Lancet* 338 (8768): 669–74.

Veatch, Robert M. 1976. *Death, Dying, and the Biological Revolution.* New Haven, Conn.: Yale University Press.

———. 1981. *A Theory of Medical Ethics.* New York: Basic Books.

———. 1984. "Limits of Guardian Treatment Refusal: A Reasonableness Standard." *American Journal of Law and Medicine* 9 (4): 427–68.

———. 1989. *Death Dying, and the Biological Revolution.* Revised edition. New Haven, Conn.: Yale University Press.

———. 1991. *The Patient-Physician Relation: The Patient as Partner, Part 2.* Bloomington: Indiana University Press.

———. 1993 "Forgoing Life-Sustaining Treatment: Limits to the Consensus." *Kennedy Institute of Ethics Journal* 3 (1): 1–19.

Weir, Robert F. 1989. *Abating Treatment with Critically Ill Patients: Ethical and Legal Limits to the Medical Prolongation of Life.* New York: Oxford University Press.

Zinberg, Joel M. 1989. "Decisions for the Dying: An Empirical Study of Physicians' Responses to Advance Directives." *Vermont Law Review* 13 (2): 445–91.

Part 2

Germany

4

Clinical Perspectives on Advance Directives and Surrogate Decision Making

Johannes Gobertus Meran

Hubert Poliwoda

Problems Related to Decision Making

One of the most difficult and important challenges for medical doctors has always been the decision about the best therapy to provide to their patients. Such decisions have become more difficult in recent years, especially in the fields of hematology and oncology, where the development of immunological and molecular-biological methods has resulted in a steady increase of therapeutic options.

For good reason, therapeutic decisions in hemato-oncology are tested and compared with alternatives in controlled studies. This is the only way to determine which criteria are required for ascertaining what constitutes good and responsible medical advice. However, the ideal way of making therapeutic decisions cannot be reduced to the statistical calculation of the best possible treatment of a certain disease in general, which is difficult enough, but needs to take into account personal desires, priorities, and the psycho-social situation of the patient. These individual bases of the decision, embodied in Sass's "value profile" (Sass 1994), are accessible only through an assessment of the experiences of the patients themselves. It is they who have to bear the responsibility for and consequences of the decision, once expert advice has been given.

Increasing Autonomy

A paradigmatic change within doctor-patient relationships has been taking place from an emphasis on paternalism to a privileging of patient autonomy.

We are indebted to Professor Richard Schenk O.P. for valuable comments and help with the translation.

Yet the asymmetric relation between sufferer and helper remains. The patient is still dependent on the help and advice of the medical expert, who should grant the patient the freedom to choose among various therapeutic options. In Germany, the actual influence that the patient has in regard to his or her own treatment is probably less than is generally accepted.

From a legal point of view, however, the question of authority is clear. The prerequisite for any therapy is the approval of the patient, who must be informed about possible alternatives, side effects, and complications (Koch 1998). Informed consent is a central part of every record of therapy (Pichler 1992; Eser and Koch 1991; Franzki 1991). It should not, however, be ignored that consent given for a certain treatment that is recommended by the responsible doctor differs from the ideal of an autonomous and independent choice among various options.

Practices of Communicating Medical Information

In the case of most hospitalized patients who are found to be terminally ill, decisions must be made as to whether a therapy should be started, extended, restricted, or terminated. Such a decision is based not only on the patient's expression of desire for a certain therapy but chiefly on the prognosis.

Depending on the patient's prognosis, a characteristic difference can be noted in the practice of informing the patient and the direction in which decisions are made. As long as it is a question of beginning or increasing a therapy in the hope of finding a cure, the discussions with the patient are more extensive than when information is to be given regarding the reduction or termination of therapy (Geisler 1987; Rest 1989): "Biological death is preceded well in advance by the social death of the one who is dying" (Schmoll 1979).

The communication to a patient that a Do Not Resuscitate order (DNR) has been drafted in his or her case is the exception and not the rule. A recent study in the Netherlands has shown that only 14 percent of the patients had been involved in their DNR decisions (Delden et al. 1993). We may assume that in Germany the percentage is even less. An obvious psychological barrier exists toward telling someone that continuation of therapy in his or her case would appear to be futile and that a DNR order has been issued. The difficulty of such discussions represents a taboo area that applies to both doctor and patient (Geisler 1987; Rest 1989).

Dilemmas within Therapeutic Decision Making

The problem is not so much with clearly predictable prognostic developments as with the unpredictable ones where both the risks and the potential gains of a therapy are difficult to calculate with any certainty. For example, assessing the risks of high-dose chemotherapy involves possibilities ranging from complete cure to death induced by the therapy itself as well as the more or less unpleasant alternatives in between. The same uncertainty holds true for palliative chemotherapy, despite the chance of possible cure and the lesser risks of therapy-induced side effects. It is never a question of a simple and finalized decision but of a dynamic process involving changes in the patient's condition and feelings as new therapeutic decisions become necessary according to the course of the patient's illness.

COMPETENT PATIENTS. As long as the competent patient is able to communicate and agree to or refuse therapeutic options, the decision can be taken to be in accord with his or her autonomous wishes. However, some problems remain unsolved. Valid consent presupposes the possibility of free and competent decision making based on sufficient information.

The flow of information from doctor to patient depends upon the success of the communication process. In a recent study carried out at the Hannover University Medical School, we have determined that only a small part of the information given by the doctor is actually grasped by the patient. As many as 41 percent of patients failed to remember even a single mention of the risks involved in bronchoscopy (Bieda and Meran 1997). Were more complex procedures to be explained, it is likely that most of the patients would be able to understand and remember only part of the essential information. The comprehensive exchange of information in the physician-patient relationship is a stepwise process that develops with the changing situation and that should be carried out over a prolonged period of time.

In addition to the problem of effectively communicating information, assessing the competence of a patient whose decision is to be sought is a difficult issue. The competence of a severely ill patient seems almost always to be impaired because of fear, pain, depression, or lack of understanding. However, whether or not a patient is competent is a matter for decision rather than discovery, dependent on whether his or her capacities reach a certain socially determined standard.

INCOMPETENT PATIENTS. Decision making in the case of an incompetent patient is far more difficult. Important decisions as to the continuation, intensification, or discontinuation of therapeutic measures sometimes occur precisely at a time when the patient is in a condition severe enough to prohibit his or her cooperation. Where the decision-making process must proceed without the patient's own input, there is frequently a tendency toward making the more cautious decision. Hence, decisions tend to be delegated to doctors in superior positions and left to their judgment. In the majority of acute care cases, relatives are rarely in a position to participate in the decision-making process as representative surrogates, due to their own understandable emotional involvement.

The uncertainty of doctors, especially those in subordinate positions, about the extent to which therapy should be given increases with the degree of difficulty that the patients themselves have in participating in the decision-making process.

Case Discussion

Case 1

A young, relapsed leukemia patient was brought to the intensive care unit in an unconscious condition. The continuation of chemotherapy would have further reduced the already insufficient production of blood and fostered severe infections. The patient, a father of three small children, had recently agreed reluctantly to continue hospital treatment in order to maximize every possible remaining opportunity. Also hopeful, the family too wanted to have everything possible done. While the condition of the patient grew worse from day to day, infections, paralysis, and epileptic cramps appeared. He had to be resuscitated several times and needed high doses of medication to ensure the continuation of his circulation. On the basis of the wishes expressed by his wife, who was accepted informally as the patient's surrogate, and on the basis of his own previously expressed desire for therapy, a comprehensive antibiotic treatment and further resuscitation with defibrillation and artificial respiration were carried out. However, the experienced nursing staff and some of responsible doctors considered further therapy futile. The question could no longer be answered as to whether the patient himself would have wanted further therapy in this previously unforeseeable condition. It seems unlikely that an advanced declaration of the patient's wishes could have been so detailed as to have solved this dilemma.

Case 2

A professor of internal medicine at the clinic was admitted to the intensive care unit in the final stages of a quickly spreading cancerous tumor. He carried with him a letter stipulating that no exceptional therapy should be carried out beyond reasonable measures. This declaration did not actually change the course of the treatment but created the basis for a relationship of trust and reflective dialogue. In addition, he had composed a last will and testament in which he gave general directives to his family and medical colleagues as well as expressions of his specific wishes for burial.

Case 3

A patient with rheumatoid arthritis and diabetes mellitus was brought into the department of internal medicine to have her drugs reevaluated. During the initial interview, she did not address her current physical problems but showed her advance directive (*Patientenverfügung* der OMEGA e.V.). She specified what she did not want, namely, to have her life prolonged by being tethered painfully to tubes in an intensive care unit. For this patient, the advance directive was a means to face her anxiety and to begin a dialogue on questions normally considered taboo.

Case 4

A 22-year-old chemistry student was brought to the emergency room and underwent resuscitation procedures. She had taken cyanide and left behind a suicide letter in which she declared that after the death of her boyfriend in an automobile accident, her own life no longer had meaning. She asked others to try to understand this. Her life could not be saved despite two hours of attempted cardiopulmonary resuscitation and the pumping of her stomach. The question remained whether her wishes should have been honored rather than attempting to revive her.

Case 5

A 44-year-old woman was brought to the emergency room. She had induced severe poisoning by toxins mixed according to the instructions published by the German Association for Humane Death (DGHS). She carried a form (*Freitodverfügung* from DGHS) stipulating her desire to commit suicide, her refusal to consent to resuscitation, and her intention to initiate a lawsuit if any attempts were successful. While starting the resuscitation, the district attorney was consulted; he concluded that the letter was not legally binding, because it could not be proven whether it represented her wishes at the present moment. Her stomach was pumped, antidotes were administered, and for several days artificial respiration was carried out. Upon awakening, the woman became enraged and aggressive toward the hospital staff and the doctors. She had to be forcibly restrained from harming herself again. After her physical recuperation she was committed to a locked psychiatric unit. Later it was determined that this was her fifteenth attempt at suicide after the death of her husband. The question remained here as well as in the previous case whether this woman, who could no longer find meaning in her life, was treated in the right way.

Review of the Literature

There are at least two essential differences between the American and the German situations regarding advance directives and surrogate decision making.

Legal Emphasis

The discussion of these topics in Germany and Austria is mostly restricted to the field of law (see Uhlenbruck 1989; Füllmich 1990; Eser and Koch 1991; Pichler 1992; Schöllhammer 1993; Bernat 1993, 1995; Bernat, Koch, and Meisel 1996; Memmer 1996, 1997). Erwin Bernat is certainly right to point out that in these countries, those obligations of the physicians that are subject to criminal prosecution dominate the discussion, whereas in the United States the rights of the patients are stressed, particularly the right of autonomy, the right to privacy, and the right to die.

Prominence of Advance Directives

The second difference is that in Europe, advance directives and surrogate decision making are hardly used in practice and therefore are not widely known in the clinical setting. In a questionnaire, we asked our clinical colleagues whether they had encountered patients with advance directives (Meran 1996). Less than a third had ever experienced a patient with anything analogous to an advance directive. However, almost all of those questioned thought it would be helpful to them for the patients to have one. In addition, our survey revealed widespread uncertainty as to the legal obligation to follow such an advance directive. Most of the physicians questioned said that the advance directive would be an important indication of the patients' wishes but not an absolute obligation for determining the medical procedure to be utilized. Although the legal situation seems unclear, the majority thought that the legal obligation to perform CPR (cardiopulmonary resuscitation) would have first priority in unclear situations.

Rainer Füllmich distinguishes three legal opinions in the judicial discussion in Germany (Füllmich 1990; see also Schöllhammer 1993; Eser and Koch 1991):

1. The advance directive is to help determine the patient's will and no more.

2. The advance directive is an absolute obligation, as long as it is not revoked.

3. The advance directive is obligatory in certain situations, if it is precisely formulated in advance in full knowledge of the consequences.

Typical of the unsolved judicial questions are the court decisions to date. The two best-known decisions in German law are the Wittig and Schwarza cases (Bernat et al. 1996; Meran 1996). On the bases of a very informal advance directive (a suicide note) and his long acquaintance with the patient, Dr. Wittig respected the wishes expressed in the note by opting to forgo any attempt to resuscitate her. The court ignored the question of the advance directive altogether but acquitted the doctor in light of the critically ill situation of the patient and the likely brain damage that had probably occurred before he had arrived (Füllmich 1990; Eser and Koch 1991; Illhardt 1992). In the most recent Schwarza decision, the German Supreme Court held that advance directives are important evidence of the patient's presumed wishes but have no binding legal power per se (Bundesgerichtshof, 13 Sept. 1994; NJW 1995, 204). Other evidence has to be taken into account as well. Thus, the Supreme Court recognized a kind of "substituted judgment" standard.

Although the German literature concerning advance directives and surrogate decision making has focused on judicial questions (particularly on criminal law), only a few physicians have contributed information from the medical perspective (Lutterotti 1985, 1991; Geisler 1987; Sass and Kielstein 1992, 1993, 1997; Meran 1996, 1997).

Origin of Advance Directives

Most patients enter the hospital with the intention of seeking therapy and are generally predisposed to accept treatment without additional assurances that their wishes will be followed. The real problem begins with a concern about the time when they might not be able to express their preferences, especially in regards to the termination of therapy. It is interesting to note that anxiety differs significantly between patients who are still in a relatively good physical condition and patients who are in an advanced stage of the dying process. Patients close to death not only fear an especially painful death but are also apprehensive about becoming a burden to others, as well as being separated from their loved ones (Geisler 1987; Rest 1989). Patients further from death more often fear future overtreatment and would like heroic measures to be limited (Lutterotti 1985). Not without reason, many of these patients fear being treated with excessive therapy. Certain procedures are clearly acknowledged to be difficult to terminate once begun (e.g., artificial respiration).

However, the opposite fear exists, if less frequently, that too little will be done when (owing perhaps to reasons of age or financial restrictions) therapy might be denied to those not in a position to demand it (Menikoff, Sachs, and Siegler 1992). More common concerns among those who are less acutely ill include a general fear of the technology utilized in intensive care treatment, fear of an impersonal or anonymous atmosphere, and the feeling of being just another case number. Such fears seem less rational to acutely ill patients who experience intensive care more as a relief (Lutterotti 1985; Geisler 1987). Markus von Lutterotti (1985) points out the practical problem that the much criticized medical heroism is most often recognized as such only after the fact, especially if it has proved to be in vain or had undesirable results.

Advance directives originate in the conviction that only the person him- or herself can truly authorize medical decisions. Every competent patient should have the right to determine his or her medical treatment, especially in regard to the possible refusal of measures that prolong life such as artificial respiration and artificial nutrition.

It could be important, as the previous case reports show, to distinguish groups of patients and types of sicknesses, since different anxieties, demands, and needs arise according to different illnesses. At least the following groups would need to be differentiated: (1) patients with tumors, (2) chronically ill patients, (3) acutely ill patients (e.g., heart attack victims), and (4) a group generically different from the other three (all possessing advance directives clarifying their wishes in the event that their status declines precipitously): patients with perpetual suicidal intentions seeking to use advance directives as a means of carrying out their objectives.

The Situation in Germany and Austria

Written expressions of a patient's wishes regarding future therapy have only started to appear in Germany in the last sixteen years. Albeit very different in form, they tend to be termed collectively "the patient's testament." They tend to stress somewhat one-sidedly the desire to forgo measures designed to prolong life, but these directives may also legitimately express the patient's desire for maximum therapy.

Although in Germany and Austria most of the decisions on therapeutic questions are made by the physicians themselves, the written consent of the patients is at least formally obtained, if only due to the law requiring such consent for diagnostic and therapeutic treatment. In Austria, it is a criminal offense to conduct any treatment without the consent of the patient except where a delay of treatment would lead to serious danger for the patient. Similarly in Germany, the rules of the German Medical Association demand that the right of every patient to self-determination be respected and that every treatment be undertaken only after consent is given. It is a criminal offense to undertake any unauthorized treatment that compromises the bodily integrity of a patient. Even successful therapeutic treatment without prior consent is considered a crime of battery (*Körperverletzung*). However, a signed consent form is no proof that valid consent was given, meaning that the patient was competent and adequately informed and could freely decide. Evaluation would be difficult, but we think that most patients follow the advice of their doctors without further discussion or consideration of other options. We could show that even if patients are properly informed about specific risks of a certain procedure, most of them cannot reproduce even the essentials (Bieda and Meran 1997). Furthermore we suspect that, particularly in rural areas, the influence of family members often tends to be more decisive than the patients' own participation in medical decision making.

Specific legislation for advance directives such as the United States's Patient Self-determination Act has not yet been formulated. However, since the will of the patient is the legal authorization, no written declaration of a patient's wishes made in a credible way will be ignored by the physicians without reason (Eser and Koch 1991; Pichler 1992; Füllmich 1990; Lutterotti 1988; Lutterotti 1991; Lutterotti 1992; Schöllhammer 1993).

Advance Directive Forms Available in Germany

1. *Patientenverfügung* from OMEGA e.V.: This is a short advance directive form from an association with close ties to Christian churches that tries to assist those who are near the end of life. OMEGA is one of the leading institutions that have established ambulatory and stationary hospices. These hospices accompany and care for the dying, offer help in domestic settings, and provide support for relatives. OMEGA is opposed to assisted suicide and active euthanasia.

2. *Freundschaftsvertrag* from OMEGA e.V.: This is a form of durable power of attorney, a contract between the patient and his or her "friend" who consents to care for and accompany the patient and who is given the right to be informed about and to influence the course of treatment.

3. *Wertanamnese und Betreuungsverfügung* from H. M. Sass and R. Kielstein: This document contains short narratives of episodes involving serious illness to help patients think about and formulate their own wishes for medical care at the end of life. Such a formulation is meant to be combined with a form of durable power of attorney. Unlike analogous American advance directives (e.g., the Medical Directive in Emanuel and Emanuel 1990), the narrative form helps a patient understand the possible situations and options involved, while avoiding language that is too technical. A preformulated evaluation form provides easy interpretation for physicians (Kielstein and Sass 1997).

4. *Patientenverfügung* from DGHS e.V.: The German Association for Humane Death is currently lobbying for active euthanasia. During the first year of membership, a form declining heroic measures to prolong life is provided to members.

5. *Freitodverfügung* from DGHS e.V.: This form declares that the holder wants to commit suicide, that no treatment should be provided, and that should treatment be provided, the DGHS is empowered to sue the physicians and their institution. Materials for carrying out assisted suicide are made available after one year of membership.

6. *Patiententestament* from W. Uhlenbruck: One of the first German living wills, this document was formulated in judicial language by a court judge in 1978.

7. *Eine Christliche Patientenverfügung* from the Evangelisch-Lutherische Kirche in Bavaria: This short living will declares that the holder desires neither active euthanasia nor the prolonging of life at any price. The holder wishes to die in peace with Christian solace, with sufficient pain medication, and, if possible, at home. A person may be given a durable power of attorney if this is required by law.

8. *Patientenanwalt-Verfügung* from J. Hackethal: This form looks quite similar to the California advance directive if somewhat shorter, but it differs in two important ways (Füllmich 1990). The patient may delegate decision-making authority even during times when he or she is able to communicate, and the revocation has to be written, not oral.

9. *Persönliche Willenserklärung* from the Ärztekammer Hamburg: This is a short proposal for an advance directive requesting the suspension of life-

prolonging treatment in cases of terminal illness. Sufficient pain medication is requested even if such medication would accelerate the dying process. The declaration must be personally handwritten and witnessed by two signatories.

Special Issues

How Are Advance Directives and Durable Powers of Attorney Assessed within Your Profession in Your Country?

As noted above, advance directives and durable powers of attorney are hardly known in Germany and are used only by a small minority of patients. The recent survey at our institution showed that few doctors have had experience with advance directives and that uncertainty about the legal implications is widespread (Meran 1996). A number of suggested forms and procedures, described above, are available.

How Could or Should They Be Used?

This question will be taken up at the end of this chapter.

What Influence Does Law and Regulation Have on the Conduct of Your Profession and on Patients' Attitudes and Goals?

The influence of legislation upon advance directives and durable powers of attorney appears to be minimal at this time. There are no specific statutes on advance directives and durable powers of attorney that can be the basis for criminal or professional proceedings. On the other hand, the general principle of patients' self-determination is guaranteed by criminal law and supported by the regulations of the medical associations (Eser and Koch 1991; Pichler 1992; Lutterotti 1991; Füllmich 1990; Schöllhammer 1993).

In the case of incompetent patients, the physician is required to make decisions in accord with the subjective interests of the patient at the time. In extreme cases, this can come into conflict with the objectively best medical interest of the patient. In addition, the physician has the obligation to consult the relatives and to weigh their statements in the context of the situation. The relatives' statements are considered to be an indication of the patient's preferences insofar as no conflicts of interest, such as property disputes or noncredible statements by the closest relatives, exist.

Most physicians are not well informed about the details of the actual legal situation. Correspondingly, the patients themselves know as little as the physicians about the possibilities and the legal status of advance directives and durable powers of attorney. We think that in general physicians rather decide in favor of life-saving treatment to be "on the safe side." This sometimes may result in undesired overtreatment, even against previously announced wishes. However, the law in Germany seems reluctant to provide legal safeguards that could remove the fear of criminal prosecution if doctors limit life-saving measures following advance directives.

What Role Could or Should Law Play in Supporting Important Professional Goals or Cultural and Moral Values in Caring for Those Who Are Terminally Ill and Incompetent?

Laws should seek to eliminate uncertainty for patients and doctors, providing a framework of reasonable rules within a sufficient scope. They should define and support the autonomy due both patients and physicians.

Where Do You See Areas or Subjects That Need Resolution of Conflict between Law and Actual Behavior, between Patients' Interests, Professional Conduct, and Legal Parameters?

There are few conflicts within the clinical setting due to the scarcity of advance directives or durable powers of attorney and the ambivalent judicial situation. The central problem of advance directives is to be found in the possible conflict between an earlier statement of preference and the actual interest of a patient who has become incompetent. The basic assumption of the affirmation of autonomy is that a person can provide information as to his or her own interests and priorities and that this person is best suited to represent such interests. In the case of advance directives, this competence must be assumed to be binding for the future. It is thus presumed that future interests can be foreseen and weighed against each other.

The problem appears to be that values and interests formulated in light of a conscious and healthy condition might no longer remain the same once the patient has become incompetent, which is to say, precisely when the advance directive is meant to come into effect. We agree with Robertson, who pointed out that the needs of a patient alter radically as soon as he or she reaches a condition of acute illness (Robertson 1991). Conflicts may arise between desires expressed while competent and the actual interests of an incompetent patient (comatose patients, apoplectics, etc.). Taking advance directives into consideration means treating incompetent patients as if they continue to hold the same values and interests as before. Every clinician knows that the subjective perception of fears and interests varies according to the development of physical sickness itself (Meran 1996).

A decision based on formerly held values might be reversed under the constraint of concrete facts and conflicts previously unforeseen. A further problem occurs, or rather the borderline of advance directives is reached, when the patient desires active euthanasia. Here we agree with Callahan, who says, "Euthanasia is thus no longer a matter only of self-determination, but of a mutual, social decision between two people, the one to be killed and the other to do the killing . . . and a complicit society to make it acceptable" (Callahan 1992, 52).

The limits of advance directives show themselves on other points as well, where the will of the patient and the judgment of the physician contradict each other significantly. This can occur in cases both where further treatment appears useless from a medical point of view but is desired by the patient or conversely where precisely those measures are refused by the patient that appear necessary from a medical perspective. In the first case, the physician is not obliged to meet every wish. The term "futile medical treatment" was coined for such situations. The difficulties in reducing or discontinuing therapy in the case of relatives acting as surrogate decision makers were demonstrated in case 1 above. By contrast, the refusal of therapy by a competent patient is to be respected, even if this will have fatal results such as in the case of blood transfusions for Jehovah's Witnesses (Eser and Koch 1991).

The following formal reservations should also be noted. The majority of advance directives are formulated too generally to provide precise directives for medical conduct. The desired conclusions can no longer be drawn when the presuppositions remain a matter of interpretation. For example, in the case of form No. 1, the physician has to answer the question as to what is to be understood by "artificial methods" and, even more difficult, what kind of situation constitutes a fatal prognosis for recovery. The same problem happens with forms Nos. 4, 6, 7, 8, 9. Still, it is clear that these advance directives at least give the responsible physician a general guideline. Still other advance directives are formulated using legal terminology, which is incomprehensible for the patient and insensitive to clinical realities (e.g., No. 6 uses "decerbration" and "intensive therapy" without further specification). Even if attempts are made to simplify the language and the problems involved, such as in the materials by Sass and Kielstein (1993) mentioned above, a prolonged period of time and supervision is required along with close consultation with the physicians involved. Even then, the process results in ambiguous statements that will require normative interpretation (Meran 1996).

In the context of the practical realization of the Patient Self-determination Act, it has been shown in the United States how problematic the timing of the composition of the advance directive can be. At the time the patient is admitted to the hospital, there is little time or space to carry out an extensive and composed discussion of the possible directions therapy might take. As Menikoff stated, the time when one is admitted to the hospital "is probably the worst time anyone could choose to undertake a thoughtful discussion of advance directives" (Menikoff et al. 1992, 165). The scenario becomes almost grotesque when we imagine a physician asking a patient just admitted to the emergency room with an acute heart attack if he or she would care to receive artificial respiration and artificial nutrition. Such questions would be better posed in the context of a longer course of care by the family physician.

There are several possible reasons for the limited acceptance of advance directives. In spite of their legal foundation, advance directives have attained little acceptance, even in the United States (Emanuel and Emanuel 1993). In Germany, the main reason for this lack of acceptance lies in the scarcity of advance directives offered, although the American experience shows that this reason alone is not decisive. Another reason might be that the necessity of advance directives is simply not recognized since the normal therapeutic procedures generally accord with the presumed preferences of the patient. Many people would rather do without heroic therapeutic measures toward the end of their lives. Still, only a few of them have been prepared to declare this in a binding written form (Menikoff et al. 1992). There appear to be reservations on the part of both patients and physicians. Our research has shown that most physicians would not be prepared to follow previously drafted directives without further reflection and judgment (Meran 1996). Similar views have been voiced in the United States.

Apart from these formal points of criticism, certain emotional factors also play a role. It is a question of how we face our own mortality, perhaps even conceptualizing our own inevitably approaching death as a taboo. Every advance directive confronts us with a reality we would rather forget and asks about the conditions under which we would prefer to die. This discomfort with the question of death is at least one reason for the lack of will and testaments expressing inheritance preferences.

In our view, here lies a positive and essential basis for advance directives. Clarification must precede any attempt to formulate our own personal desires and priorities. Raising the question of an advance directive also provides an opportunity to come to a clear and less anxious realization of the possibility of serious illness and the reality of our own mortality. A discussion of the possible development of a sickness can reduce unfounded anxiety. The knowledge that one will have an influence on the choice of therapy, even if one seems to be hopelessly passive, can be a significant emotional relief.

Which Areas and Matters Require Further Transdisciplinary and Transcultural Study; How Should Those Studies Be Conducted?

AUTONOMY. The principle of the autonomy of the patient, which is at the root of informed consent, has not yet been internalized or consequently applied in medical practice in Germany. The rights and obligations of the patients need to be more clearly publicized. Particularly within the new states of the former East Germany, the principle of autonomy should be promoted and the awareness of self-determination increased.

INFORMATION. The extent to which a patient can absorb information regarding the possible future course of his or her illness needs further study to avoid utopian claims. Our own initial studies of the question have shown that only relatively small concrete units of information are understood and remembered (Bieda and Meran 1997). In any case, a written augmentation of the information is desirable, especially one adapted to different stages and developments of the disease involved.

COMPETENCE. There needs to be a realistic evaluation of the extent to which a patient can potentially make a free and competent decision. The realistic spectrum of a patient's freedom of decision needs closer examination, as does the question of what minimum level of competence is required for such decision making (McKnight 1993; Gillon 1993; Meran 1996).

ALTERATION OF PREFERENCE. The further question as to possible changes in the preferences of a patient during the course of the disease becomes especially acute with the transition from competent to incompetent status. A study should be undertaken to investigate patient wishes beginning from a baseline compared to intra-individual changes. The results of studies we have undertaken to evaluate the quality of life in patients with testicular cancer have shown that important attitudinal changes take place as a response to even small changes in the patient's physical condition.

MEDICAL JUDGMENT. Quite often, the incentive to draft an advance directive or durable power of attorney is the anxiety that one will not be treated in the way desired. The causes and roots of such anxiety deserve closer study. Widely published reports in newspapers and magazines should take more care to be accurate and responsible. Patient information sessions should take place in the offices of the family doctor wherever possible. The psychological effects of advance directives should be investigated in order to determine whether the security and confidence aimed at is realized.

An overlegislation of the relation between doctor and patient, as it seems to have occurred in the United States with the corresponding increase of suits and evaluatory processes, is not only undesirable from the physician's point of view (Meisel 1992). The relationship between the physician and patient should remain a matter of trust (fiduciary) and not be reduced to a relationship fixed by contract. Courts, where personal tragedies are thrown into public view, seem to be the wrong place to discuss and decide ethical questions. Nevertheless, a certain judicial framework to define the rights and obligations of physicians is necessary.

What Do You Expect to Be Prime Future Questions in This Area? How Would You Go about Resolving Them? Which Principles Should Govern Surrogate Decision Making and Advance Directives?

We would fear that the allocation of resources would influence the relationship of physician, family, and patient in a negative way. The temptation to save money could dangerously influence decisions to carry out active euthanasia, coloring the medical decision about hospital resources and the family's decision about its own family resources, as well as the patient's perception of his or her burden on those same resources.

The distinction between an advance directive preventing excessive treatment and an advance directive ensuring the success of suicidal measures, perhaps for the benefit of a third party, is of greatest importance here.

Availability of advance directives and durable powers of attorney should be integrated into the exchange of information in the physician-patient relationship, helping the current information process become a more sensitive form of communication.

The ideal form of advance directive has yet to be found. A dynamic type of advance directive should be sought that allows it to adapt to the changing interests and desires of the patients. We think that solutions to decision-making problems can best be expected from representatives entrusted with durable powers of attorney. However, as Menikoff et al. (1992, 1167) point out, "Surrogates can never make exactly the decision that the patient would have made." Therefore a "higher degree of scrutiny" is appropriate, at least for unusual decisions. We agree with Robert Veatch, who claims that surrogate decisions should remain within a range of reasonableness (Veatch 1998).

What Primary Goals Would You Recommend for the Future?

Awareness of problems involving self-determination at the end of life should be increased. There is a need to improve the relationship between patient and physician, and the advance directive can facilitate the beginning of a serious conversation. Themes once taboo can be verbalized more easily in a narrative context, such as that proposed by Sass and Kielstein (1992). There is a need to further verbalize and apply the principle of autonomy in Germany. The use of advance directives and surrogate decision making will, at least in the near future, reach only a small group, but it could prove to be a vehicle for more widespread patients' rights and autonomy.

References

Bernat, Erwin. 1993. "Das Recht an der Grenze zwischen Leben und Tod." In *Ethik und Recht an der Grenze zwischen Leben und Tod,* ed. E. Bernat, 141–95. Graz: Leykam.

———. 1995. "Behandlungsabbruch und mutmasslicher Patientenwille." *Recht der Medizin* 2:51–61.

Bernat, Erwin, Hans-Georg Koch, and Alan Meisel. 1996. "Das Patiententestament und der Stellvertreter in Gesundheitsangelengenheiten: Ein Vergleich des deutschen, amerikanischen und japanischen Rechts." *Jahrbuch für Recht und Ethik* (Annual Review of Law and Ethics) 4:445–64.

Bieda, Katja, and Johannes G. Meran. 1997. "Aufklärung zwischen rechtlicher Forderung und Patientenwunsch." *FORUM der Deutschen Krebsgesellschaft* 2: 112–16.

Bundesgerichtshof. September 13, 1994, NJW 1995, 204.

Callahan, Daniel. 1992. "When Self-determination Runs Amok." *Hastings Center Report* 2 (2): 52–55.

Delden, Johannes J. M. van, Paul J. van der Maas, Loes Pijnenborg, and Casper W. N. Looman. 1993. "Deciding Not to Resuscitate in Dutch Hospitals." *Journal of Medical Ethics* 19:200–205.

Emanuel, Ezekiel J., and Linda L. Emanuel. 1990. "Living Wills: Past, Present and Future." *Journal of Clinical Ethics* 1:9–19.

Emanuel, Linda L., and Ezekiel J. Emanuel. 1993. "Decisions at the End of Life: Guided by Communities of Patients." *Hastings Center Report* 23:6–14.

Eser, Albin, and Hans-Georg Koch. 1991, *Materialien zur Sterbehilfe: Eine internationale Dokumentation.* Freiburg: Eigenverlag Max-Planck-Institut für ausländisches und internationales Strafrecht.

Franzki, Harald. 1991. "Ärztliche Aufklärung aus juristischer Sicht." *Diskussionsforum Medizinische Ethik in Wiener Medizinischer Wochenschrift* 2:ix–x.

Füllmich, Rainer. 1990. "Der Tod im Krankenhaus und das Selbstbestimmungsrecht des Patienten." Frankfurt: Peter Lang.

Geisler, Linius. 1987, *Arzt und Patient: Begegnung im Gespräch*. Frankfurt: Pharma Verlag.

Gillon, Ranaan. 1993. "Autonomy, Respect for Autonomy and Weakness of Will." *Journal of Medical Ethics* 19:195–96.

Illhardt, Franz Josef. 1992. "Ich will zu meinem Peterle." *Diskussionsforum Medizinische Ethik in Wiener Medizinischer Wochenschrift* 11/12:lxvi–lxxi.

Kielstein, Rita, and Hans-Martin Sass. 1997. "Die Wertanamnese: ein narrativer Ansatz zur Erstellung und Interpretation von Betreuungsverfügungen." *Wiener Medizinische Wochenschrift* 147:125–29.

Koch, Hans-Georg. 1994. "The Decision to Aid Dying and Related Legal Issues: 'Advance Directives' and 'Durable Powers of Attorney' under German Law." In *Advance Directives and Surrogate Decision Making in Health Care,* ed. H. M. Sass, R. M. Veatch, and R. Kimura, 114–35. Baltimore: Johns Hopkins University Press, 1998.

Lutterotti, Markus von. 1985, *Menschenwürdiges Sterben.* Freiburg: Herder.

———. 1988. "Sterbehilfe, lex artis und mutmasslicher Patientenwille: Ärztliche Überlegungen zu juristischen Vorschlägen." *Medizinrecht* 2:55–58.

———. 1991. "Patiententestament." *Diskussionsforum Medizinische Ethik in Wiener Medizinischer Wochenschrift* 3:xiii–xiv.

———. 1992. "Der Arzt und das Tötungsverbot." *Medizinrecht* 1:7–14.

McKnight, Christopher J. 1993. "Autonomy and the Akratic Patient." *Journal of Medical Ethics* 19:206–10.

Meisel, Alan. 1992. "The Legal Consensus about Forgoing Life-Sustaining Treatment: Its Status and Its Prospects." *Kennedy Institute of Ethics Journal* 2:309–45.

Memmer, Michael. 1996. "Das Patiententestament." *Recht der Medizin* 3:99–107.

———. 1997. "Patientenverfügungen im österreichischen Recht." *Wiener Medizinische Wochenschrift* 147:135–38.

Menikoff, Jerry A., Greg A. Sachs, and Mark Siegler. 1992. "Beyond Advance Directives: Health Care Surrogate Laws." *New England Journal of Medicine* 327: 1165–69.

Meran, Johannes G. 1996. "Advance Directives and Surrogate Decision Making: Ethical Questions, Legal Response and Clinical Summary; A Critical View." *Jahrbuch für Recht und Ethik* (Annual Review of Law and Ethics) 4:381–444.

———. 1997. "Patientenverfügungen aus ärztlicher Sicht." *Wiener Medizinische Wochenschrift* 147:117–20.

Pichler, Johannes W. 1992. "*Internationale Entwicklungen in den Patientenrechten.* Vienna: Böhlau Verlag.

Rest, Franco. 1989, *Sterbebeistand, Sterbebegleitung, Sterbegeleit.* Stuttgart: Kohlhammer.

Robertson, John A. 1991. "Second Thoughts on Living Wills." *Hastings Center Report* 6:6–9.

Sass, Hans-Martin, and Rita Kielstein. 1992. "Die Wertanamnese." In *Medizinethische Materialien des Zentrum für Medizinische Ethik* 76. Bochum: Zentrum für Medizinische Ethik Bochum.

———. 1993. "Wertanamnese und Betreuungsverfügung: Instrumente zur Selbstbestimmung des Patienten und zur Entscheidungshilfe des Arztes und Betreuers." In *Medizinethische Materialien des Zentrum für Medizinische Ethik* 81. Bochum: Zentrum für Medizinische Ethik Bochum.

———. 1997. "Akzeptanz und Validierung von Betreuungsverfügungen: ethische und klinische Überlegungen." *Wiener Medizinische Wochenschrift* 147:121–24.

Schmoll, Hans-Joachim. 1979. "Sterben als sozialer Prozess: Über das soziale Umfeld des Sterbenden." In *Sterbebeistand bei Kindern und Erwachsenen,* ed. E. Engelke, H. J. Schmoll, and G. Wolff, 40–48. Stuttgart: Enke Verlag.

Schöllhammer, Lutz. 1993, *Die Rechtsverbindlichkeit des Patiententestaments.* Berlin: Duncker & Humblot.

Uhlenbruck, Wilhelm. 1989. "Patiententestament." In *Lexikon Medizin, Ethik, Recht,* ed. A. Eser, M. von Lutterotti, and P. Sporken, 782–91. Freiburg: Herder.

Veatch, Robert M. 1994. "Ethical Dimensions of Advance Directives and Surrogate Decision Making in the United States." In *Advance Directives and Surrogate Decision Making in Health Care,* ed. H. M. Sass, R. M. Veatch, and R. Kimura, 66–91. Baltimore: Johns Hopkins University Press, 1998.

5

The Decision to Aid Dying and Related Legal Issues

Advance Directives and Durable Powers of Attorney under German Law

Hans-Georg Koch

Introduction

Issues pertaining to aid in dying are among the most widely discussed problems in medical law and ethics in Germany.[1] The word *euthanasia* is avoided for the most part to prevent associations with Nazi atrocities. This chapter cannot and does not seek to cover all aspects of this topic. Instead, it focuses on legal issues concerning the medical decisions to be made when the patient has become legally incapable of expressing his or her wishes with respect to medical action or nonfeasance. For a more comprehensive overview of the legal situation and question of reform concerning aid in dying in Germany, the reader may consult my report on the Federal Republic of Germany (H.-G. Koch 1991, 31ff.).

Issues that relate to the decision-making power over one's own life are significant to the aid in dying discussion. As background for the following discussion, my remarks summarize succinctly certain basic premises in German law. On the one hand, every act that actively shortens life—at least in the form of killing on demand (216 StGB [*Strafgesetzbuch*]: *Tötung auf Verlangen*)—gives rise to criminal penalties. On the other hand, an ill person is basically under no obligation to undergo medical treatment, even when the omission of such treatment would cause death. This means that acts of medical assistance do not become legitimate merely because of the existence of an illness that requires treatment and can be treated. Rather, these acts may be justified only by reference to the procurement of the patient's consent (or the consent of the patient's legal surrogate).

This rule of thumb is deviated from in order to preserve life in the case of patients who are incapable of making decisions. Under these circumstances, the legal representative's obligation of maintaining the patient's well-being is typically understood to mean that the representative must seek out available means of prolonging the patient's life. Such a duty also applies to the representative of a suicide patient. Further, until now, the German courts have required—under a great deal of criticism—the conscious suicide patient to accept lifesaving medical treatment, even though the act of suicide is not explicitly prohibited by law. Finally, German law provides for a special type of authority for treating mentally ill patients who threaten to put themselves in danger. This legal situation creates problems—to be discussed later—whenever instances of suicide coincide with aid in dying situations.

The first part of this chapter presents several cases in which issues concerning advance directives or third-party decision making are raised. In all of these cases, the courts have to grapple with these issues in various ways, in part by "questioning" the physician's decision, at least after the fact. Clearly, we are not just dealing with textbook cases. A short description of the facts of each case is followed by a presentation of the legal issues involved. These cases should immediately elucidate what types of predominantly extraordinary cases the courts have reviewed to date. In contrast to the United States, Germany has not yet evolved a body of case law on highly relevant and frequently encountered problems involved, for example, in the case of the long-term comatose patient. In this sense, it is difficult to reach any definite conclusions on the state of the law, and therefore uncertainty exists among many in the medical profession.

The second part of this chapter provides a comprehensive overview of the legal situation, and the third part is an attempt to summarize the pertinent legal literature on this topic. Finally, the fourth part is a compilation of general theses on individual issues, particularly to the extent that these issues bear on the international character of this project. To render this exposition complete, the appendix contains documents that exemplify failed attempts to create a statutory solution to the problem of aid in dying. The attempt by members of the legal profession to formulate a model advance directive is also included.

Case Studies

The Wittig Case

FACTS. Dr. W. was Ms. U.'s doctor. Ms. U. was a 76-year-old woman who suffered from various illnesses and was weary of life after the death of her husband. She wrote the following request to her doctor: "In full possession of my faculties I ask that my doctor not admit me to a hospital or a nursing home, place me in an intensive care unit or administer any medication to me which would prolong my life. I desire to die with dignity. I neither want to be hooked up to a machine nor do I want to receive any organ transplants."

When Dr. W. paid a scheduled visit to his patient on November 28, 1981, he found her unconscious on the couch with a note in her hand that she herself had written: "To my doctor: please, no hospital! Relieve me!" Judging from the many medication bottles scattered about, Dr. W. realized that Ms. U. had taken an overdose of morphine and sleeping pills with the intention of committing suicide. She was hardly breathing and appeared to have no pulse. Dr. W. estimated that Ms. U. could no longer be saved and, even if this were possible, she would have to live with permanent injury. As a result, Dr. W. did nothing to attempt to save her life. Instead, he waited in her apartment until Ms. U. had died.

LEGAL ISSUES PRESENTED. The issue in this case involves the problematic role of a physician when the act of suicide and aiding such an act intersect. Was it permissible for the physician to refrain from attempting to save the patient's life, or was he under a duty to forgo such measures? Did he commit a criminal act by failing to meet his statutory obligation of providing assistance to an injured person, or is he criminally liable for homicide?

Because an acquittal of Dr. Wittig was to be expected, the prosecuting attorney obviously pursued the accusation with the goal of bringing about a reform in the case law of the Federal Court of Justice on issues concerning suicide, which in certain respects had been controversial and highly criticized. Dr. Wittig was indeed acquitted by each court that reviewed the case. The Federal Court of Justice had great difficulties in conceiving the event in question as involving suicide; it was, thus, unable to provide legal clarification of the issue regarding voluntary suicide. Moreover, the court's opinion did not explicitly address questions related to advance directives (BGHSt [Entscheidungen des Bundesgerichtshofs in Strafsachen] 32, 367ff.).

The Respirator Case

FACTS. Mrs. M. suffered from an incurable disease of the spinal cord that would ultimately cause death due to progressive paralysis. When Mrs. M. was admitted to the hospital on July 2, 1985, she was unconscious and in the process of "dying." Prior to developing this condition, she had made it known that she did not want to be hooked up to a respirator in the terminal stage of her disease. Although the attending physicians wanted to respect her wishes, Mrs. M.'s son, a doctor, arranged for her to receive artificial respiration. She regained consciousness, although her state was no more than a prolongation of the dying process. Mrs. M. described her condition as "unbearable torture" and on July 3, 1985, wrote the following declaration "in full possession of all her faculties" with the assistance of a special electric typewriter that was the only means by which she was still able to express herself: "I want to die because I can no longer bear my condition. The sooner, the better. This wish comes from the bottom of my heart." Subsequent to the drafting of Mrs. M.'s declaration, her husband—with the approval of her son—switched off the machine in a moment when they were not being observed. Mrs. M. died an hour later. She would have continued to live at least another 24 hours, had the respirator not been turned off.

LEGAL ISSUES PRESENTED. As in the case described above, the court here (Landgericht [District Court] Ravensburg, *Neue Zeitschrift für Strafrecht* 1987, 229ff.) also acquitted the defendant of the charge of killing on demand (216 StGB). In its obiter dicta, the court addressed only marginally the requirements for an effective advance directive. The unusual fact that the respirator had been switched off by a person other than the attending physician raised special questions. The court's holding was supported by an overwhelming majority of legal scholars and professionals; this case was not appealed.

The Extended Surgery Case

FACTS. Mr. X. consented to neurological surgery due to unclear but potentially critical test results. The surgery was initially intended to be exploratory; however, in the event that during the exploratory surgery it was deemed that further surgery would be medically necessary, the physicians were to discuss the matter with Mr. X.'s wife who was to be available at all times. Mr. X. gave his wife a power of attorney "to consent to or decline further surgery." Despite this agreement, the doctors failed to consult with the patient's wife when further surgery became necessary. Later, Mr. X. sued for damages on account of the partial blindness that had been caused by the subsequent surgery. The court awarded Mr. X. damages (Landgericht Göttingen, Versicherungsrecht 1990, 1401ff. with commentary by E. Deutsch; not final).

LEGAL ISSUES PRESENTED. This is not a case involving aid in dying. Nonetheless, it is the only ruling of a German court thus far that deals with the issue of the authorization of a proxy to make a decision regarding a medical procedure. Legal commentators criticize in part the possibility of a legally operative power of attorney intervening in utmost personal matters and draw parallels, for example, to the prohibition against the performance of a marriage ceremony by an agent or representative. Despite this argument, the regional court in Göttingen held that an agreement that authorizes the spouse to consent to the performance of further surgery that has a therapeutic goal is legally permissible. The court's opinion is correct insofar as legal representatives may—and under certain circumstances must—consent to medical procedures on behalf of the patient. Nonetheless, this dictum does not necessarily pertain to the authority of a legal or legally appointed representative with discretionary power in aid in dying cases.

The Apallic Syndrome Case

FACTS. Relatives of a patient who had been comatose for nearly two years sought the consent of the guardianship court to terminate medical treatment as well as a court order to constrain the use of further treatment in the event of new complications. The relatives alleged that the patient's existence was "inhumane." The court (Amtsgericht [Municipal Court] Berlin-Neukölln, *Neue Juristische Wochenschrift* 1987, 2933ff.) did not concur with this view. It concluded that a future improvement in the patient's condition—the costs of which would be covered by health insurance—could not be ruled out. Moreover, it could not be determined to what extent the patient was suffering. The court was unable to establish the grounds upon which it could justifiably interfere with the authority of the appointed welfare officer who had decided to continue the patient's treatment. The court stated that it was not a question of whether the patient's preference would have been to terminate the treatment because in this case such a decision to terminate would violate the constitutional guarantee of human dignity pursuant to Article 1 of the Basic Law. The court reasoned that even if the patient were conscious it would not be legally obliged to observe such a will. The relatives appealed the municipal court's decision, but the patient died before a court of appeals could decide the case.

LEGAL ISSUES PRESENTED. This opinion is probably the only pertinent decision of a German guardianship court—at least the only one that has been released thus far. This is also the only decision that has dealt with issues pertaining to passive aid in dying during the lifetime of a patient. In its decision, the court seems to have been guided conceptually by the effort to protect life by preserving human existence. Considering the sweeping euthanasia program of the Nazi regime, it is understandable that governmental bodies today are extremely reluctant to put their "seal of approval" on conduct aimed at terminating life. Moreover, the current debate in Germany is often characterized by repeated arguments against suicide that are based on the forcible tactics of the Nazis that completely eliminated an individual's free will. German history thus continues to encumber significantly the current debate over aid in dying.

Conflict among Surrogate Decision Makers

FACTS. Patient P. suffered a stroke on February 15, 1985, that left him in a comatose state unable to breathe independently. On March 6 and 7, 1985, the patient's wife and legal representative attempted to persuade the attending physicians at the university clinic to disconnect the respirator so that her husband could "die a natural death with dignity." The doctors did not comply with her request immediately, but waited to disconnect the machine until 6 P.M. on March 7, 1985, when the patient's brain activity could no longer be measured. Complaints by each party about the other's conduct led the prosecuting authorities to commence a preliminary investigation that involved charging the attending doctors with personal injury and charging the wife with attempted instigation of manslaughter. Both charges were dropped (see H.-G. Koch 1991, 128ff.).

LEGAL ISSUES PRESENTED. This case clearly demonstrates several important problems typical of decision making in aid in dying cases. For example, doctors and relatives may assess the chances of success of further medical treatment differently. It is not unusual for a dispute to arise in determining what constitutes a dignified existence for a patient. Finally, it is interesting to note that in this case the relationship between the patient's wife and the attending physicians dramatically deteriorated as the patient's medical condition worsened. Lawyers remain unaware of the background of these events, however, since the case never went to trial.

The Stopping of Artificial Nutrition Case

FACTS. A 70-year-old female patient, who suffered from serious, irreversible brain damage caused by a 1990 cardiac arrest, was unable to express her wishes intelligibly, much less to enforce them. As she could not swallow, she had to be fed artificially through a tube. Since the end of 1990 the patient had not reacted when spoken to, she could not walk or stand, and her response to visual, acoustic/aural, and mechanical stimuli was to wince or grunt. There was no indication that she felt pain. In March 1993, her doctor and her son, who was her guardian, decided to bring an end to her hopeless condition and ordered the nursing staff to discontinue artificial feeding. The staff refused to carry out the order, however, and informed the guardianship court, which, in turn, informed the prosecutor. As a result, doctor and son were prosecuted for attempted manslaughter (BGHSt 40, 257ff.).

LEGAL ISSUES PRESENTED. The German Supreme Court (BGH), among other things, had to clarify the legal significance of the *presumed* will of the patient (who had died in late 1993 of unrelated complications), both in terms of its immediate legal consequence and in terms of its effect on the legality of actions undertaken by her guardian. The BGH restricted itself to a great extent to reflections on the legal authority of her physician and her guardian to withdraw treatment; the court did not have to judge first and foremost whether termination of the life-saving treatment was in fact called for.

Finally, the BGH was induced to broach the following question: Which criteria are determinative if the available information is insufficient to determine the presumed will of the patient? In this case, in the Court's opinion, one could and must fall back upon common values. To be sure, such an analysis must be engaged in carefully; if there is any doubt, preservation of life must have priority over personal considerations of the physician, family members, and other involved persons. Naturally, the decision will depend considerably on the medical prognosis and on the proximity of death: "The less likely that a life of human dignity will be restored (according to common values) and the more immediate the impending death, the more justifiable the termination of treatment."

The expression "advance directive" does not appear in the BGH decision, but between the lines one can almost hear the sigh of the judge who wrote the judgment: "How much easier this case would have been had the patient had made use of an advance directive!" With good reason the BGH did not accept as a sufficient indication of her current presumed will an oral declaration of the patient, made some eight or ten years earlier after watching a television program about a bedridden patient with stiff joints and bedsores. According to the facts as established by the trial court [LG Kempten, Bavaria], the patient affirmed that "she would not like to end like this." But in designating presumed consent as a generally available ground of justification, the BGH gave the defendants a hint that they successfully followed at the retrial: they presented a multitude of witnesses who testified that the patient had made similar declarations on various other occasions as well. This testimony allowed the presumed will of the patient to be established despite the absence of a formal (e.g., written) advance directive. As a result, the judges in Kempten did not have to resort to "common values," an alternative that the BGH had suggested but that would have required further substantive concretization.

When the decision of the German Supreme Court refers to the presumed will of a patient permanently incapable of making a decision, it is certainly correct that her presumed will is determinative only if she cannot express herself at the very moment the decision concerning continuation or termination of treatment is made. Otherwise, she could (and must) be asked what she prefers. The BGH obviously—and correctly—wants the woman's (presumed) will at the moment she became incapable of consenting to be decisive. The woman's thoughts immediately before she became incapacitated must be determined. It is evident that a formal advance directive would be a useful expedient to answer that question. Regrettably, however, the BGH did not have occasion to comment in detail on the requirements of such an advance directive. In the German legal literature, no uniform opinion on this subject has yet developed.

Another question, and one that is not clearly answered by the BGH decision, is the significance of the legal instrument of presumed consent in cases where a statutory guardian (*Betreuer*) has begun making decisions on behalf of the patient. There are many arguments—most importantly that expressed in § 1901 I, 1 and 2 Civil Code—for avoiding "competition" between a guardian and a (formal) living will. It seems proper that, when a guardian has been appointed, the presumed will of the patient should be the basis of the guardian's decision. He or she must inquire into this presumed will—which could be documented in a (formal) living will—and must implement it. According to this view, the final decision of the LG Kempten leaves much open for further (judicial) thought. Of course, this affects neither the finality nor the legitimacy of the acquittal of the two defendants.

Summary of the Legal Issues

The Recognition of Advance Directives

As the cases presented above clearly demonstrate, German courts have not paid much attention to advance directives. Only a handful of cases that are considered pertinent have been published. It is typical, instead, for the issues to be examined from the perspective of penal codes. The main issue, however, is whether life-sustaining measures can be terminated, not whether they must be terminated. Until now, the German courts have not been presented with a case in which a doctor is held liable for not having acted in accordance with a patient's request to allow him or her to die. In Germany, there are no statutes to date that specifically address the issues of advance directives or durable powers of attorney. At the same time, literature and commentary pertaining to the law and ethics of medicine have covered extensively the issue of aid in dying in general as well as the subissues addressed here in particular. My personal impressions, which are not necessarily representative, were gleaned from many lectures and discussion rounds on this subject and are as follows: the audience's interest—especially that of older people—was decidedly marked by a concern that in a critical situation the patient's desire to die with dignity might not be respected. At the same time, audience members expressed little concern that a patient in such a situation might be "given up" too early.

Current German Law on Aid in Dying

In general, the issues pertaining to decision making and the criteria necessary for decision making in cases involving aid in dying have been widely dealt with in legal articles and commentary. There have also been private attempts to draft legislation based on concepts central to the aid in dying debate (e.g., J. Baumann et al. 1986; see also the appendix). However, governmental bodies in Germany have continuously espoused the view that legislation sui generis on aid in dying is not necessary. Although the topic unleashed extensive political debates in the mid 1980s, recent attempts to create statutory regulation of this area have begun to taper off. At present, it is not to be expected that the legislative bodies in Germany will devote their time to the topic of aid in dying either as a whole or in terms of a particular subissue such as advance directives. Like many legal issues that relate to medicine, the issue of aid in dying will not be expressly regulated by statute in the near future or beyond, despite the fact that various newly enacted laws concerning the care of persons of legal age may provide insight into the problems of aid in dying (see below). Therefore, the requirements for and limits on permissibility must be deduced from general rules of law, such as acts of criminal homicide. In principle, this does not promote legal certainty; moreover, it creates greater uncertainty in the assessment of special issues such as advance directives and powers of attorney.

As early as 1979, the German Medical Association attempted to develop "Guidelines for Aid in Dying" ["Guidelines"] (*Bundesärztekammer* 1979) in order to counteract legal uncertainty. However, these guidelines are not tantamount to actual rules of the profession; they merely serve the purpose of facilitating interpretation or construction. The Guidelines themselves only address indirectly the issues focused on here: they propose that the presumed preferences of a person who is unconscious or otherwise unable to make a decision are to be taken into account and that close relatives or friends are to be consulted. According to the commentary that accompanies the Guidelines, previous declarations of a patient's wishes in which the patient indicates a refusal of any form of artificial life sustenance can provide an important indication of his or her wishes. However, a patient's current presumed preferences are dispositive and can only be determined through careful consideration of all the given circumstances of a case. Previous declarations are not binding insofar as they can be revoked at any time. The decisive question is whether or not the patient would revoke the previous declaration in the present situation (Guideline No. II b and comment No. III.3).

Case Study from a Legal Perspective

It is obvious from the cases described above that the issue of aid in dying is a multifaceted one. References to terminology comport with legal distinctions:

—Mitigated dying: occurs by means of palliative medical attention or care as well as personal care;

—Passive aid in dying: the omission of life-sustaining measures for a terminally ill patient;

—Indirect aid in dying: for example, the administering of pain killers with the possible outcome of a hastened death;

—Active aid in dying: intentionally and actively causing death pursuant to the patient's express demand;

—(Actively) aided suicide: helping a person kill him- or herself, typically occurring in cases related to aided dying, in order to put an end to intolerable suffering;

—Nonprevention of suicide: occurs despite an existing opportunity to hinder the suicide; such a case is associated with aid in dying issues as a result of the motive of the person wanting to commit suicide.

A particularly important issue concerns the limits of a physician's duty to treat seriously disabled newborn babies.

These cases raise various issues with regard to decisions in individual cases. In the present context, our attention is focused on the discontinuation of treatment and indirect aid in dying; direct, active aid in dying is a crime pursuant to 216 StGB and, thus, constitutes illegal physician conduct.

Summary of Literature on Advance Directive and Authorization Issues

Current Legal Opinion on Issues of Aid in Dying

It would be an insurmountable endeavor to try to provide a summary of all the positions that legal scholars hold on the issue of aid in dying. There are an enormous number of special publications that address these issues from the perspective of legal and political theory; for example, legal commentaries and textbooks often deal with this subject area.

Even within the fields of philosophy, ethics, and theology, including the literature on questions pertaining to medical ethics, there is an abundance of written positions and opinions on aid in dying issues (see, e.g., Illhardt and Koch 1985; Lutterotti 1987; Eser et al. 1989/92). Naturally, this topic is also widely discussed in articles and texts intended for persons outside the profession (see, e.g., Kübler-Ross 1983) including extensive coverage by the media. By contrast, there are comparably far fewer empirical studies dedicated to the research on these issues (see Schöne-Seifert 1989, 156ff.).

The vast array of positions that are argued range from those explicitly in favor of sustaining life (see, e.g., Bockelmann 1968, 112ff.; Schöttler 1990, 105ff.) to those willing to recognize a compromise (e.g., Ehrhardt 1965; Eser 1977) to those clearly advocating the right to self-determination and free will. Those aligning with the latter position urge in particular that killing on demand be legalized as a means of aid in dying (see Hoerster 1986; 1988; Singer 1984; Kuhse 1990). The majority consensus, which is by no means extreme, contends that the physician's right to provide treatment should be linked, at least minimally, with the alleged consent of the patient (cf. Leonardy 1989).

On the whole, there has been a flood of literature covering issues of aid in dying and suicide from legal (including criminal), medical, ethical, philosophical and theological perspectives. Of special significance are discussion-oriented case studies (Troschke and Schmidt 1983, 71ff.; Anschütz, Jahrmärker, and Toellner 1989; Anschütz, Wellmer, and Laufs 1990; Ruhrmann et al. 1990) and, in particular, interdisciplinary compilations (Blaha, Gutjahr-Löser, and Niebler 1978; Eser 1976; Eid 1985; Hiersche 1975; Leist 1990; Schöch 1987; Winau and Rosemeier 1984) that are intended to promote an exchange of ideas and points of view across the boundaries of each particular field. Although incomplete, detailed bibliographies that itemize legal publications may be found (see, e.g., Bade 1988; Bottke 1982; Dellingshausen 1981; G. Koch 1984; H.-G. Koch 1991; Otto 1986).

Advance Directives and the Appointment of a Representative

Since the end of the 1970s, legal literature in Germany has increasingly turned its attention to the question of the extent to which and under what conditions a patient may prepare a declaration for the contingency of an aid in dying situation. Regional Court Judge Uhlenbruck (Uhlenbruck 1978), whose interests are geared toward issues of medical law, was probably the first member of the profession in Germany to dedicate comprehensive research to this particular subject area (possibly influenced by a report by the American Luis Kutner, see Kutner 1976). Until now, mainstream legal commentary has unfortunately addressed this topic in a more generalized fashion. Even the criminal law section of the Fifty-sixth German Law Congress (Berlin 1986), which dealt with aid in dying issues in detail, did not focus on these particular issues; this was also true of the alternative draft legislation on aid in dying ("Alternative Draft") from the same year. In a vote, the majority of the German Law Congress expressed its reluctance, agreeing that the relevance of advance directives needed to be "examined critically." The use of powers of attorney would not guarantee an improvement of the patient's situation under German law and, furthermore, did not appear to be suited to reduce in the long-term distrustful attitudes toward conduct ostensibly aimed at the welfare of the patient. The resulting Alternative Draft proposed that the solution to more specific problems should be left to actual practice (see Baumann et al. 1986, 6).

In the past few years, there has been a more intense debate in the legal literature on issues pertaining to advance directives. The majority of positions advocate the binding nature of advance directives (e.g., Füllmich 1990, 71ff.; Uhlenbruck 1992, 134ff.; Schöllhammer 1993, 29ff.) and even the criminal liability of physicians who violate such declarations (Sternberg-Lieben 1985; Rickmann 1987). Rickmann offers a more balanced and differentiated solution to the problem of advance directives: she categorizes a group of cases in which a patient's advance directive should be considered binding. This group includes the directives of informed testators who are concretely approaching death (e.g., terminal cancer patients, but also people who experience the decay of old age as a terminal illness) as well as directives from patients—even healthy ones—who are capable of making decisions and contemplate the onset of a "total irreversible comatose state." Rickmann emphasizes the immanent weakness of preformulated forms and points to the superiority of an individually drafted declaration (see similar conclusions in Harder 1991). Directives by healthy patients and those that arise under other circumstances should be viewed, by contrast, as a mere indication of the patient's wishes (see Rickmann 1987; Saueracker 1990).

In addressing the binding force of an advance directive, Schöllhammer goes even further and claims that, ultimately, the patient must bear the risk of a wrong diagnosis (Schöllhammer 1993, 150ff.). However, he concedes that it is the responsibility of the doctor to determine whether the patient has changed his or her position or whether there is any other reason to question the patient's directive.

Mandatory form requirements do not exist under German law. Therefore, it is incorrect to say that a patient must have his or her declaration countersigned by two witnesses (e.g., Kleinsorg 1983). Moreover, it is incorrect for the Deutsche Gesellschaft für Humanes Sterben (German Society for Humane Dying) to validate directives, which are based on their own standard forms, only upon demonstrated proof of membership contribution. In practice, however, an advance directive is generally written and, as such, provides the doctor with concrete evidence of the patient's wishes (Uhlenbruck 1992). Some patients attempt to corroborate the binding nature of their declarations by having the declarations or at least their signatures notarized. In individual cases, such formalities might indeed reinforce the evidentiary nature of the declaration in the eyes of the physician. However, where there are substantive defects with regard to the actual wishes of the patient, no formalities will be able to correct such deficiencies.

In response to certain immanent limitations of advance directives, an increasing number of German academics and professionals are beginning to advocate "representation by appointment in health matters" for aid in dying situations; in some respects, such a power of attorney is actually considered superior to the written advance directive of a patient (e.g., Uhlenbruck 1978, 568; Koch 1988, 22; Füllmich 1990, 80ff.; Uhlenbruck 1992, 139). Current welfare law, which has brought about fundamental changes in the statutory provisions on the guardianship of persons of legal age since it became effective on January 1, 1992, is cited in recent articles proposing that the appointment of a welfare officer is impermissible when the declarant has already made prior arrangements. This is particularly the case when the declarant has manifested his or her wishes by means of a declaration with respect to a situation in which a welfare officer would otherwise be appointed (Schöllhammer 1993, 137).

Current welfare law also includes a provision to allow a person to manifest his or her wishes by self-appointing a welfare officer. This type of declaration falls under the scope of the recently enacted 1987 para. 4 BGB (German Civil Code) according to which a German guardianship court must comply with the declaration provided that it does not jeopardize the welfare of the declarant. The new 1901a BGB also appears to be applicable to this set of cases. According to this provision, documents in which a person has articulated the selection of a welfare officer or the desired scope of care in the event of a welfare situation must be presented to the guardianship court without delay.

The welfare officer has a duty to comply with the requests of the declarant; his or her decisions must take into account the welfare of the declarant (cf. 1901, para. 2 BGB). This obligation entails taking seriously and adhering to obviously relevant dispositions made by the declarant prior to the impairment of his or her ability to communicate treatment preferences. Therefore, the new statutory provisions on welfare care can certainly be construed as an implicit recognition of the validity of drafting an advance directive and appointing a representative (Schöllhammer 1993, 137ff.). The guardianship court must approve discretionary decisions made by a representative in his or her capacity as welfare officer (cf. 1904 BGB) that concern medical treatment that might hasten death (as in the case of some forms of indirect aid in dying).

In the Kempten case (see above), the German Supreme Court argued for an application mutatis mutandis of this rule in cases of passive euthanasia, at least if the process of dying has not yet begun. This opinion has justifiably been the subject of criticism in the literature. Although a detailed discussion of these issues cannot be entered into here, some differences between the approaches taken by judges in American and German guardianship courts—based on the aforementioned BGH decision—should be mentioned. American judges must examine the tenability of the guardian's proposed decision; in contrast to their German colleagues, however, in most jurisdictions they need not formally approve the guardian's decision of letting the patient die, if the case is not in dispute. Accordingly, American courts, and thus the state, are less directly involved in the fatal events, a fact that may be of psychological significance in the decision-making process.

In addition, the role of the court obviously makes a difference: In a criminal proceeding the court (in the aforementioned case the BGH) makes an ex post facto determination. In a civil procedure, however, where the judge is involved during the patient's lifetime, the court shares the responsibility for his or her death. In any case, it is noteworthy that the interpretation of the German legal situation comes from a criminal court that in traditional fashion passes judgment over completed events—ex post—but does not make decisions that may lead to the subsequent death of a human being.

Positions on Individual Issues

1. The prevailing position in German legal literature is one critical toward the advance directive. However, support is increasing for the position that this instrument is a generally appropriate means for an individual to articulate his or her preferences with regard to the type and scope of medical treatment that he or she would desire in the event that he or she becomes unable to make such decisions. Such a provision for the expression of preference is particularly applicable to cases of terminal illness.

2. Doubts about the utility of advance directives, such as those presented in the chapter in this volume by Meran and by Poliwoda, basically do injustice to this instrument. Although it is certainly true that the advance directive is not a panacea to decision-making problems related to medical treatment at the end of an individual's life, it is also necessary to make distinctions when evaluating this instrument. What is decisive is whether the advance directive can be regarded as relevant in an individual case or whether doubts as to the effectiveness of the directive can be raised due to a particular set of circumstances.

3. An advance directive should elucidate the fact that the declarant is aware of the state of his or her illness and its likely progression. The instrument should contain concrete and unambiguous language and should avoid abstract terminology (such as "a dignified death"). For this reason, currently available advance directive models from a variety of institutions (see also the paper by Meran and Poliwoda) are not always adequate. The special "Do Not Resuscitate orders" that hospitals offer patients prior to scheduled complex operations in the United States are not yet customary in Germany.

4. Concerns about the binding nature of a directive can be eliminated through the clear confirmation at regular intervals that the previously drafted directive has remained valid. This verification can be best achieved by an explicit reference within the instrument. However, if the directive is actually in the possession of the patient, this fact should be construed as a manifestation of the declarant's present intent to recognize the continued validity of the directive. A similar example is that of an organ donor identification card. In the event that the declarant's state of health should drastically decline, the directive should be altered to reflect this.

5. When such steps are followed, the declaration by a patient should not merely be construed as an indication of his or her alleged preferences but also as a manifestation of free will.

6. Even when an advance directive is considered to be binding, life-sus-

taining measures that are taken in spite of the disposition should not constitute punishable conduct. On the other hand, as further treatment constitutes a violation of the patient's right of self-determination, in serious cases claims for damages may be sought. Treatment that is administered contrary to the binding will of the patient—expressed by any means whatsoever—is not included within the parameters of the physician-patient relationship; therefore, neither the patient nor his or her insurance should be liable for remuneration in such a case.

7. In general, it is the patient's responsibility to ensure that the treating physicians are aware of the existence of his or her directive. The advance directive is not a legal instrument whose purpose is to execute the governmental correction of allocation problems. Under German law, a physician is under no duty to inform the patient—for example, before an operation—about the option to prepare such a declaration. Nonetheless, in the course of treating progressively, terminally ill patients, doctors should, more than they have done in the past, inquire about patients' wishes and assist them with developing a directive at a sufficiently early stage so that critical decisions regarding treatment can be more easily made at a later point. The form of documentation of the patient's wishes is, by contrast, of secondary importance. At present, there does not seem to be a need in Germany for a centralized public advance directive register like the one recently introduced in Denmark.

8. The issue of continued treatment can also be addressed in an advance directive. The physician is bound by these instructions only to the extent that they fall within the general scope of medical obligation. For example, a doctor cannot be required by the directive to implement measures that are not regarded as medically indicated.

9. The private sector should facilitate the creation of institutions whose purpose is to assist patients in preparing such directives and to assume the responsibility for delivering the instrument to an attending physician in a "critical situation."

10. In comparison to the static nature of the written advance directive, the appointment of a representative has various important advantages. It should be clarified, however, that such an authorization requires that a stable relationship of trust exist between the appointee and declarant. The term *durable power of attorney,* commonly used in Germany, has the tendency to be misleading. Special legal knowledge is not a requirement for such a position; consequently, a long-term family doctor is a viable option.

11. As in the case of a decision left to the discretion of an appointed representative, an advance directive should only entail legally permissible con-

duct that does not violate the defensible interests of the patient. For this reason, although a patient may legitimately decline life-sustaining measures, he may not stipulate measures that actively cause death. The principle of the priority of the patient's welfare that regulates the conduct of legal representatives should also apply here. At the same time, it must be considered that the patient's welfare, in terms of both length and quality of life, may also be determined by the will of the patient.

12. The medical diagnosis and the patient's personal circumstances may render the patient unable or unwilling to make use of such legal instruments as the advance directive or an appointed representative. To the extent that the patient's alleged will is legally dispositive in such situations, a previous "anamnesis," or value history, as described by Sass and Kielstein (1996) can be useful as an "aid in inquiry." The anamnesis can also be helpful to the designated representative. If, however, the anamnesis was not established in connection with the particular illness or medical condition that is at issue, doubts could be raised about this instrument's validity.

13. The Hospizbewegungen (organizations dealing with terminal care) as well as aid in dying organizations concentrate on various aspects of dignified death. Their main objectives—good medical attention and care for the dying patient as well as the promotion of the patient's right to free self-determination at the end of life—should not be construed as mutually exclusive counterparts but rather as complementary aspects of the protection of a dying patient's integrity. The symbiotic nature of these objectives does not, however, prevent individual activities or objectives of these institutions from being subject to critique.

14. As is customary with legal medical issues, the political issues raised by aid in dying and, in particular, decision making with regard to the treatment of terminally ill patients must continue to be discussed on an interdisciplinary level. The experience and solutions of foreign countries that have confronted these issues could be of great value. For example, Germany still lacks considerable information on the United States' years of experience with advance directives and legally appointed representatives. Decision making by physicians in Germany about the treatment of the terminally ill patient currently involves many unanswered questions and, therefore, could benefit greatly from urgently needed empirical research.

15. Although the attempt in Germany to implement legislation on aid in dying issues is not a political priority at the moment, the debate should continue to build momentum. An attempt must be made to create legislation on

advance directives and durable powers of attorney. The requirements of and limitations on the various forms of aid in dying must ultimately be formulated into comprehensive statutory regulation.

Appendix

1. German Draft of an Act Enabling Aid in Dying (AE-Sterbehilfe) proposed by a Criminal Law Professors' Working Group (to be incorporated into the section of Crimes against Life in the German Penal Code)

211 Murder

212 Homicide

213 Homicide under mitigating circumstances

214 Terminating or omitting life-sustaining measures

(I) A person who terminates or omits life-sustaining measures does not act unlawfully when

1. the person concerned expressly and earnestly demands that treatment be terminated or omitted, or

2. the person concerned, according to good faith medical judgment, has irreversibly lost consciousness or, in the case of a most seriously damaged newborn, will never gain it, or

3. the person concerned, according to good faith medical judgment, is otherwise unable to decide on initiating or continuing medical treatment and if, on the basis of reliable indications, it may be assumed that with regard to the duration and course of his hopeless state of suffering, in particular because of his terminal illness, he would decline this treatment, or

4. in case of terminal illness of the person concerned, with respect to his state of suffering and the hopelessness of a treatment, according to good faith medical judgment the initiating or continuing of life-sustaining measures is no longer indicated.

(II) Section (I) also applies in the case where the person's condition is caused by an attempt of suicide.

214a Measures to mitigate suffering

When a physician, or a person acting under a physician's authority, in the case of a terminally ill person with that person's express consent, or whose consent may be assumed from the circumstances, takes measures to mitigate grave states of suffering which otherwise cannot be relieved, he does not act unlawfully, even though, as an unavoidable side effect, the occurrence of death may be hastened.

215 Nonprevention of suicide

(I) A person who omits to prevent another person's suicide does not act unlawfully when the suicide is based upon a decision which, as expressly declared or as can be concluded from the circumstances, has been chosen earnestly and in free will.

(II) Such a decision to commit suicide shall not be considered as chosen in free will when, in particular, the person concerned is under the age of 18 years or when his will is affected by circumstances comparable to those which would provide a defense of insanity.

216 Killing on demand

Original provision:

(I) If a person has killed the victim because of the latter's express and earnest demand to do so, he is to be sentenced to imprisonment for a period ranging from 6 months up to 5 years [instead of otherwise 5 to 15 years (in case of homicide: 212) respectively for lifetime (in case of murder: 211)].

Draft amendment:

(II) The court may refrain from rendering a sentence (although the defendant has been found guilty by verdict according to Section (I)) if the killing was designed to terminate a most severe and permanent state of suffering which for the victim was no longer tolerable and which could not have been relieved or mitigated by other measures.

Note

1. The widely used word *Sterbehilfe* is not a very precise term. Depending on the context it could mean active or passive euthanasia, palliative care, or comfort care for the dying.

References

Anschütz, Felix, Hans Jahrmärker, and Richard Toellner. 1989. "Fall und Kommentare: Leidensminderung mit Todesfolge (Hildegard L.)." *Ethik in der Medizin* 1:162–68.

Anschütz, Felix, Hans-Konrat Wellmer, and Adolf Laufs. 1990. "Fall und Kommentare: Therapiebeschränkung durch Patientenwillen? (Gertrude F.)." *Ethik in der Medizin* 2:90–93.

Bade, Ulf. 1988. *Der Arzt an den Grenzen von Leben und Recht: Über die Erlaubtheit ärztlicher Sterbehilfe unter besonderer Berücksichtigung des 216 StGB*. Dissertation. Lübeck, Würzburg.

Baumann, Jürgen, et al. 1986. *Alternativ-Entwurf eines Gesetzes über die Sterbehilfe (AE-Sterbehilfe)*. Stuttgart: Thieme.

Blaha, Herbert, Peter Gutjahr-Löser, and Engelbert Niebler, eds. 1978. *Schutz des Lebens: Recht auf Tod*. Munich: Olzog.

Bockelmann, Paul. 1968. *Strafrecht des Arztes.* Stuttgart: Thieme.

Bottke, Wilfried. 1982. *Suizid und Strafrecht.* Berlin: Duncker & Humblot.

Bundesärztekammer. 1979. "Richtlinien für die Sterbehilfe." *Deutsches Ärzteblatt* 76 (14): 957–60.

Dellingshausen, Ulrike Baronin von. 1981. *Sterbehilfe und Grenzen der Lebenserhaltungspflicht des Arztes.* Düsseldorf: Mannhold.

Ehrhardt, Helmut. 1965. *Euthanasie und Vernichtung "lebensunwerten" Lebens.* Stuttgart: Enke.

Eid, Volker, ed. 1985. *Euthanasie oder soll man auf Verlangen töten?* 2d ed. Mainz: Grünewald.

Eser, Albin. 1977. "Lebenserhaltungspflicht und Behandlungsabbruch aus rechtlicher Sicht." In *Zwischen Heilauftrag und Sterbehilfe,* ed. Alfons Auer, Hartmut Menzel, and Albin Eser, 75–147. Cologne: Heymanns.

———, ed. 1976. *Suizid und Euthanasie als human- und sozialwissenschaftliches Problem.* Stuttgart: Enke.

Eser, Albin, Markus von Lutterotti, Paul Sporken, Franz Josef Illhardt, and Hans-George Koch, eds. 1989/1992. *Lexikon Medizin-Ethik-Recht.* Freiburg: Herder.

Füllmich, Reiner. 1990. *Der Tod im Krankenhaus und das Selbstbestimmungsrecht des Patienten.* Dissertation, University of Göttingen. Frankfurt: Peter Lang.

Harder, M. 1991. "Voluntas aegroti suprema lex: Bemerkungen zum sogenannten 'Patiententestament.'" *Arztrecht* 26:11–20.

Hiersche, Hans-Dieter, ed. 1975. *Euthanasie: Probleme der Sterbehilfe—Eine interdisziplinäre Stellungnahme.* Munich: Piper.

Hoerster, Norbert. 1986. "Rechtsethische Überlegungen zur Freigabe der Sterbehilfe." *Neue Juristische Wochenschrift* 39:1786–92.

———. 1988. "Warum keine aktive Sterbehilfe?" *Zeitschrift für Rechtspolitik* 21: 1–4.

Illhardt, Franz Josef, and Hans-Georg Koch. 1985. *Medizinische Ethik: Ein Arbeitsbuch.* Heidelberg: Springer.

Kleinsorg, Hans. 1983. "Die ärztliche Entscheidung." In *Das Patiententestament,* ed. Erwin Deutsch, Hans Kleinsorg, and Josef-Georg Ziegler, 7–22. Hildesheim: Bernward.

Koch, Gerhard. 1984. *Euthanasie—Sterbehilfe: Eine dokumentierte Bibliographie.* Erlangen: Palm und Enke.

———. 1988. "Sterben im Krankenhaus." *Deutsche Gesellschaft für Chirurgie: Mitteilungen* 1:17–23.

———. 1991. "Landesbericht Bundesrepublik Deutschland." In *Materialien zur Sterbehilfe,* ed. Albin Eser and Hans-Georg Koch, 31–193. Freiburg: Eigenverlag des Max-Planck-Institut für ausländisches und internationales Strafrecht.

Kübler-Ross, Elisabeth. 1983. *Was können wir noch tun?: Antworten auf Fragen nach Sterben und Tod.* 6th ed. Stuttgart: Kreuz.

Kuhse, Helga. 1990. "Warum Fragen der aktiven und passiven Euthanasie auch in

Deutschland unvermeidlich sind." *Deutsches Ärzteblatt* 87:783–88.

Kutner, Luis. 1976. "Die Verfügung zu Lebzeiten: Zur Bewältigung des historischen Vorgangs Tod." In *Suizid und Euthanasie als human- und sozialwissenschaftliches Problem,* ed. Albin Eser, 360–67. Stuttgart: Enke.

Leist, Anton, ed. 1990. *Um Leben und Tod: Moralische Probleme bei Abtreibung, künstlicher Befruchtung, Euthanasie und Selbstmord.* Frankfurt: Suhrkamp.

Leonardy, Helmut. 1989. "Zum rechtlichen Rahmen der Sterbehilfe." In *Aktuelle Probleme und Perspektiven des Arztrechts,* ed. Heike Jung, Richard Johannes Meiser, and Egon Müller, 14–33. Stuttgart: Enke.

Lutterotti, Markus von. 1987. *Menschenwürdiges Sterben.* 2d ed. Freiburg: Herder.

Otto, Harro. 1986. *Recht auf den eigenen Tod? Strafrecht im Spannungsverhältnis zwischen Lebenserhaltungspflicht und Selbstbestimmung. Gutachten D für den 56. Deutschen Juristentag,* in *Verhandlungen des Deutschen Juristentages Berlin,* vol. 1 (Gutachten). Munich: C. H. Beck.

Rickmann, Sabine. 1987. *Zur Wirksamkeit von Patiententestamenten im Bereich des Strafrechts.* Frankfurt: Peter Lang.

Ruhrmann, G., Eduard Seidler, Ulrich J. Niemann, and Felix Anschütz. 1990. "Fall und Kommentare: Leidensminderung. Wunsch nach aktiver Tötung? (Säugling T.F.)." *Ethik in der Medizin* 2:200–205.

Sass, Hans-Martin, and Rita Kielstein. 1996. *Die medizinische Betreuungsverfügung in der Praxis.* Bochum: Zentrum für Medizinische Ethik; 3d revised edition, 1997.

Saueracker, Luise. 1990. *Die Bedeutung des Patiententestaments in der Bundesrepublik Deutschland aus ethischer, medizinischer und juristischer Sicht.* Frankfurt: Peter Lang.

Schöch, Heinz, ed. 1987. *Gibt es ein Recht auf einen würdigen Tod?* Hofgeismarer Protokolle, Tagungsbeiträge aus der Arbeit der Evangelischen Akademie Hofgeismar, vol. 231. Hofgeismar.

Schöllhammer, Lutz. 1993. *Die Rechtsverbindlichkeit des Patiententestaments.* Berlin: Duncker & Humblot.

Schöne-Seifert, Bettina. 1989. "Verzicht auf Lebenserhalt: offene Fragen." *Ethik in der Medizin* 1:143–61.

Schöttler, Rudolf. 1990. *Menschenrechte für jeden oder "Sterbehilfe" vom Anfang bis zum Ende: Eine liberale Antwort.* Krefeld: Sinus.

Singer, Peter. 1984. *Praktische Ethik.* Stuttgart: Reclam.

Sternberg-Lieben, Detlev. 1985. "Strafbarkeit des Arztes bei Verstoss gegen ein Patienten-Testament." *Neue Juristische Wochenschrift* 38:2734–39.

Troschke, Jürgen von, and Helmut Schmidt, eds. 1983. *Ärztliche Entscheidungskonflikte: Falldiskussion aus rechtlicher, ethischer und medizinischer Sicht.* Stuttgart: Enke.

Uhlenbruck, Wilhelm. 1978. "Der Patientenbrief: die privatautonome Gestaltung des Rechts auf einen menschenwürdigen Tod." *Neue Juristische Wochenschrift* 31: 566–70.

———. 1992. "Vorab-Einwilligung und Stellvertretung bei der Einwilligung in einen Heileingriff." *Medizinrecht* 10:134–41.

Weissauer, Walther, and Hans Wolfgang Opderbecke. 1995. *Behandlungsabbruch bei unheilbarer Krankheit aus medikolegaler Sicht, Medizinrecht* 13:456–62.

Winau, Rolf, and Hans Peter Rosemeier, eds. 1984. *Tod und Sterben.* Berlin: de Gruyter.

6

Images of Killing and Letting-Die, of Self-determination and Beneficence

The Ethical Debate on Advance Directives and Surrogate Decision Making in Germany

HANS-MARTIN SASS

Case Discussion

Making a Case for Cases

Debates about professional ethics in Germany quite often are overshadowed, even dominated, by unproductive theoretical quarrels and controversies arising from (1) academic controversies among schools of philosophy and theology, (2) legal disputes that might not accord with the issues under debate, or (3) general public reaction to issues that are so new to moral reasoning that emotional rather than ethical responses guide the answer. The analysis and assessment of new scenarios of moral challenge that confront professionals and laypersons by means of a scenario-based case-study approach allows one to (1) draw on the day-to-day experiences of those confronted with new technical and ethical challenges and (2) discuss ethical parameters together with technical and legal ones as they develop within complex technical, legal, and moral situations, thereby permitting (3) a direct prima facie analysis and assessment of cases based on dormant but functional values-and-wishes preferences, (4) a fresh view on traditional contexts of law as well as human behavior that is guided by principles other than legal ones, and (5) the development of strategies of moral assessment and legal adjustment concerning new situations that challenge both human behavior and the law.

Progress in predictive medicine and in acute care and intensive care intervention have contributed to the development of new scenarios in decision making for demented, comatose, or terminally ill patients and new challenges to balance the self-determination of laypersons and patients with the ethos of Hippocratic beneficence and paternalism and with the requirements of professional responsibility. Changes in technical parameters call for analyzing the situational interrelatedness of technical, legal, and ethical microprinciples and midlevel principles, for example, for what I elsewhere have called (Sass 1991a, 1992a, b) a method of *differential ethics,* rather than for the development of new general concepts in professional, social, or individual ethics. New technical developments ease some traditional moral and legal problems while sharpening others and posing new ones. The study of advance decision making and proxy decision making in health care, therefore, should include an analysis of the interrelatedness of law and behavior as well as a look at how law and behavior, independent or interrelated, react or should react to those new scenarios.

The risks of the situational method of assessment in case studies and scenario assessment include the possible confusion of customary, accepted, or traditional behavior with morally good, right, and justifiable behavior, whereas the risks of the theoretical approach based on conviction, belief, metaphysics, theology, or schools of thinking include a blindness for real-life challenges and the links between finely tuned technical, legal, cultural, and ethical midlevel principles. General theories might be clumsy in grasping the facts of life and concrete situational challenges; situational ethics might be blind in recognizing basic conflicts that have not been made a subject of critical and emancipationist theory. The scenario assessment and case study approach, using the bottom-up method starting with midlevel moral principles and prima facie individual or societal assessment, as compared to the top-down method of starting with theoretical, often ideological reflections on basic moral principles, does not represent the mainstream method in current value- and emancipation-oriented German public debate (Sass 1992b) but has a long and well-established tradition in pre-Kantian, Aristotelian, and Thomist moral reasoning (ThAq. STh. I–II, art. 4: *quanto magis ad particularia descenditur*). The following five cases represent different scenarios for implementing advance directives and utilizing surrogate decision making in contemporary health care where values and wishes, principles and virtues clash and where they are interrelated with technical, medical, and legal parameters.

As each of us will eventually die one's own death and experience one's own suffering and finitude, there are compelling reasons to become aware of one's own story as it is webbed into a net of interacting stories. It is essential to review one's own plans, wishes, values, and preferences for the future story of one's life in the hermeneutical light of the stories of others by establishing for interpretation by others one's own value anamnesis and advance directive, and by signing one's own durable power of attorney (Kielstein and Sass 1993a–c).

Cases

WHO SHALL DECIDE? Mr. B. is 79 years old and dependent on others. His eyesight and hearing have become impaired. He seems to have lost all interest in life. At times he is very confused and does not recognize others. He has pain in his legs and can walk only short distances because of poor blood supply to his legs, which is caused by years of smoking. Blood vessel surgery might improve mobility and reduce pain, thus improving his quality of life. Mr. B. does not understand the situation and cannot express preferences. He does not have an advanced directive. Two sons and the physician favor surgery, but one son is opposed (Kielstein and Sass 1993a, 320).

This case demonstrates the basic problem for surrogate decision making in scenarios where no overwhelming support for one technical solution over alternative courses of action can be established on the grounds of expert decision making or clear evidence of "benefit" to the patient. In cases such as the one described above, limited medical benefits and quality-of-life improvements can be identified, but there are also medical risks and uncertainties regarding the patient's best interests and presumed preference. In the absence of an oral or written value anamnesis or advance directive that might guide decisions, or of a durable power of attorney, the bioethical principles of beneficence, utility, and even justice become void. Therefore, other secondary maxims that are not directly patient-oriented, such as low-cost care or easy-care aspects, might determine proxy decisions. Additional risks of paternalistic and heteronomous reasoning include the identification of moral agents for making decisions, such as medical experts, ethical experts, or individuals or teams of the patient's family members. Conflicts among proxy decision makers cannot be resolved in the absence of reliable and resourceful information and directives on behalf of the incompetent; resorting to a "best and widely used standard" does not resolve the conflict but rather replaces it by using a measurement other than consensus formation regarding the individual case. This is a "worst case scenario" in terms of facilitating patient-oriented, individualized treatment as well as efficacy and utility in the use of widely accepted standards in clinical ethics; Mr. B. did not have a value anamnesis or an advance directive, nor had he executed a durable power of attorney.

WHAT IS THE "BEST TREATMENT POSSIBLE"? Mrs. L. (age 56) had various surgeries and chemotherapy related to metastatic cancer during the last twenty months; recent diagnosis confirmed the existence of inoperable abdominal cancer. When renal failure occurred she was put on dialysis and promised a new round of chemo-"therapy." Six weeks later she died of ovarian cancer (Kielstein and Sass 1993a, 320).

Mrs. L.'s story represents one of those sad scenarios in which no clear information on terminal status has been given to the patient and in which the physicians might actually lie to the patient, raising unjustified hopes for a possible remission. There are many similar stories in which physicians reduce their professional reasoning exclusively to technical probabilities of prolonging life without recognizing the patient as a person: her values, hopes, wishes, and preferences in quality-of-life issues. According to Wolff's (1989, 193–204) prominent and widely accepted lists of prima facie professional obligations—readiness to accept responsibility and accountability, discretion and secrecy, truthfulness (*Verantwortungsbereitschaft, Verschwiegenheit, Wahrhaftigkeit*) —and prima facie professional virtues—patience, understanding, compassion, helpfulness, sacrifice (*Geduld, Einfühlungsvermögen, Mitempfinden, Hilfsbereitschaft*)—physicians in this case violated at least the obligations of truthfulness and accountability and all professional virtues. Such behavior results in professional violation of the principle of beneficence, as all forms of beneficence have to balance the two principles of *primum nil nocere* and *bonum facere* and the two principles of patient self-determination and professional responsibility. Such balancing is essential in order to define and to implement the best possible care and to develop and strengthen the principle of trust as the fundamental principle guiding expert-lay interaction (Sass 1992a, 134). When this balance is neglected, as in the case described above, the principle of beneficence has become an empty shell hurting rather than comforting the patient.

This is not a case in which principles of self-determination and beneficence clash, as it might be viewed from the perspective of American bioethics; rather it is a case of poor, narrow-minded, and technology-oriented beneficence conflicting with responsible, caring, compassionate, and patient-oriented beneficence that integrates differential ethics into a respectfully communicated diagnosis (Sass and Viefhues 1989).

LEGALLY, INDIVIDUAL WISHES SHOULD COME FIRST. In 1994 the German Supreme Court (Bundesgerichtshof 1995) heard a case in which the son and the physician of a severely demented bedridden elderly woman decided to discontinue artificial feeding after the existing supply of nutrition was used up. On this occasion the court ruled that decisions regarding withholding or providing life-sustaining treatment have to be based on the "presumed will of the patient at the actual moment," and that for determining the presumed actual will "previous oral or written statements of the patient as well as his religious conviction, his age-related life expectancy, other personal value concepts [*Wertvorstellungen*], or the suffering from pain, all have to be taken into consideration." The court further ruled that so-called rational or normal decisions, based on so-called objective criteria of a best interests standard may not be used, and that criteria that "represent general commonly shared values" (*allgemeine Wertvorstellungen*) may only be used as a default position in the total absence of any indication of what the patient's presumed will might be. The court thus affirmed the right to self-determination in personal and private matters as the most important expression of the constitutionally guaranteed "human dignity" (*Würde des Menschen*). Kutzer, a Supreme Court judge, makes a strong point in the support of self-determination at the end of life as an expression of "human dignity" in life unto its end in death, and in defining a constitutional right to be cared for in the final hours of life (Kutzer 1996).

This Supreme Court decision and Judge Kutzer's article stand in stark contrast to attitudes and regulation by the German Chamber of Physicians, which hold that "previous written directives or information given to those close to the patient may only serve as hints [*Anhaltspunkte*]" to determine the presumed will of the patient; these guidelines suggest that physicians need not recognize oral or written directives as a general and mandatory rule and that physicians are free to decide based on their assumption of what the actual will of the patient presumably might be (Bundesärztekammer 1993).

CHANGING VALUES AND WISHES. Mr. D., 44 years old and a diabetic for more than 30 years, has to inject himself with insulin daily and obey a strict diet. Four years ago he became blind, a late result of diabetes. Two years ago he became a patient in his neighborhood dialysis center and had to be connected to an artificial kidney machine three times a week for a couple of hours. When he became a dialysis patient, he initially refused treatment and expressed his wish to die. A year ago, his left leg had to be amputated. He consented to surgery because it would allow him to live long enough to be present at his daughter's wedding and to see his first grandchild. Now, lifesaving amputation of his left arm is mandated. This time he refuses surgery and the continuation of dialysis treatment against the strong and repeated recommendations of his physicians. He slowly glides into a coma and dies, as he had wished, ten days after his last dialysis treatment (Kielstein and Sass 1993a, 321).

D.'s story is evidence of the fact that patients adjust to reduced quality-of-life parameters and that their will to live depends on social and familial contacts as well as on personal goals and aspirations. He is an educated and autonomous patient, experienced and disciplined by three decades of managing his own insulin treatment. His will to live and his expectations and goals for the quality of his life change within the altered (reduced) parameters of his health status. At one time he refuses further life-sustaining treatment, but then he reconsiders; years later he refuses again but sticks to his decision against the physician's advice, who respects D.'s decision as a competent expression of self-determination. One might question whether or not D. was still competent to make those last decisions and, thus, whether to substitute the "new person's" request with a reasonable standard of best care or, alternately, with clinical hermeneutics of the "old patient's" preferences, wishes, and standards. How should one handle the dilemma posed by the choice to respect the wishes of patients compromised in their capacity to make decisions: respect their wishes at all, or respect only "good" or "reasonable" wishes?

The second dilemma of changing preferences, wishes, and values relates to the influence of new experiences on a person's reasoning about his or her quality of life and goals. Situations that are unthinkable to healthy and active individuals become livable once they occur, such as in the case of Frank Williams (age 30). An active sportsman and successful racecar driver, he had a severe accident on his way home from a race and has been a quadriplegic ever since. If he had possessed an advance directive at the time of the accident, it would have instructed his physicians to let him die; if his wife had been his legal proxy she might have decided accordingly. Now he can speak and enjoys being driven to racing events and coaching the racing team he owns. His wife Ilona described their story in a book entitled *A Different Kind of Life,* which was published under the German title *Dein Schmerz geht durch mein Leben* (Your Pain Goes through My Life; Williams and Cockerill 1992), to underline the impact of compromised persons on their environment.

Frank had no previous experience of severe trauma or compromising health conditions, although both Ilona (age 39) and her mother (age 61) had. Ilona, who had been a dialysis patient for 22 years, and her mother, who had cared for Ilona during that time, were invited by a physician to discuss the establishment of advance directives. During those discussions and in her written statements and directives Ilona took the position that nearly everything possible should be done to keep her alive, whereas her mother expressed opposite views and wishes for future medical interventions, even rejecting dialysis treatment for herself. How much weight should prospective surrogate decision makers give to the statement of Ilona's mother who "knew" what she was talking about as compared to Frank who "should have known" the risks of car racing, if both had drafted advance directives refusing lifesaving intensive care in dialysis treatment or in severe trauma treatment?

LOSING THE WILL TO LIVE. Mrs. S., 80 years old, is alert and competent but suffers from heart pain, arthritis, and Crohn's disease. Her two sons live in another state. Since her husband Peter died two years ago, she has lost the will to live and has asked her physician to respect her decision to commit suicide at some point. Now she calls the doctor and tells him that she has taken the necessary pills and wants to die in peace and not be revived or admitted to the hospital. When the doctor makes a house call a few hours later, he finds her lying on the couch unconscious and a note on the table reading "Please, let me die. I want to be with my Peterle." The doctor follows her wishes (Kielstein and Sass 1993a, 321, adopted from Eser and Koch 1991, 90–98 [BGH 4. Juli 84-3StR 96/84] and Uhlenbruck 1992).

The dominant principle determining action in this case is that of self-determination; Mrs. S. does not want to live without her beloved spouse or to suffer the increasing multimorbid complications associated with old age. Consequently, she has lost the will to live and commits a predetermined suicide at a time that she herself has chosen. One could argue that a state of depression caused her to do what she had talked about for a long time but never done before; would the possibility that she may have been depressed obligate others (neighbors, the physician, family) to initiate lifesaving intervention? She had repeatedly expressed a strong preference for suicide to the physician she trusted and who had known her for a long time; would her decision to commit suicide have been less autonomous if she had discussed it with her doctor only once or never before? Did the physician, by not making a house call immediately and by honoring her wish to be spared further intervention, violate the professional principle of beneficence and the virtues of accountability, helpfulness, and sacrifice? Did he violate the trust she had put into their relationship by not counseling strongly enough against suicide during previous visits? As far as we know, Mrs. S. had never discussed the technicalities of dosage and drugs for successfully committing suicide with her physician; might he have been obligated not to refuse to have such a conversation and to give information or prescribe drugs more adequate than those that would be available to the patient?

What are the arguments for and against nondirective counseling in the preparation of advance directives, particularly in cases of suicide or assisted suicide, and how could such counseling be carried out successfully? If Mrs. S. had been in Frank Williams' position, she would have needed assistance in suicide; if all other medical parameters were identical, would the slippery-slope argument or an awareness of professional ethos have prevented the physician from giving her the lethal dose with his own hands? What is the principal difference between killing and letting someone die, for the medical professional and for the lepers? Would it have made a difference if he had allowed or instructed someone else to do it, or if Mrs. S. had drafted a value anamnesis, an advance directive, or a durable power of attorney—or all of them? If trust is the fundamental principle encompassing each and every expert-lay relationship, is trust more eroded by allowing the patient's suicide or assisting in it or by being evasive in communicating information and by failing to help when suicide becomes an option?

Professional Guidelines and Professional Behavior

The professional standard for physicians in recognizing advance directives is the *Guidelines for Assisting the Dying* (Bundesärztekammer, *Richtlinien für die Sterbehilfe,* 1993). These guidelines stress the priority of the "actual presumed will" of the patient over past oral or written directives or expressed values, wishes, and preferences: "A previous written document refusing artificial prolongation of life may become an important indication for the patient's will. Important, however, is the actual presumed will which can only be established as a result of careful assessment of all aspects of the case. Previous statements cannot be already binding for the simple reason that they may be withdrawn at any time."

The guidelines address scenarios that highlight the experiences of terminally ill patients and allow the reduction of life-prolonging interventions and concentration on palliative and other forms of care to ease suffering, but not the intentional hastening of death. In the prevailing culture of clinical decision making they are rarely recognized and integrated into the pool of information on which intervention decisions are based. The guidelines recommend that those closest to the patient be consulted but make it clear that final responsibility to decide rests with the physician. Without consent of a court-appointed proxy, the physician may not reduce or stop treatments against the will of the patient. The same is true for parents of minors. Durable powers of attorney are more a legal instrument than a means of improving the determination of the "best possible" treatment or "presumed will" of the patient.

The Bochum Questionnaire for Medical-Ethical Practice (Sass and Viefhues 1992) was originally developed in 1987 for single-case management and its stresses, for trust-based physician-patient interaction, and for partnership in decision making. It is used in clinical decision making and in clinical ethics education but has not been officially supported by any professional organization. In regard to clinical decision making at the end of life, the questionnaire addresses issues of quality of life, self-determination, the capacity of the patient to understand and to decide or participate in decision making, and expert obligations, expressed in a list of six questions for patient-oriented care:

> (1) Does the patient request palliative care, even if this might be harmful or reduce his [or her] life expectancy? (2) Does the patient request or has he or she been offered medical relief from symptoms of the dying process? (3) Are wishes or requests of the patient clear and distinct? (4) How does he/she express the wishes? (5) How can the physician morally justify not following a patient's requests? (6) What options does the physician have? (Sass 1990, 24)

This checklist works within the accepted and established culture of beneficence and pressures the physician to consider palliative care and the easing of the symptoms of the dying process as obligations distinctly different from the obligations of healing, aiding chronically ill patients, or saving lives. The checklist tries to corner the physician into a position where he or she has to justify his or her own arguments and actions if they are not in accord with the patient's presumed or expressed wishes and values.

Review of the Literature

Professional behavior seems to be very much in line with the *Guidelines* and a prevailing culture of "treating to the end," which often results in overtreatment and prolongation of suffering. Calls to replace "therapeutic activism" with "emphatic companionship" (Nolte 1993) are rare; discussion of the benefits and disadvantages of advanced directives and durable powers of attorney or of their acceptability is absent from professional medical journals, with a handful of exceptions. The value profile approach has only recently been introduced into the German debate (Kielstein and Sass 1993a–c; Sass et al. 1996), and it is too early to assert that methods of value anamnesis or value history will be accepted by health care professionals, the lay community, and the courts. No major public movement is visible that would be strong enough or would grow strong enough to change things by introducing suitable forms and procedures for advanced directives and durable powers of attorney. Palliative care (Klaschik and Nauck 1993) as well as studies of the clinical and psychological parameters of the dying process (Rosemeier 1993) are being carried out and may contribute to the development of an awareness of the advantages of value anamneses, advance directives, and durable powers of attorney. The hospice movement is small, but growing, and will expand within its niche; some more concerned individuals who are scared of being admitted to and "tortured" in intensive care units might join the DGHS (Deutsche Gesellschaft für Humanes Sterben, 1993a–c; Atrott 1990).

Changes in the law that would allow medical intervention for the hastening of death if requested by terminally ill and suffering patients have been suggested by legal experts (Baumann et al. 1986; Eser 1976; Schreiber 1986, 1993; Hoerster 1989), but have not found strong support either in the medical profession, among legislators, or in public debate. Single spectacular cases are reported routinely (Bönisch and Leyendecker 1993) and brought to court (Eser and Koch 1991), but so far no broad-based movement is in sight that would bring to the forefront of public debate a discussion of whether there is a right to have value anamneses, advance directives, and durable powers of attorney.

The recent "Care Law" (*Betreuungsgesetz*) recommends that people utilize all three of these instruments; promotional material provided by the Federal Ministry of Justice (Bundesministerium für Justiz 1992; see also Jürgens and Kröger 1992; Brückner 1989; Helmrich 1993) even contains drafts and recommended language for both instruments. However, their authority in court and their recognition by the medical community have not been tested; moreover, some legal experts claim that these forms would not be enforceable (Schick [1993] discusses the Austrian scenario; Wassermann [1993] argues that hastening death would be illegal in Germany; while Uhlenbruck [1992] holds to the contrary) and that legal frameworks have to be changed in the direction of the *Alternative Proposal Assistance in Dying* (Baumann et al. 1986) or other proposed language (Hoerster 1989). In 1991 the federal association of legal experts was close to supporting changes in the law, but those discussions were very negatively influenced by a recent and well-publicized spectacular case of a controversial physician who had given his terminally ill patient a lethal dose of cyanide and who had submitted as evidence and for his own protection her self-delivered videotape.

Issues in need of clarification, such as whether to accept patients' wills in advance or at all or whether to make a firm distinction between hastening death and allowing one to die, are discussed at the crossroads of several areas of intellectual, cultural, moral, and legal debate, which can be highlighted by the keywords *mercy killing, dying with dignity, autonomy, Hippocratic ethos,* and *the Holocaust.* These keywords flag landmarks of the moral and intellectual discourse and overshadow the scenarios of analyzing, accepting, and implementing advance directives and living wills. In the absence of a well-established body of literature and debate on specific issues related to drafting, accepting, and reviewing advance directives, these keywords determine the field in which a more specific discussion will have to take place.

As far as the literature shows, it is not so much a tension between the law and actual behavior of professionals and laypersons as the absence of a moral and clinical culture in which prevailing attitudes would allow discussion of those specifics that mark the actual debate in the United States (Bernat 1993; Cate and Gill 1991; Cogan et al. 1992; Doukas and McCullough 1991; Doukas and Gorenflo 1993; Emanuel and Emanuel 1991; Emanuel 1993; Finucane et al. 1993; Gibson 1990; Grundstein-Amato 1992; Pearlman et al. 1993; Sehgal et al. 1992; Veatch 1993; Walker 1993). The literature proves that professional attitudes and public and individual behavior have not been shaped around an awareness of issues of death and dying in light of the fact that these issues do not constitute a part of a culture of self-determination and success. This repression of such significant issues persists even though a prudent implementation of the principle of self-determination would seem to highlight the importance of having advance directives and trusted surrogates for future scenarios where personal identity and individual concepts of life and its values are at stake.

Mercy Killing

Advance directives and living wills are not widely discussed as a means of avoiding unnecessary suffering at the end of life but rather are considered to be most relevant to issues of "mercy killing." Mercy killing, performed either by nurses (who are called "angels of death" with a mixture of fear and admiration) or by family members (compassionate individuals close to the dying person who often take such action as a last resort), seems to occur more often than not without the "victim"'s consent and, thus, instantly gains intense media attention for a few days. Media attention then becomes intensive again during subsequent court hearings and sentencing. The media focus primarily on emotional issues such as patients who undergo prolonged suffering, patients neglected by family and not cared for by physicians in a humane way, and overworked nurses left alone to care for the severely demented and other sufferers by uncaring doctors. Periodic mercy killing seems to be an indication that neither public culture in general nor attitudes and cultures of families, suffering persons, nurses, and physicians provide for more acceptable—morally, legally, and ethically—means of dealing with unbearable suffering or the imminent and irreversible dying process.

The Deutsche Gesellschaft für Humanes Sterben (German Society for Humane Dying, or DGHS), a lay organization without significant support in the medical or legal community, provides its members with forms of advance directives, living wills, organ donation cards, and powers of attorney so that the DGHS may sue professionals and institutions who do not honor requests expressed in these documents (DGHS 1992a–c). In addition, this organization published a numbered-copy booklet containing prescriptions and advice for self-delivery (Atrott 1990). This limited edition booklet is said to contain prescriptions similar to those given by Humphry (1992), whose book has been translated into German and is available in bookstores. The society came under criticism and media attention when its president was sentenced for privately selling cyanide to the group's members at exorbitant prices (Bönisch and Leyendecker 1993).

Others take the position of criticizing the entire modern concept of intervening in the dying process and suffering, as this would not allow the dying person to experience life to its fullest potential. Bartholomäus-Leggewie (1993) asks whether the Christian response to the severe suffering and terminal illness of one's fellow humans should be "slaughtering by necessity or blessing" and refers to the Christian tradition of the *ars moriendi* and the awareness of the finitude of life. She also makes reference to the Benedictine Rule, which calls for making it a custom and a rule of a free life to have the permanent and unpredictable threat of death daily before one's eyes, *morem cotidie ante oculos suspectam habere* (RB 4,47). Spaemann (1992) holds that there is a taboo surrounding death and dying that should not be broken; therefore we should refrain from having even rational discussions about the advantages or disadvantages of interfering with the dying process.

Dying with Dignity

Death and dying, as well as reflections on death and dying, occur in the gray zone between the conscious and the unconscious, as Heimann (1976) understands it. This might explain the difficulties involved in the attempt to address the issues of death and dying, more specifically and technically issues of advance directives and living wills, in a logical and reasonable fashion. Spaemann (1992) argues that "we shall not give up the taboo" of even discussing issues of euthanasia and should therefore avoid embarking on the slippery slope of differentiating rationally between voluntary or involuntary, active or passive euthanasia. Therefore, as Spaemann argues, arguments advanced by the philosophers Singer (1984) and Kuhse (1990) or alternatives to the existing legal and regulatory system as they were put forward by a group of legal experts, *Alternativentwurf Sterbehilfe* (Assistance in Dying; Baumann et al. 1986), should not even be discussed in academic or professional circles.

A number of publications (Atrott and Pohlmeier 1990; Böckle 1979; Hahn and Thoms 1983 [East German publication]; Salomon 1991; Schwartländer 1976 [which includes contributions by Auer, Doelle, Eser, Heimann, Juengel, and Schulz]) educate health care professionals and lay readers about how to cope with suffering and dying. Sporken (1984) was the first to compassionately communicate "what the dying need"; those who followed sometimes had different priorities and came from different philosophical and religious perspectives but united in challenging "therapeutic activism" (Kehl 1989; Koch 1992; Mattheis 1993; Muschaweck-Kürten 1993; Salomon 1991).

Many writers emphasize the importance of communicative interaction with the dying (Haarhaus 1993; Muschaweck-Kürten 1993), either referring to the Christian tradition (Ebert and Godzik 1993; Buckman 1990) or basing their conclusions on Apel's (1988) and Habermas's (1983) theory of discursive interaction. A few specialized contributions discuss dying with dignity in intensive care and dialysis units (Windels-Buhr 1990), care of cancer patients (Stiefel and Senn 1993) and patients receiving only palliative care (Klaschik and Nauck 1993), special care parameters in geriatrics (Sass 1991b), quality-of-life assessments in cancer patients (Muthny, Koch, and Stump 1993), psychiatric considerations when a patient requests the hastening of death (Helmchen 1993), or issues involved with withholding nutrition or hydration from the dying (Strebel et al. 1993).

Respect for the dying process, according to Kurt Schobert, the general secretary of the DGHS (1993), can only be fostered when "help in distress" (*Leidhilfe*) as well as "liberty to choose" (*Freiheit der Wahl*) are implemented. Looking at the issue from the other side of the spectrum and representing a conservative position, Jonas (1984/85) argues for the "right to die" in a humane way, which in his understanding does not call at all for active euthanasia but rather for "allowing one to die" by forgoing intensive care that merely prolongs suffering. The position of Auer (1976), a Roman

Catholic moral theologian, is similar to that of Jonas; he presses for a change in attitudes toward clinical behavior and respects the "right to a 'natural' death." Similar moral arguments for "dying with dignity" are voiced by Roman Catholic theologian Böckle (1979) and members of the Roman Catholic Bishops Conference (Deutsche Bischofskonferenz 1975, 1993). Although the bishops argue harshly against any form of euthanasia, they hold views similar to the previously mentioned "Guidelines of the German Chamber of Physicians" (*Bundesärztekammer* 1979) that not everything possible has to be done or should be done to artificially prolong the lives of terminally ill patients. A more liberal Roman Catholic position on euthanasia and suicide based on the Christian "dying with dignity" argument has been voiced by Ranke-Heinemann (1987).

Jüngel (1976), a Lutheran theologian, holds that above all a "life community" (*Lebensgemeinschaft*) with the dying and the frail has to be implemented, a community that includes personal and physical nearness but also the "word," for example, communication by speaking, reading, and listening to the word of God in psalm reading and prayer. He quotes Luther: "God as a person and His word make us qualify as creatures with whom God has determined to speak to eternity and as immortals" (Luther, WA43, 481). Thus, in Jüngel's conception, mercy killing would be contrary to the Christian message of a merciful God and to moral principles of compassion, helpfulness, patience, and sacrifice.

Autonomy

Looking at the concept of autonomy characteristic of the Age of Reason from the point of view of the American tradition, one might conclude that Hume's arguments in favor of euthanasia and suicide and Thomas Morus's well-developed moral theological reasoning for devising procedures for carrying out voluntary euthanasia would be the single option in critical and emancipation theory and in advancing rational arguments of moral theology. Not so in the German history of ideas. Morus's theological and moral arguments in favor of euthanasia were never discussed widely enough within theological circles, where the debate stressed that killing someone was a sin against natural law (ThAq II–II, 64, 5). Timmermann (1993, 20–21) argues that Morus's support of the practice of euthanasia was well argued within the scenario of the religious and moral values of the Utopia but that his reasoning should not be transported out of that Christian context, in which it was valid, "consequent and reasonable, to offer the patient suffering badly under chronic or terminal diseases, to end her or his life earlier than it would normally occur."

For the sake of asserting the morality of euthanasia within pluralistic societies, Morus's results would not be as convincing as a belief in the immortality of the soul, and other features cannot be presumed to be commonly shared. However, Timmermann stresses that Morus's method of careful argumentation and balancing arguments pro and contra euthanasia can and should be looked at as good paradigms for a differentiated analysis and assessment of suicide and euthanasia.

The use of the autonomy principle to justify suicide has been criticized by clinical psychiatrists, who argue that most or all suicidal intentions and acts are a result of mental disorders or diseases (Holderegger 1979; Helmchen 1993). Wolf (1991, 252) argues against that position, asserting that the capability for risk-aware rational reasoning, a realistic understanding of reality, and adequate information are the three necessary preconditions under which a free and rational decision maker might prefer suicide over other options. In other words, the decision to commit suicide cannot always be termed "sick" from the point of view of heteronomous psychiatric beneficence. Although certain suicidal behavior definitely is not an expression of liberty but rather an indication of severe mental disease, there seems to be a fine line between other forms of "depression" as clinically observable mental disorders and sentimental weltschmerz, which is a healthy, often eccentric, bizarre, and strange, but not mentally and rationally sick, behavior.

On the one hand, categorizing weltschmerz within a classification scheme for mental disorders that encompasses civil disorder, aggressive or dominant attitudes, and other forms of socially unacceptable behavior is in some sense unacceptable diagnostic paternalism, the terrorizing of others by means of medicalization and pseudo-scientific definition. On the other hand, real mental disorders might be tolerated for reasons of political correctness or lack of societal or professional will or capacity to define perversions and harmful behavior toward oneself and others as what they are: disorders, and not expressions of autonomy and self-determination. Whining males are accepted in one culture, not in others; in Europe they were accepted during the Romantic period, not before that point or after, and rarely today.

Does a free and open society, with a plurality of values and a tradition of allowing individuals to have different, even eccentric priorities among values and in lifestyles, have the right to medicalize (and therefore treat) or to determine to be illegal (and therefore punish) morally or politically incorrect forms of behavior? Do all forms of depression, auto-aggression, or negative attitudes toward life have to be medically and legally controlled for the sake of the (sick) person, or only some forms? Which types of suicidal behavior have to be accepted as genuine and legitimate forms of self-determination, and which not? Which advance directives that mention suicide as one among other rational options will have authority over the presumed obligations of others to save the lives of those who have committed suicide; will arguments of those who intervene have to be based on analyzing the advance directive or on analyzing the situation in which the suicide was executed?

Most prominently, it was Immanuel Kant, the arch-authority on critical reasoning and autonomy, who came out strongly against Hume and the theory that the "regulative idea" of liberty and the principle of autonomy ever could justify self-killing (Kant 1785, 395–96; 1797, 422ff.; Römpp 1988; Wolf 1991, 252). In his view, euthanasia would severely compromise the respect for persons and the dignity of humans; it would also be a perverse form of heteronomous ethics violating the Age of Reason concept of autonomy by ending the life of an autonomous person. *Selbsttötung* and *Selbstmord,* self-killing and self-murdering, are the words used in German for the Latin *suicide,* but the term *Selbstmord* (self-murdering) is the most commonly used. It is Kant's argument that, as life is the precondition for dignity, autonomy, and self-determination, life itself cannot be at the disposal of the autonomous individual; therefore, self-killing would be an expression of not being free, that is, driven by self-pity, desperation, or fear, rather than an expression of free self-determination.

Wolf (1991, 252) calls Kant's argument sharp but not convincing; he argues that Kant does not address cases in which suicide would protect human dignity and liberty that otherwise might be annihilated through torture, disgrace, or degradation. Influenced by classical Indian thought, Schopenhauer (Birnbacher 1985; Zentner 1988), in his *Die Welt als Wille und Vorstellung* (The World as Will and Representation), took issue with Kant on various topics; however, like Kant, he argued that suicide is an inappropriate instrument for self-redemption from suffering. However, Schopenhauer's disciple Mainländer (1876, 1886) stressed suicide as the logical and appropriate means for self-deliverance from unnecessary medical suffering and weltschmerz.

The philosophers Amery, in *Laying Hands on Yourself* (1976), and my teacher Kamlah, in *Meditatio mortis* (1976), both understood and argued for suicide as the final expression of self-determination and the final victory over the limits, sufferings, and shortcomings of life. Both ended their lives accordingly when they felt that the time had come. Their arguments for suicide can be understood not as a type of advance directive but instead as advance explanations of actions they had logically and morally considered long before these actions were executed. In order to rebut prosuicide arguments on the basis of autonomy, Schwartländer differentiates between two types of autonomy: "power to execute" as dominance-being and "moral-legal autonomy" as responsibility-being; he concludes that autonomy is the "mystery" of life, whereas death is life's "enigma" and that therefore rational arguments for a "right to die" cannot be given, as the scenario of death and dying surpasses utility and the capacity of rational calculations (Schwartländer 1976, 31–33). Schwartländer's position is close to that of Jonas (1984/85), who for similar reasons refused to accept logical reasoning supporting brain-death criteria.

Positions taken by philosophers range from Singer's to Spaemann's (Doelle-Oelmueller 1993) without much compromise or consensus. On the basis of such arguments, the philosophical debate concerning the right to request euthanasia or to commit suicide is inconclusive, in part as a result of Kant's position against "taking lives." But a majority of positions, including those that have been influenced by Kant (Pieper 1993; Wolf 1991) and all positions influenced by or representing utilitarian arguments (Koller 1993; Kuhse 1990; Leist 1989), favor the honoring of rational decisions to commit suicide. A majority of philosophers would agree. Pieper (1993, 98) summarizes this perspective: "A physician bound by his ethos of care may not become a representative of death by actively supporting a patient's wish to die. But he can respect the autonomy of someone competent and determined to commit suicide by omitting all life-prolonging interventions, i.e. by not forcing him to continue living against his will."

Hippocratic Ethos

The quote from Pieper's analysis of the principle of autonomy can serve as a description of professional behavior by health care personnel that could find clinical support. There are two arguments in clinical ethics: one stresses healing and the alleviation of pain as the sole professional obligations, whereas the other uses the slippery-slope argument. Lutterotti (1992, 1993) recollects from his clinical experience that the overwhelming interest of terminally ill and suffering patients is the improvement of their remaining quality of life, not the end of life. His five arguments against a watering down of the Hippocratic ethos of not killing and not assisting in or advising on killing are the following: (1) Life is not at one's disposal, therefore utilitarian arguments are not valid; (2) the medical ethos of healing and alleviating suffering is incompatible with killing; (3) the best interests of the vast majority of patients does not call for a debate on killing, although an extremely small number of cases might call for such debate; (4) any kind of killing will initiate a slippery slope, which then—a utilitarian argument—will cause angst and reduction of trust in the medical profession; and (5) a ban on killing cannot be based on utilitarian arguments, as they might at other times call for killing on utilitarian grounds (Lutterotti 1992, 13). Lutterotti's arguments represent the mainstream of the profession's value concepts and behavioral preferences very well. This system of professional ethics and associated behavior seems to be very powerful, no matter what the law says or what the patients request in oral or written form.

At most, those who agree with Lutterotti will concede that the scenarios of terminality and dying require a consideration of other priorities, such as compassion, personal attention, communication, and palliative care. But even given the reluctance of health care professionals to consider special obligations and virtues in caring for the dying or to honor preferences, wishes, and values of the severely and irreversibly compromised, there is an increasing number of medical and ethical studies and recommendations (Klaschik and Nauck 1993; Nolte 1993; Mattheis 1993; Rosemeier 1993; Eid 1993; Storck 1993; Muschaweck-Kürten 1993) that explore changing attitudes within the framework of traditional paternalistic beneficence. These studies identify a shift toward more compassion, attention, and individualized patient-oriented special care for those in the dying process. Proposals of new forms of value anamneses and advance directives that would give the physician additional and essential information about the patient's values and wishes and that would not negate the responsibilities of beneficence, but rather would allow for better-informed decision making as essential, nontechnical individual expressions, are becoming available and work as well in the context of prevailing beneficence as in the context of self-determination (Kielstein and Sass 1993a–c).

For practical reasons, there seems to be a "consensus in general" supported by WHO, the Austrian and German professional organizations of physicians, and the Christian churches that the medical ethos does not call for "extraordinary means" and that purely life-prolonging interventions should not be used when terminally ill but competent patients do not accept them. In those cases "human facts have simply to be accepted" and the forgoing of extraordinary means does not constitute suicide (Wolkinger 1993, 48–53; Evangelische Kirche in Deutschland 1989; Bundesärztekammer 1979; Bischofskonferenz 1975, 1993). It has been argued that continued support of the principle of self-determination might broaden the acceptance of a renewed euthanasia debate in Germany. In particular, concern has been voiced that support for, and information about methods of, conducting euthanasia in the neighboring Netherlands might spill over into Germany. As Schimtz holds (1993, 38), "Sensibility for the complexities of life and the need for the protection of life might disappear under the unilateral support of the right to self-determination. The language of the debate on euthanasia becomes less controllable and more brutal."

Holocaust and Euthanasia

In Germany, it is not possible to evaluate the moral, legal, and clinical dimensions, including benefits and risks, associated with the term *euthanasia* without being aware of the use of the term in Nazi language as a means and a goal to exterminate millions of fellow human beings. The killings of "others" during the Third Reich still overshadows all discussions on euthanasia and will do so for a long time. A sick paternalism devised by a group of demagogues concluded that other fellow humans were racially or genetically "of inferior nature" or of compromised mental or physical status and lived a "life unworthy of living"; therefore, these demagogues took action to "liquidate" or "euthanize" those unfortunates (Binding and Hoche 1920).

An extensive and ongoing debate about the immorality of the Nazi killings and exterminations documents the long-lasting effect of what can be called a Holocaust syndrome in German public culture. On the one hand, this causes shamefulness and an atmosphere of taboo in which it is ethically incorrect to discuss issues of killing others, while on the other hand the Nazi past serves not only as an impressive example of outrageous forms of discrimination against "cripples" and "inferior races" but also as a blueprint for "slippery-slope" arguments against euthanasia (see von Engelhardt 1993; Schmuhl 1992; Hasiba 1993). This history of discrimination may explain why for the foreseeable future a rational debate on euthanasia can never be held in Germany as in the neighboring Netherlands. German media and public culture are so strongly aware of the Nazi cruelties that during recent years every attempt by Singer (1984) or Kuhse (1990) to speak in Germany or Austria had been prohibited or protested (Schöne-Seifert 1991).

Euthanasia originally meant a good and peaceful dying process free from pain and not influenced by any human intervention (Rainer 1993) in the nature of a generous gift from the gods. While involuntary killing of the sick or frail, even of slaves, has not been reported in the classical Greek and Latin literature, *eulogos exagoge,* self-delivery of irreversibly ill, educated individuals was understood as a high and most exemplary form of culture, education, and liberty. Only our century changed the meaning of euthanasia to suggest an instrument of killing—for example, *to euthanize* (von Engelhardt

1993; Schmuhl 1993). *Euthanasia* has become an ambiguous term, burdened by a history of vague ideological definition and inhumane, discriminatory actions; therefore it has the potential to instigate confrontational and ideological exchange and conflict. Also problematic is the fact that, used as a general term, it does not contribute to the rational analysis of moral, behavioral, cultural, medical, and legal parameters of scenarios in which advance directives and surrogate decision making have to be evaluated.

A differentiation in the use of the term euthanasia and scenario-based usage does reduce the risk of misunderstanding and misappropriating (Wassermann 1993; Winau 1993b). Von Engelhardt offers such a differentiation and summarizes seven different ways to understand euthanasia that have been developed during moral and intellectual debates (von Engelhardt 1993) and that have also been dealt with in novels and dramas (Viefhues 1991):

> 1. physical (external) and intellectual (internal) euthanasia, a perversion of the concept of man that at any time can introduce actions of ethnic cleansing, mercy killing, abortion, and so on;
>
> 2. active and passive euthanasia, where the latter could be justified only if "informed, legal, and moral consent" is clearly given;
>
> 3. direct and indirect euthanasia, where the first poses the severest risks to a trust-based physician-patient relationship;
>
> 4. euthanasia with or without the direct hastening of death;
>
> 5. heteronomous and autonomous euthanasia;
>
> 6. euthanasia executed by the physician, friend, family, or in the form of suicide;
>
> 7. euthanasia in response to terminal illness, social distress, political suppression, loss of mental and intellectual orientation and sense, or emotional distress. (von Engelhardt 1993, 23–24)

Other specifications are offered by Koller (1993, 87), who differentiates between active ("doing something") and passive ("abstaining from doing something") scenarios and in each set of scenarios distinguishes further between voluntary, involuntary, and nonvoluntary letting one die and killing: (1) allowing a competent person to die on his or her request, (2) allowing a terminally ill and incompetent person to die, (3) letting a competent person die against his or her will, (4) killing a competent person on request, (5) killing a terminally ill and incompetent person, and (6) killing a competent person against his or her will.

Winau (1993a) differentiates between "assistance in dying" (*Hilfe im Sterben*) such as palliative care and care that reduces the symptoms of the dying process itself and "assistance to die" (*Hilfe zum Sterben*), such as hastening or causing the death of persons who are not near death yet. He further makes a distinction between subjective arguments for "assistance to die" (*Hilfe zum Sterben*), which can either be suicide or assisted suicide or killing on request, and objective arguments for "eradicating objectively worthless life."

Making these kinds of differentiations is extremely helpful in an attempt to (1) discuss different clinical and personal scenarios on their own merits and not within the general framework of "killing," (2) develop clinical and technical scenarios for further rational and transdisciplinary evaluation, (3) prepare medically possible and ethically acceptable models that can be used to rewrite laws, regulations, or professional guidelines wherever necessary, and (4) develop concepts and language for use in advance directive forms and for the education and instruction of surrogates. Each scenario sheds a different light on killing and suicide, and all scenarios directly or indirectly answer the question of how we humans understand ourselves and how we understand and deal with disorder and suffering.

Von Engelhardt holds that issues of euthanasia are primarily issues to be addressed in terms of culture, not within the technicalities of civilization and medicine. Winau, in addition to the already proposed differentiation among forms of euthanasia, further differentiates the previously mentioned assistance in dying and assistance to die by distinguishing between "assistance" and "care" for the dying; he emphasizes that "care for the dying has always a high priority" and includes "attitudes in accompanying a dying's last journey" and "allowing for the dying's own death" (Winau 1993a, 21).

Special Issues

How Are Advance Directives and Durable Powers of Attorney Assessed?

As there have not yet been detailed professional or public debates on either advance directives or durable powers of attorney, this question can be answered only indirectly. Philosophical debates are still relatively theoretical and address issues of suicide (self-delivery, *Selbsttötung*) and care and assistance in the process of dying (*Sterbehilfe*). Philosophers representing or influenced by utilitarian thought strongly present arguments in favor of both (Hoerster 1989; Leist 1989; Wolf 1991), as do Amery (1976) and Kamlah (1976), who use classical eudaemonistic and existentialist arguments in their promotion of individual human dignity and the implementation of self-determination. On the other side of the spectrum are positions more closely associated with the official reasoning of the Roman Catholic church, calling for either a taboo on the mere discussion of differences between active and passive euthanasia (Spaemann 1992) or the consideration of the moral obligation to withhold intensive treatment from terminally ill or dying patients (Boeckle 1979; Eid 1993; Storck 1993; Wolkinger 1993). Both positions argue in a paternalistic fashion. Positions critical of accepting the self-determination principle for making life-and-death decisions emphasize strongly the quest for better personal, humane care for the dying, whereas the utilitarian and similar positions rarely address issues of improved personal attention and compassion with the frail and dying.

Whereas professional ethicists and philosophers take general positions on both sides of the spectrum and rarely discuss the specifics of advance directives and durable powers of attorney, there is a clear preference in favor of *Sterbehilfe,* "assisting the terminally ill and suffering at their explicit request in the process of dying," among the German population. Polls conducted in 1993 (Sb 1993) confirm this: 68 percent demanded that *Sterbehilfe* be permitted, whereas 30 percent were opposed to its authorization and 2 percent were undecided; only 58 percent of those supporting *Sterbehilfe* were voters for the conservative Christian Democratic Union, but those who aligned with socialist or green parties were more supportive.

Wedler distributed questionnaires to participants of the Hessen Chamber of Physicians' academy meeting, "Prevention of Suicide and Care for The Dying"; 27 out of 80 experts answered (Wedler 1996). Twenty-six accepted the "double effect" of palliative medication shortening life (1 against), 25 would discontinue life-supporting machinery (2 against), 9 would discontinue artificial feeding (15 against), but only 2 would directly hasten death by providing an overdose of medication (24 against); 7 would welcome initiatives to improve the legal standing and acceptance of advance directives (5 against). Eighteen declared that the patient should decide about prolonging or discontinuing life-sustaining treatment (9 against), 8 wanted those decisions made by physicians alone (13 against), 10 by family members (12 against), and 18 by the physician together with persons close to the patient (5 against). Sehgal et al. (1996) and Rothenberg et al. (1996) reviewed physicians' attitudes in Germany, Japan, and the United States and found that in Germany and Japan the reluctance by physicians to share decision making with patients is much lower than in the United States and that the prevalence of advance directives in those two countries is extremely low.

May, Gawrich, and Stiegel (1997) discuss results of interviews and trials with physicians, nurses, patients, and students regarding value-and-wish profiles and preferences in end-of-life care and treatment. They stress the wide variety of individual narrative responses and the competence of laypersons to differentiate clearly between what they would want to be done at the present and how that would be different from what they would wish or request for a later stage. Wishes requesting first-class palliative care and the withdrawal of life-sustaining treatment in conditions of prolonged coma and severe dementia and during the last stages of terminal illness ranked highest, in particular among physicians and nurses. Palliative treatment is insufficient, due to many physicians' unfamiliarity with the basics of modern palliative care and overbureaucratization of palliative care paperwork and regulation in Germany. This insufficiency is in part responsible for the request to make physician-assisted suicide and mercy killing more accessible. It has also been recognized by intensive care specialists (Donner and Zenz 1994). The German Society of Surgeons was the first to issue specific guidelines addressing end-of-life or multimorbidity situations in which the medical ethos and obligation to intervene and to treat should be considered on a case-by-case decision-making process and should take the patient's value-and-wish profile into account (Deutsche Gesellschaft für Chirurgie 1996).

How Could or Should Value Anamneses, Advance Directives, and Durable Powers of Attorney Be Used?

All of these instruments cannot and should not be seen as easy solutions for complex clinical and personal decision making in the face of multimorbidity and dying. However, they can and will be valuable, even indispensable, instruments when used to (1) improve the overall trust-based client-expert interaction in health care matters, (2) assist the layperson in reflecting on future situations of disease and dying, (3) define goals, values, and wishes for such situations, and (4) give caretakers and proxies information and direction that will serve, together with other clinical and laboratory information, to establish what would be the best possible treatment for each individual. The most prudent combination would be the triad of integrated forms of advance directives, durable powers of attorney, and value anamneses, which contain information on the individual's actual values, preferences, and wishes and his or her own perspective on how those actual statements should govern future proxy decisions (Kielstein and Sass 1992a–c).

Advance directives should not command the use or refusal of certain technical procedures such as dialysis or minor or major surgery (Doukas and McCullough 1991; Emanuel and Emanuel 1991; Kielstein and Sass 1993c,

9–13, 21) but should, rather, display and discuss those individual values, wishes, and preferences (Kielstein and Sass 1993c, 46) that, in future clinical situations, will direct clinical decision makers, caretakers, and proxies to integrate information on values and wishes into clinical judgment. The availability of personal and individual information on values, wishes, and preferences does not take any responsibility away from caretakers but rather gives practitioners an increased opportunity to broaden clinical hermeneutics and clinical judgment, as they can be based on more accurate and essential information. Refusal lists of specified medical interventions seem to be neither helpful in the clinical setting nor in the patient's best interest; they should be replaced by lists of specified preferences, values, and wishes, which will then become a part of differential diagnosis and individualized clinical hermeneutics and decision making. A wide variety of advance directive instruments (see the appendix for different forms and models), many yet to be developed, and the promotion of advance medical care planning by physicians and cultural and religious organizations seem to be instrumental in furthering the use and acceptance of advance directives.

Recently, quite a few committees and conferences of Protestant and Catholic churches have started to address the issue (Beck 1996; Bischofskonferenz 1993; Evangelische Kirche 1989; Koch 1992). A combination form of an advanced directive has been developed recently by Kielstein and Sass (Sass and Kielstein 1996). It primarily provides information regarding the person's system of beliefs and wishes and a value profile. It also provides a limited number of medical directives for palliative care and treatment decisions for situations of prolonged coma, severe dementia, and the final stages of terminal illness. It has been widely tested and modified in cooperation with patients, nurses, physicians, and legal experts.

The Influence and Role of Law

Although philosophers and ethicists tend to reason and to propose independently from the law, experienced clinical ethicists and hospital chaplains are more aware of legal parameters than are university-based philosophers. Physicians, who experience a special responsibility and ethos, do not care much about the law either, but this does not motivate them to publicly advocate or implement active euthanasia or to argue publicly or within the profession in favor of strongly supporting advance directives, value anamneses, or durable powers of attorney.

Traditional forms of paternalistic attitudes on the part of physicians, nurses, patients, family, and legal experts seem to be stronger forces in protecting the status quo than is the legal framework, which has not yet been tested as to whether or not modifications in the law would be necessary for some or all options and directions that would be requested in advance directives, value anamneses, and durable powers of attorney, or for simply accepting these instruments as strong or weak sources of guidance (Uhlenbruck 1992; Wassermann 1993; Eser and Koch 1991). If the influence of the law and regulations on the professional attitudes of physicians and nurses and on the lay public are weak, then changes in the law would have no strong influence on changing attitudes. The implementation of proposed modifications in the penal law that would allow the hastening of death on request might reduce the reluctance of physicians to follow patients' wishes somewhat, but if the former really wanted to, there would be opportunities to hasten death in many cases without leaving evidence of the intention or the actual attempt to intervene.

Definitely more important would be legal, regulatory, or administrative actions that would advocate the concept and initiate the drafting of forms for value anamneses, advance directives, and durable powers of attorney; this would stimulate the creation of such informational materials as that produced by the Federal Ministry of Justice about the Care Law (*Betreuungsgesetz;* Bundesministerium der Justiz 1992). Making advance directives and durable powers of attorney mandatory in a weak or strong way, similar to legislative and administrative initiatives in the United States (Cate and Gill 1991), would be a test of how strong, albeit dormant, the population's acceptance of or demand for these instruments would be and how the medical establishment would react to it.

It might be that other reasons, such as the economic consideration of saving money in the costly intensive care of terminally ill patients, might be more compelling than the acceptance of hastening death by 60 percent of the population, as demonstrated in the polls (sb 1993). From an ethical point of view, however, economic considerations favoring the introduction of advance directives and durable powers of attorney would be less acceptable than considerations of patient-oriented treatment and of self-determination.

I do not foresee major conflicts between the law and behavior of professionals and laypersons. The law does not require or even recommend that people draft advance directives and durable powers of attorney, health care professionals do not recognize them as valid, and only a minority of people actually have these instruments in place. It might be the case that, regardless of what the law or the lawyers say, physicians have a comfortable leeway to choose to follow the course that is best for their patients, or their pocketbooks, or that is compatible with the wishes of patients or insurers. Because the review of possible forms of malpractice (which might include treatment against the expressed will or presumed wishes of the patient) is technically difficult and often inconclusive, strengthening and educating professional and lay cultures might be the preferred way to improve the quality of the health care delivery system.

Eisenbart (1997) recently proposed changes in the law that would improve the legal standing of advance directives and make it mandatory for physicians to base their decisions on these instruments. Uhlenbruck (1996) has developed a model that would give proxy decision making in personal and private matters a higher legal authority, if the designated proxy is bound to act within the framework of wishes and values provided by the designee. Hof (1996), however, questions the authority and power of modifications in the legal system to change well-established attitudes of making end-of-life decisions in medical and lay culture.

Transdisciplinary and Transcultural Studies

The weak spot in German debate about such questions seems to be public and political preoccupation with a weltanschauung-based general and confrontational approach to issues of euthanasia and suicide. One of the prerequisites of introducing the details of value anamneses, advance directives, and durable powers of attorney, and their own inherent moral, clinical, and legal problems, into professional and public debates and into the physician-patient interaction would be to conceptually and semantically differentiate between total forms of killing, letting one die, hastening death, or prolonging life or suffering, and also between different forms of weak and strong directives, wishes, and recommendations. German public and professional culture seems to be in need of a more precise and differentiated ethics to replace fragmented ideological discussions and an often nebulous general moralism (Sass 1992b). This might be brought about by increased interdisciplinary and transcultural exchanges and a new appreciation of prima facie moral values and cultural attitudes within the community. As there is hardly an established platform of discourse with legal and clinical experts, so legislators and judges also seem to be in need of more intense communication with philosophers and clinicians. This might be brought about by confronting not only ethicists and legal experts, but also intellectuals in the media and fields other than theology and philosophy.

Conflict Resolution: Law and Behavior and Forms of Behavior

It seems to be more of an educational challenge than a legal one to change attitudes of experts and laypersons toward advance directives and to break the taboos surrounding hard decisions at the end of life or in cases of incompetence. Therefore, the process of working on and reviewing value anamneses, advance directives, and durable powers of attorney from time to time, alone or with family, the trusted proxy, or the family physician, is an end in itself as well as a means of improving the quality of the forms and their content. If the attitudes of all involved parties have changed dramatically enough, then the law of the state and self-regulations by professional organizations will respond with changes if necessary. As long as physicians are reluctant to honor advance directives and to respect proxy decision makers, for whatever reason, there is no need to change the law; on the other hand, changes in the legal and regulatory approach could influence physicians in a positive way, if supported by a strong public movement or individuals of highest professional and moral public reputation.

The quest to change the educational scenario and attitudes before changing the law has been addressed recently by Kielstein in an "action guide" (Kielstein 1994) consisting of eight rules, four for the layperson and four for the health care professional. Rules for the patient:

1. Find a health care professional whom you trust, who takes you seriously as a person, and with whom you can discuss a wide range of issues related to health, disease, and dying.

2. Recognize both the benefits and limits of medicine, in the areas of prevention and treatment, assisting the chronically ill, and caring for the dying.

3. Be grateful for being healthy, prevent health risks, and experience quality of life that comes with old age and morbidity as transformed, not reduced.

4. Discuss with family, friends, and a trusted health care expert those values, wishes, and preferences that should direct caretakers and proxies in making decisions for care in life-and-death situations and when you are incompetent; draft a living will and an advance directive and review these forms frequently, as you might want to change them or add unto them.

Rules for the health care professional:

1. Treat your patient as a person, not just as a compilation of his or her symptoms and diseases.

2. Preventing and healing, assisting the chronically ill, and caring for the frail and dying are distinctly different professional challenges; meet them.

3. Provide information and education for your patient so that he or she can become risk-competent in health care matters.

4. Assist your patients in establishing value anamneses, advance directives, and durable powers of attorney.

Among the primary future questions that would certainly need careful attention in the German context in order to improve the conceptualization, acceptance, and distribution of value anamneses, advance directives, and durable powers of attorney would be the following sets of five questions:

1. *Change:* (a) How can attitudes toward death and dying be changed so that self-determination and respect for the self-determination of others, which are basic principles determining action in other areas of life, will be exercised via value anamneses, advance directives, and durable powers of attorney? (b) Who are the prime agents for change—physicians, citizens, legal experts, legislators, insurers, the media? (c) Who wants change? and which changes? (d) What role in particular can the law or the legal system play in facilitating change among individuals, families, institutions, the medical community, the political or economic communities? (e) What are the necessary features of the law, the legal system, or the legal establishment that will support change?

2. *Values, Wishes, and Directives:* (a) What are the interactions between actual values or wishes and directives for prospective situations in which the set of values and wishes might differ from the present one? (b) What do we know about how individual and generalized or objective limits and capacities enable us to assess and control risk associated with future events? (c) Which strategies or forms can be developed to give the individual and his or her trusted proxy, or both, a say in the clinical hermeneutics of value anamneses and advance directives? (d) What role does anxiety about pain play in attitudes toward dying, refusal and request of intervention, and advance directives; how will promises for, and convincingly demonstrated benefits of, palliative care and attention to a patient's anxiety about pain influence attitudes toward advance di-

rectives? (e) To what extent can full palliative care and attention to anxiety be considered part of routine medical service? Must decisions about these treatments be based on the patient's self-determination, or can they be arrived at by a joint decision of the patient or proxy with the expert and the expert team?

3. *Surrogate Decision Makers:* (a) Which virtues and capacities are characteristic of a good surrogate decision maker and which moral, legal, and medical principles should guide surrogates? (b) Who qualifies as a proxy, who does not; how are proxies chosen, and how do they establish their authority? May committees or experts substitute for proxies in cases in which no durable powers of attorney have been written? (c) What types of contributions can a surrogate make in sharing, cosharing, advising, or reviewing decision making or decision-making procedures? (d) What are the limits up to which health care experts are allowed to follow suggestions or directives of surrogates? (e) How are medical, legal, and ethical responsibility and liability split or integrated in joint decision making?

4. *Development and Implementation:* (a) What are the optimal goals and designs of further research exploring how best to improve quality, introduction, and acceptance of value anamneses, advance directives, and durable powers of attorney? (b) What are the specific requirements, problems, and risks for specific populations or groups of patients and how can they be dealt with in specialized value anamneses, advance directives, and durable powers of attorney? (c) In particular, what methods are available or able to be developed to establish the wishes and values of the semicompetent or noncompetent individual; what other means would become available to allow for individualized treatment of borderline competent or incompetent patients? (d) How flexible do patients, professionals, or both prefer the language and format of advance directives to be? (e) Which quality controls and implementation and interpretation controls can serve as devices to guarantee that values, wishes, and directives will be respected and integrated into differential diagnoses?

5. *Transculturality and Comparative Law:* (a) To what extent are attitudes related to disease, dying, and death determined by the nature of suffering and dying and to what extent by cultural or legal conditions? (b) Which challenges associated with value anamneses, advance directives, and durable powers of attorney are common to all cultures and legal parameters? Which are specific to those of different perspectives?

(c) Which areas and subject matters would allow for transcultural approaches? Which would not? (d) Which areas and subject matters would benefit from a global legal harmonization, and how should a dialogue on such matters be started? (e) How does academic deliberation on such matters relate to real-life situations in hospitals, families, and courts, and how could the results of such discussion be transferred into individual experiences, public culture and attitudes, and the medical and legal settings in which death, dying, and surrogate decision making constantly take place?

References

Amery, Jean. 1976. *Hand an sich legen: Diskurs über den Freitod.* Stuttgart: Klett.

Apel, Karl-Otto. 1988. *Diskurs und Verantwortung: Das Problem des Übergangs zur postkonventionellen Moral.* Frankfurt: Suhrkamp.

Atrott, Hans H. 1990. *Menschenwürdiges und selbstverantwortetes Sterben.* A not publicly available brochure for members of the Deutsche Gesellschaft für humanes Sterben e.V., Postfach 110529, W-8900 Augsburg 11, each copy numbered.

Atrott, Hans H., and Hermann Pohlmeier, eds. 1990. *Sterbehilfe in der Gegenwart.* Regensburg: Roderer.

Auer, Alfons. 1976. "Das Recht des Menschen auf einen 'natürlichen Tod.'" In *Der Mensch und sein Tod,* ed. Johannes Schwartländer, 82–93. Göttingen: Vandenhoek und Ruprecht.

Bartholomäus-Leggewie, Lore. 1993. "Notschlachten oder segnen?" *Zeitschrift für medizinische Ethik* 39:90–94.

Baumann, J., et al. 1986. *Alternativentwurf Sterbehilfe.* Stuttgart: Vandenhoek und Ruprecht.

Beck, Joachim, ed. 1996. *Patiententestament: Eine Hilfe für alle?* Colloquium of the Evangelischen Akademie Bad Boll, January 22, 1996. Protokolldienst 1/96. Bad Boll: Evangelische Akademie.

Bernat, Erwin. 1993. "Das Recht an der Grenze zwischen Leben und Tod, Zum Stand der Diskussion in den USA." In *Ethik und Recht an der Grenze zwischen Leben und Tod,* ed. Erwin Bernat, 141–95. Graz: Leykam.

Binding, Karl, and Alfred Hoche. 1920. *Die Freigabe der Vernichtung lebensunwerten Lebens: Ihr Mass und ihre Form.* Leipzig: Meiner.

Birnbacher, Dieter. 1985. "Schopenhauer und das ethische Problem des Selbstmordes." *Schopenhauer Jahrbuch* 66:115–29.

Bischofskonferenz, Deutsche. 1975. *Das Lebensrecht des Menschen und die Euthanasie.* Bonn: Hirtenschreiben der Deutschen Bischöfe.

———. 1993. *Die Hospizbewegung: Profil eines hilfreichen Weges im katholischen Verständnis.* Bonn: Hirtenschreiben der Deutschen Bischöfe.

Böckle, Franz. 1979. *Menschenwürdig sterben.* Theologische Meditationen 52. Zurich: Benziger.

Bönisch, Georg, and Hans Leyendecker. 1993. *Das Geschäft mit der Sterbehilfe.* Göttingen: Steidl.

Brückner, Christian. 1989. "Was leisten Patientenverfügung und Freitoderklärung das Kommunikationsmittel zwischen Unterzeichner und Drittperson?" *Schweizerische Ärztezeitung* 70:1149–58.

Buckman, Robert. 1990. *Was wir für Sterbende tun können: Praktische Ratschläge für Angehörige und Freunde.* Zurich: Kreuz Verlag. Translation of *I Don't Know What to Say: How to Help and Support Someone Who Is Dying.* Toronto: Key Porter, 1988.

Bundesärztekammer. 1993. "Richtlinien für die Sterbehilfe." *Deutsches Ärzteblatt* 90 (37): 1628–29.

Bundesgerichtshof. 1995. Urteil vom 13.09.1994: 1 StR 357/94 (Zulässigkeit des Abbruchs einer ärztlichen Behandlung bei mutmasslichem Einverständnis). *Neue Juristische Wochenschrift* 1995: 204–7.

Bundesminister für Justiz. 1992. *Das neue Betreuungsgesetz.* Bonn: Bundesministerium für Justiz.

Cate, Fred H., and Barbara A. Gill. 1991. *The Patient Self-determination Act: Implementation Issues and Opportunities. A White Paper of the Annenberg Washington Program.* Evanston, Ill.: Communications Policy Studies, Northwestern University.

Cogen, R., B. Patterson, S. Chavin, J. D. Cogen, L. Landsberg, and J. Posner. 1992. "Surrogate Decision Maker Preferences for Medical Care of Severely Demented Nursing Home Patients." *Archives of Internal Medicine* 152:1885–88.

Deutsche Gesellschaft für Chirurgie. 1996. *Leitlinie zum Umfang und zur Begrenzung der ärztlichen Behandlungspflicht in der Chirurgie.* Paper presented at the 113th Plenary Session of the Deutschen Gesellschaft für Chirurgie.

Deutsche Gesellschaft für Humanes Sterben. 1992a. *Betreuungsverfügung: Formblatt.* Augsburg: DGHS.

———. 1992b. *Patientenschutzbrief: Formblatt.* Augsburg: DGHS.

———. 1992c. *Freitodverfügung: Formblatt.* Augsburg: DGHS.

Doelle-Oelmueller, Ruth. 1993. "Euthanasie—philosophisch betrachtet: Ein Diskussionsbeitrag zu Argumenten von Spaemann und Singer." *Zeitschrift für medizinische Ethik* 39:41–54.

Donner, B., and Michael Zenz. 1994. "Medikamentöse Schmerztherapie." *Deutsches Ärzteblatt* 91 (24): A1703–8.

Doukas, David J., and Daniel W. Gorenflo. 1993. "Analyzing the Values History: An Evaluation of Patient Medical Values and ADs." *Journal of Clinical Ethics* 4 (1): 41–45.

Doukas, David J., and Lawrence B. McCullough. 1991. "The Values History: The Evaluation of the Patient's Values and ADs." *Journal of Family Practice* 32 (2): 145–53.

Ebert, Andreas, and Peter Godzik, eds. 1993. *Verlass mich nicht, wenn ich schwach werde: Handbuch zur Begleitung Schwerkranker und Sterbender.* Hamburg: Rissen.

Eid, Volker. 1993. "Ethische Aspekte der Sterbehilfe: aus katholisch-theologischer Sicht." *Zeitschrift für ärztliche Fortbildung* 87:55–65.

Eisenbart, Bettina. 1997. "Patienten-'Testament' und Stellvertretung in Gesundheitsangelegenheiten." Dissertation, University of Göttingen.

Emanuel, Ezekiel J., and Linda L. Emanuel. 1991. "Living Wills: Past, Present, and Future." *Journal of Clinical Ethics* 1 (1): 9–19.

Emanuel, Linda. 1993. "ADs: What Have We Learned So Far." *Journal of Clinical Ethics* 4 (1): 8–16.

Engelhardt, Dietrich von. 1993. "Euthanasie in historischer Perspektive." *Zeitschrift für medizinische Ethik* 39:15–25.

Eser, Albin. 1976. "Der manipulierte Tod: Möglichkeiten und Grenzen der Sterbehilfe aus rechtlicher Sicht." In *Der Mensch und sein Tod,* ed. Johannes Schwartländer, 61–81. Göttingen: Vandenhoek und Ruprecht.

Eser, Albin, and Hans G. Koch. 1991. *Materialien zur Sterbehilfe.* Freiburg: Max Planck Institut für ausländisches und internationales Strafrecht.

Evangelische Kirche in Deutschland, Deutsche Bischofskonferenz. 1989. *Gott ist ein Freund des Lebens: Herausforderungen und Aufgaben beim Schutz des Lebens.* Gütersloh: Mohn.

Finucane, Thomas E., B. A. Beamer, R. P. Roca, and C. H. Kawas. 1993. "Establishing Advance Medical Directives with Demented Patients: A Pilot Study." *Journal of Clinical Ethics* 4 (1): 51–54.

Gibson, John M. 1990. "Reflecting on Values." *Ohio State Law Journal* 51 (2): 451–71.

Grundstein-Amato, Rivka. 1992. "Value Inquiry: A Method of Eliciting Advance Health Care Directives." *Humane Medicine* 8:31–39.

Haarhaus, Friedrich. 1993. "Anleitung zum Gespräch über das Kranken- und Schwerverletzten-Testament." *Die Schwester/Der Pfleger* 32:814–16.

Habermas, Jürgen. 1983. *Moralbewusstsein und kommunikatives Handeln.* Frankfurt: Suhrkamp.

Hahn, Susanne, and Achim Thoms. 1983, *Sinnvolle Lebensbewahrung—humanes Sterben: Auseinandersetzung mit dem ärztlichen bewahrungsauftrag gegenüber menschlichem Leben.* Berlin: VEB Verlag der Wissenschaften.

Hasiba, Gernot D. 1993. "Euthanasie im Dritten Reich." In *Ethik und Recht an der Grenze zwischen Leben und Tod,* ed. Erwin Bernat, 27–42. Graz: Leykam.

Heimann, Hans. 1976. "Bewusstes und Unbewusstes über Tod und Sterben." In *Der Mensch und sein Tod,* ed. Johannes Schwartländer, 34–43. Göttingen: Vandenhoek und Ruprecht.

Helmchen, Hanfried. 1993. "Tötung auf Verlangen." *Zeitschrift für ärztliche Fortbildung* 87:36–41.

Helmrich, Herbert. 1993. *Rechtliche Aspekte einer humanen Sterbebegleitung.* Unpublished manuscript. Konrad Adenauer Haus, Bonn.

Hoerster, Norbert. 1989. "Tötungsverbot und Sterbehilfe." In *Medizin und Ethik,* ed. Hans-Martin Sass, 287–95. Stuttgart: Reclam.

Hof, Hagen. 1996. *Rechtsethologie: Recht im Kontext von Verhalten und ausserrechtlicher Verhaltensregelung.* Heidelberg: Decker.

Holderegger, Adrian. 1979. *Suizid und Suizidgefährdung.* Freiburg and Vienna: Universitätsverlag.

Humphry, Derek. 1992. *In Würde sterben: Praxis Sterbehilfe und Selbsttötung.* Hamburg: Carlsen. Original edition 1991, *Final Exit.* Eugene, Ore.: Hemlock Society.

Jonas, Hans. 1984–85. "Das Recht zu sterben." *Scheidewege: Jahresschrift für skeptisches Denken* 14:10–22.

Juengel, Eberhardt. 1976. "Der Tod als Geheimnis des Lebens." In *Der Mensch und sein Tod,* ed. Johannes Schwartländer, 108–25. Göttingen: Vandenhoek und Ruprecht.

Jürgens, Andreas, and Detleve Kröger. 1992. *Das neue Betreuungsrecht.* Munich: Beck.

Kamlah, Wilhelm. 1976. *Meditatio mortis.* Stuttgart: Klett.

Kant, Immanuel. 1785. *Grundlegung zur Metaphysik der Sitten. Akademie Ausgabe,* vol. 4.

———. 1797. *Metaphysik der Sitten. Akademie Ausgabe,* vol. 6.

Kehl, Robert. 1989. *Sterbehilfe, Ethische und rechtliche Grundlagen.* Bern: Zytglogge.

Kielstein, Rita. 1994. "Wertanamnese—Methoden zur Erkennung des Patientenwillens." *Zeitschrift für ärztliche Fortbildung* 88: 743–54.

Kielstein, Rita, and Hans-Martin Sass. 1993a. "Using Stories to Assess Values and Establish Medical Directives." *Kennedy Institute of Ethics Journal* 3:303–25.

———. 1993b. *Wertanamnese und Betreuungsverfügung: Instrumente zur Selbstbestimmung des Patienten und zur Entscheidunghshilfe des Arztes und Betreuers.* 2d ed. Bochum: Zentrum für Medizinische Ethik.

———, eds. 1993c. *Materialien zur Erstellung von wertanamnestischen Betreuungsverfügungen.* Bochum: Zentrum für Medizinische Ethik.

Klaschik, Eberhard, and Friedemann Nauck. 1993. "Erfahrungen einer Palliativstation." *Deutsches Ärzteblatt* 90 (Heft 48): 3226–30.

Koch, Traugott. 1992. "Sterbehilfe als Thema der Ethik." *Diakonie* 18:230–36.

Koller, Peter. 1993. "Personen, Rechte und Entscheidungen über Leben und Tod." In *Ethik und Recht an der Grenze zwischen Leben und Tod,* ed. Erwin Bernat, 71–95. Graz: Leykam.

Kuhse, Helga. 1990. *Menschliches Leben und seine Würde.* Bochum: Zentrum für medizinische Ethik.

Kutzer, Kurt. 1996. "Die Würde des Menschen ist unantastbar: bis zuletzt, Sterben und Sterbehilfe in der Rechtsprechung." In *Leben bis zuletzt: Sterben als Teil des*

Lebens, 21–26. Bonn: Sekretariat der Deutschen Bischofskonferenz, and Hannover: Kirchenamt der Evangelischen Kirche in Deutschland.

Leist, Anton, ed. 1989. *Leben und Tod: Moralische Probleme bei Abtreibung, künstlicher Befruchtung, Euthanasie und Selbstmord.* Frankfurt: Suhrkamp.

Lutterotti, Markus von. 1992. "Der Arzt und das Tötungsverbot." *Medizinrecht* 1:7–14.

———. 1993. "Grenzen ärztlicher Behandlungspflicht und passive Sterbehilfe." *Zeitschrift für medizinische Ethik* 39:3–14.

Mainländer, Philipp. 1876/86. *Philosophie der Erlösung.* 2 vols. Frankfurt.

Mattheis, Ruth. 1993. "Ethische Aspekte der Sterbehilfe: aus ärztlicher Sicht." *Zeitschrift für ärztliche Fortbildung* 87:68–70.

May, Arnd, Stefan Gawrich, and Katja Stiegel. 1997. *Empirische Erfahrungen mit wertanamnestischen Betreuungsverfügungen,* Bochum: Zentrum für Medizinische Ethik

Muschaweck-Kürten, Petra. 1993. "Sterbebegleitung." *Zeitschrift für ärztliche Fortbildung* 87:90–93.

Muthny, Fritz A., Uwe Koch, and Sylvia Stump. 1993. "Praxis und Bedeutung der Lebensqualitätsforschung für die Onkologie." In *Onkologie im psychosozialen Kontext,* ed. F. Muthny and G. Haag. Heidelberg: Asanger.

Nolte, Stephan H. 1993. "Emphatische Begleitung und Beratung statt therapeutischem Aktionismus." *Deutsches Ärzteblatt* 90 (40): C1773–75.

Pearlman, Robert A., K. C. Cain, D. L. Patrick, M. Appelbaum-Maizel, H. E. Starks, N. S. Jecker, and R. F. Uhlmann. 1993. "Insights Pertaining to Patients Assessment of States Worse than Death." *Journal of Clinical Ethics* 4 (1): 33–41.

Pieper, Anemarie. 1993. "Stichwort "Autonomie." *Zeitschrift für medizinische Ethik* 39:95–98.

Rainer, J. Michael. 1993. "Zur Euthanasie in der griechischen und römischen Antike." In *Ethik und Recht an der Grenze zwischen Leben und Tod,* ed. Erwin Bernat, 19–25. Graz: Leykam.

Ranke-Heinemann, Uta. 1987. "Selbst- und Femdtötung im Urteil der katholischen Moraltheologie." *Humanes Leben—Humanes Sterben* 7 (2): xx–yy.

Römpp, Georg. 1988. "Der unfreie Tod. Kant und die ethische Dimension des Suizids." *Freiburger Zeitschrift für Philosophie und Theologie* 35:415–31.

Rosemeier, Hans-Peter. 1993. "Zur Psychologie des Sterbens und des Todes." *Zeitschrift für ärztliche Fortbildung* 87:76–100.

Rothenberg, L. S., J. F. Merz, N. S. Wenger, M. Kagawa-Singer, D. R. J. Macer, N. Tanabe, S. Fukuhara, K. Kurokawa, H. L. Fuenzalidas-Puelma, J. G. Meran, E. Bernat, T. Hosaka, and G. N. Marshall. 1996. "The Relationship of Clinical Perspectives Regarding Medical Treatment Decision-Making in Four Cultures." *Jahrbuch für Recht und Ethik* (Annual Review of Law and Ethics) 4:335–79.

Salomon, Fred. 1991. *Leben und Sterben in der Intensivmedizin: Eine Herausforderung an die ärztliche Ethik.* Lengerich: Pabst.

Sass, Hans-Martin. 1990. *Training in Differential Ethics and Quality Control.* Bochum: Zentrum für Medizinische Ethik.

———. 1991a. "Ethische Expertise und Güterabwägung." In *Güterabwägung in der Medizin,* ed. Hans-Martin Sass and Herbert Viefhues, 116–36. Heidelberg: Springer.

———. 1991b. *Geriatrische Forschung und Ethik in der Medizin.* Bochum: Zentrum für Medizinische Ethik.

———. 1992a. "Risiko aus der Sicht der Medizinethik." In *Risiko,* ed. Klaus Giel and Renate Breuninger, 125–74. Ulm: Humboldt Studienzentrum der Universität.

———. 1992b. "Generalisierender Moralismus und Differentialethik." In *Politik und Kultur nach der Aufklärung, Festschrift für Hermann Lübbe,* ed. Kurt Röttgers, 186–205. Basel: Schwabe.

Sass, Hans-Martin, F. O. Bonkovsky, A. Akabayashi, R. Kielstein, and R. S. Olick. 1996. "Advance Health Care Documents in Multicultural Perspectives." *Jahrbuch für Recht und Ethik* (Annual Review of Law and Ethics) 4:465–508.

Sass, Hans-Martin, and Rita Kielstein. 1996. *Die medizinische Betreuungsverfügung in der Praxis.* Bochum: Zentrum für Medizinische Ethik; 3d revised edition, 1997.

Sass, Hans-Martin, and Herbert Viefhues. 1989. "Bochumer Arbeitsbogen für die medizinethische Praxis." In *Medizin und Ethik,* ed. H.-M. Sass, 371–75. Stuttgart: Philipp Reclamjun.

———. 1992. *Differentialethische Methodik in der biomedizinischen Ethik.* Munich: GSF-Forschungszentrum.

sb. 1993. "Einstellung zur Sterbehilfe in der Bundesrepublik Deutschland." *Humanes Leben—Humanes Sterben* 13 (3): 1.

Schick, Peter J. 1993. "Todesbegriff, Sterbehilfe und aktive Euthanasie: Strafrechtsdogmatische und kriminalpolitische Erwägungen." In *Ethik und Recht an der Grenze zwischen Leben und Tod,* ed. Erwin Bernat, 121–40. Graz: Leykam.

Schmitz, Philipp. 1993. "'Euthanasie'—verschiedne Wege ethischer Orientierung in einem christlichen Umfeld." *Zeitschrift für medizinische Ethik* 39:27–40.

Schmuhl, Hans-Walter. 1992. *Rassenhygiene, Nationalsozialismus, Euthanasie.* Göttingen: Vandenhoeck und Ruprecht.

Schobert, Kurt F. 1993. "Die Ehrfurcht vor dem Sterben." *Humanes Leben—Humanes Sterben* 13 (4): 2.

Schöne-Seifert, Bettina. 1991. "Silencing the Singer: Antibioethics in Germany." *Hastings Center Report* 21 (6): 20–27.

Schopenhauer, Arthur. 1819/1844. *Die Welt als Wille und Vorstellung.* 2 vols. Leipzig.

Schreiber, Hans-Ludwig. 1986. "Das Recht auf den eigenen Tod: Zur gesetzlichen Neuregelung der Sterbehilfe." *Neue Zeitschrift für Strafrecht,* 337–45.

———. 1993. "Tötung auf Verlangen." *Zeitschrift für ärztliche Fortbildung* 87: 31–54.

Schwartländer, Johannes. 1976. "Der Tod und die Würde des Menschen." In *Der*

Mensch und sein Tod, ed. Johannes Schwartländer 14–33. Göttingen: Vandenhoek und Ruprecht.

Sehgal, A., A. Galbraith, M. Chesney, et al. 1992. "How Strictly Do Dialysis Patients Want Their Advance Directives Followed?" *Journal of the American Medical Association* 267:59–63.

Sehgal, A. R., C. Weisheit, Y. Miura, M. Butzlaff, R. Kielstein, and Y. Taguchi. 1996. "Advance Directives and Withdrawal of Dialysis in the United States, Germany, and Japan." 276:1652–56.

Singer, Peter. 1984. *Praktische Ethik.* Stuttgart: Reclam.

Spaemann, Robert. 1992. "Wir dürfen das Tabu nicht aufgeben." *Die Zeit,* no. 25 (June 12): 14.

Sporken, Paul, ed. 1984. *Was Sterbende brauchen.* Freiburg: Herder.

Stiefel, F., and H. J. Senn. 1993. "Euthanasie und fortgeschrittenes Tumorleiden." *Zeitschrift für medizinische Ethik* 39:99–104.

Storck, Hans. 1993. "Ethische Aspekte der Sterbehilfe: aus evangelisch-theologischer Sicht." *Zeitschrift für ärztliche Fortbildung* 87:66–67.

Strebel, U., ed. 1993. "Herbsttagung der Schweizerischen Gesellschaft für Biomedizinische Ethik 'Gilt die Pflicht zu ernähren, bis zum Tode.'" *Schweizerische Rundschau Medizin (Praxis)* 82:1025–58.

Timmermann, Jens. 1993. *Das Thema Sterbehilfe in Thomas Morus 'Utopia.'*" Bochum: Zentrum für Medizinische Ethik.

Uhlenbruck, Wilhelm. 1992. *Selbstbestimmung im Vorfeld des Sterbens.* Bochum: Zentrum für Medizinische Ethik.

———. 1996. "Die Altersvorsorge-Vollmacht als Alternative zum Patiententestament und zur Betreuungsverfügung." *Neue Juristische Wochenschrift* (Heft 24): 1583–85

Veatch, Robert. 1993. "Forgoing Life-Sustaining Treatment: Limits to Consensus." *Kennedy Institute of Ethics Journal* 3:1–19.

Viefhues, Herbert. 1991. *Das Motiv der "Euthanasie" in der fiktionalen Literatur.* Bochum: Zentrum für Medizinische Ethik.

Walker, Margret Urban. 1993. "Keeping Moral Space Open." *Hastings Center Report* 23 (2): 33–40.

Wassermann, Rudolf. 1993. "Begriffsbestimmung: Sterbehilfe, Sterbebeihilfe, Euthanasie, unterlassene Hilfeleistung, fahrlässige Tötung—aus juristischer Sicht." *Zeitschrift für ärztliche Fortbildung* 87:13–18.

Wedler, Hans-Ludwig. 1996. "Ergebnisse einer Meinungsumfrage unter Experten." In *Suizidprävention und Sterbehilfe,* ed. F. Anschuetz and H. L. Wedler, 151–58. Berlin: Ullstein Mosby.

Williams, Virginia, and Pamela Cockerill. 1992. *Dein Schmerz geht durch mein Leben.* Lübbe: Bergisch-Gladbach. Translation of *A Different Kind of Life.* London: Doubleday, 1991.

Winau, Rolf. 1993a. "Begriffsbestimmung: Sterbehilfe, Sterbebeihilfe, Euthanasie, unterlassene Hilfeleistung, fahrlässige Tötung—aus ärztlicher Sicht." *Zeitschrift für ärztliche Fortbildung* 87:19–21.

———. 1993b. "Der eigene und der fremde Tod: Überlegungen zur Geschichte der Sterbehilfe." *Zeitschrift für ärztliche Fortbildung* 87:3–12.

Windels-Buhr, Doris, ed. 1990. *Grenzen der Behandlung in der Anästhesie, Intensivmeidizin, Dialyse.* Lengerich: Pabst.

Wolf, Jean-Claude. 1991. "Sterben, Tod und Tötung." In *Praktische Philosophie: Grundorientierungen angewandter Ethik,* ed. Kurt Bayertz, 243–77. Reinbek: Rowohlt.

Wolff, Hanns-Peter. 1989. "Arzt und Patient." In *Medizin und Ethik,* ed. Hans-Martin Sass, 184–211. Stuttgart: Reclam.

Wolkinger, Alois. 1993. "Todesbegriff, Sterbehilfe und aktive Euthanasie: Ein moraltheologischer Beitrag." In *Ethik und Recht an der Grenze zwischen Leben und Tod,* ed. Erwin Bernat, 43–60. Graz: Leyklam.

Zentner, Marcel R. 1988. "Der Selbstmord als Antwort auf das Leid bei Schopenhauer." *Freiburger Zeitschrift für Philosophie und Theologie* 35:433–48.

Part 3

Japan

7

Advance Directives and the Japanese Ethos

Gen Ohi, M.D., Ph.D., M.P.H.

Introduction

Advance directives become relevant in a situation in which the following conditions coexist: (1) advanced medical technology is available, (2) the medical technology is economically affordable, and, most important, (3) the patient has no one whom he or she can truly trust or who can represent him or her in terminal stages of illness. In other words, the patient is solitary and rich enough to afford to prolong an undesirable life of wretched quality.

This is the outlook for increasing numbers of individuals in developed countries. However, in the developing countries in which I have worked, the social norm contrasts sharply with the preceding situation. The majority is poor, able to derive only minimal benefit from advanced medical science, but surrounded by caring relatives. Thus, the purpose of this introduction is to give a brief description of the type of basic ethical orientation prevalent in South and Southeast Asia and probably in the areas of the world where mutual assistance has been the central means of survival throughout the historical past. I juxtapose it with another type of basic ethical orientation, one that is most conspicuously observed in the United States. Although Japan has emerged as a member of the group of affluent countries during the past several decades, the majority (at least, its older generations) maintains the ethical orientation that has been generated, inherited, and intensified in a society characterized by poverty and mutual assistance. I am hopeful that some knowledge and sensitivity to the difference in ethical orientations might help promote understanding of the ethical sentiments of the Japanese concerning the practice of advance directives.

From a Darwinian viewpoint, human ethics may be regarded, at the level of a group, as the strategic standards ensuring the optimal continuation and prosperity of the group, and at the level of an individual as a standard of behavior patterns expected to maximize his or her survival as a constituent of the group. Each individual's ethical orientation may then be construed as the strategic direction internalized. At least two directions are conceivable and actually observable from the standpoint of the survival strategy. One involves the maintenance of good relationships with others (particularly those in the same group), and the other is characterized by autonomy in terms of observing, judging, and making decisions. In our daily life, we usually use tactics derived from one or both of the strategic directions, depending on the nature of our perception of the situation. However, the tendency to go in one strategic direction over the other appears to vary from one society to another and to be framed by the cultural and historical process of the society. More often than not, in societies adopting mutual assistance as the primary mode of survival like East and Southeast Asia, people proceed in the direction that emphasizes maintaining good relations with others. I designate this the "relation-type ethical orientation" (RTEO). Typically in the United States and some other Western countries, the other type prevails, the "autonomy-type ethical orientation" (ATEO).

Two behavioral features of RTEO merit mention here. One is the tendency to avoid outright confrontation with others. This encompasses a broad spectrum of attitudes such as a commitment not to let others lose face to equivocal expressions of denial. Providing their guests with food and presents to an extent disproportionate to their living standard may be an analogous aspect. In efforts directed toward the maintenance of good relationships with others, the ethical principles at work are those of nonmaleficence and beneficence. These behavioral patterns are sometimes puzzling to Westerners. For instance, Americans find it difficult to understand why the Japanese do not use "yes" and "no" as clearly as in American culture. In 1993, Mr. Clinton sent a note to Mr. Yeltsin cautioning him that a Japanese yes might really mean no. However, this ambiguous use of yes and no is not restricted to Japan but also prevails in East and Southeast Asia. In Thailand, Indonesia, Malaysia, Vietnam, Cambodia, China, Korea, and Taiwan, I have noted clear indications of "no" under the guise of "yes."

The other feature is an obscuring of the boundary of "person," which is clearly demarcated in American society and accompanied by an awareness of rights, self-determination, privacy, and the like. Typically, in rural Java and Japan, activities for mutual assistance are extremely intimate and frequent, hardly leaving room for privacy. A Japanese student in charge of Indonesian students at her dormitory was impressed by their practice of not knocking on the door before entering her room. She was obviously unaware of the historical fact that the Japanese of her great-grandfathers' generation did not have the habit of knocking. In both Indonesia and Japan, there is no indigenous word corresponding to *privacy.*

Although peoples in East and Southeast Asia have RTEO in common, there are variations in the method of weighing values associated with their behaviors. This may be explained on the grounds that the harsher the conditions of survival, the more of the ego (*Jibun*), as defined by T. Sugiyama Lebra (1976), has to be relinquished to survive, whereas one has the tendency to minimize unpleasant stressors within the context of maximizing one's chance of survival. For instance, the behavior of farmers in southern Thailand where nature is generous and mankind can make a living with minimal toil is distinctly more individualistic than that of Japanese farmers who have lived for generations with unstable climatic conditions perennially necessitating concerted and efficient labor.

It is not my intention to lecture on the behavioral features related to RTEO in Asia, nor do I expect the reader with ATEO to feel the emotions generated when one with RTEO makes a decision contrasting sharply with his or her sense of ethical appropriateness. Cartesians would ignore the existence of such sentiments and emotions. But I believe that it is also necessary for those with ATEO to appreciate the psychological components as well as calculations involved in "indirect and gentle" approaches in the daily communication processes in the region.

Case Discussion

The Patient May Not Be Told the Truth

A 51-year-old man gradually developed upper abdominal distress and distension. A gastroscopy revealed an advanced adenocarcinoma at the esophageo-gastric junction. He lived in a small town in the agricultural zone of northern Japan with his wife, a son, and a daughter. The family was notified by his physician, who explained the diagnosis and prognosis. Although the patient hinted that he wanted to know the name and the nature of the disease, he never straightforwardly requested that the physician reveal the diagnosis.

The family members and relatives were unable to decide whether they should tell the patient the truth. Three of them traveled to Tokyo to consult with a physician, who had spent some five years in the region near their neighborhood 40 years earlier. There were two major reasons why they could not reveal the truth: (1) they were not sure of the reaction from the patient upon his learning the truth; (2) more important, they would not know how to face him once he had been told. He might, upon learning that such a horrible fate would befall him, become a "stranger" and an incomprehensible person, different from the amiable person they were familiar with. Maintaining a pleasant and smooth relationship with him presupposes their being familiar with his mentality and the range of his emotions.

The physician advised them to reveal the truth to the patient on the grounds that he had expressed his desire to know it, if not vehemently demanded it. They thanked him without reaching a clear decision. He heard a few months later that the patient had died without knowing the true nature of his disease.

COMMENT. Although in recent years the number of people advocating the use of advance directives has been on the rise, the actual cases of writing a directive remain few. Several factors probably account for this discrepancy between the volume of the voices raised and the cases that have materialized.

1. There is no possibility for the patient to draft an advance directive, even if the intent is present, unless he or she is told the truth. As is clear in this case, it is not an accepted practice for the physician to disclose the depressing truth to the patient in Japan (or in East and Southeast Asian countries). In the ethos of RTEO, the ethical principle of nonmaleficence may bear a greater psychological weight than in regions where ATEO predominates.

It should be noted that, according to Jung's terminology, our ethical orientation is not necessarily confined to the conscious layer of our psyche. There are things we find extremely difficult to perform, even though our reasoning dictates otherwise. In 1983, when we studied physicians in three areas of Japan, the overwhelming majority (70–80%) in each area replied that they preferred to have the truth about their disease disclosed irrespective of its nature (Ohi 1989). However, at the professional level, very few regularly told the truth to the patient with incurable cancer; some of the physicians confessed that the prospect of harming the patient constitutes an insurmountable barrier to them. This suggests that their professional decision whether to impart very traumatic information is being influenced by a force other than the reasoning taking place at the rational conscious level. Its presence may be felt only when one is forced to diverge significantly from one's basic ethical orientation. Imagine a circumstance, for instance, in which you are asked by members of your society to kill your friend, who has supposedly caused unbearable damage to this society. Physicians may experience a similar internal feeling of conflicting loyalties when faced with the prospect of sharing traumatic information. Clearly, patients who, as a result of their physicians' reluctance to do harm through such truth-telling, remain ignorant of the severity of their illness are unprepared to create advance directives.

2. It is also possible that there is a culturally defined aversion to drafting a written document in the form of an advance directive. In a harmonious family setting in which its members regard verbal instruction as a sufficient means of communication, articulating one's preferences with a document might be regarded as a display of distrust to other members.

A report on the Japanese from the Ministry of Health and Welfare published in the summer of 1993 contains a chapter exploring attitudes toward advance directives. It revealed that 75 percent of the respondents were in favor of the idea, while 34 percent indicated that there was no need for "written directives," and 51 percent supported surrogate decision making (Ministry of Health and Welfare 1993).

A recent study conducted in two rural communities (one in Japan and the other in Taiwan) revealed that, should they reach a terminal stage, 89 percent and 72 percent, respectively, of respondents preferred pain control rather than life prolongation as a therapeutic strategy. When asked about the advisability of drafting advance directives to express their choice of treatment strategy, 58 percent of the Japanese and 69 percent of the Taiwanese indicated that oral expression would suffice, and 21 percent and 10 percent replied that there was no need to leave either a written or oral directive (Ohi and Chiu 1995).

Belonging

1. A 67-year-old man who had had a cancerous portion of his colon resected five years previously said that he had never discussed the nature or state of his disease with his wife because she became visibly apprehensive every time he tried to do so. He found that he would elicit similar reactions of denial or aversion from his friends when he brought up the subject. As a result, he stopped talking with his family and friends about his disease. However, concerned and curious about the nature and prospect of his disease, he joined a group formed by cancer patients and found that he could discuss a wide variety of cancer-related subjects, including advance directives, within this circle. However, he did not entertain the idea of entering a hospice. In his words, "I know the median life span of the patient at a hospice is 2.5 months. I do not want to alienate myself from my friends by becoming a hos-

pice patient." He knew very well that the turnover of his cancer support group was fairly rapid; 15 percent of the group members die annually.

2. A 56-year-old woman developed uterine cancer that had invaded the surrounding tissues. She had the uterus, bladder, and part of the rectum removed, as well as a colostomy, and the openings for ureters were made. When I saw her at the National Cancer Center in Tokyo, she was aware that her disease was probably incurable. She also told me that she was occasionally permitted to return to her apartment on the weekends to visit with her friends. The frequency of such visits had decreased considerably since her friends had been informed about the incurable nature of the disease.

She told me that she could not discuss the nature of her disease with her visiting friends, and I inquired why. "Because I can tell that they do not like the subject raised," she replied. When I inquired further, she added, "Well, for instance, my friend starts crying."

COMMENT. Without the anthropological knowledge of the penchant to maintain harmonious relationships described above, it is probably difficult to understand the attitude of the wife (and friends) toward the cancer patient in the first case. Why does his wife find it so difficult to listen to and discuss with her beloved husband the subject about which he is obviously concerned? But he has observed similar reactions among his close friends upon raising this subject. Their usual reactions are characterized by attempts to console him such as "You are healthy now, are you not? Let us not talk about such a sinister [*engidemonai*] subject."

In the second case, the response of the woman's friend is more dramatic and unambiguous. She has accurately interpreted the friend's message. The crying has a twofold meaning: one an expression of pity and sympathy, the other, a plea not to bring up the subject of her cancer. The first message is easy to see: "I am terribly sorry that your cancer cannot be cured, and I cry for you." The second, however, may need some elaboration. At the conscious level of the friend's thinking, her logic may flow this way: "Why do you have to raise such a difficult subject at this moment when we have so many other pleasant topics to discuss together, such as the events of our high-school days when our drunken teacher behaved very comically, etc.? Even if you want me to make comments on your incurable disease, I would not be able to make an appropriate remark that would not offend you. What I fear is that by virtue of suffering from incurable cancer, your feelings might have become entirely different from those of us stupid, healthy individuals; you might be thinking with an entirely different logic, etc. So please let us talk only about the pleasant subjects to which we can both relate." If the thinking process she follows is paraphrased, it will be like the following: "Because of your disease status, you are now feeling, thinking (and maybe even behaving) differently from us members of the group of which you were a member until recently. You have now become an alien, the one ostracized and expelled (*mura-hachibu*) from the group!"

To understand the deep psychological pang involved in the *mura-hachibu*, one must accept psychological dynamics in the Jungian sense, the reactivation of emotions aroused frequently in the historical past. Without an appeal to this kind of postulate, it is difficult to explain the fear that a child who has never seen a snake in its life manifests against an innocuous reptile. Likewise, one needs to know some historical aspects of the typical Japanese occupation of farming. In the past, relying on a tropical plant like rice for subsistence in the Japanese archipelago was a relatively unstable way of life. During the Edo Period, which lasted some 300 years up to the end of nineteenth century, the Japanese population is estimated to have remained relatively constant at around 30 million. Cold summers, droughts, and floods punctuated the period, causing frequent famines and millions of deaths. It is easy to envision that in such an environment the *mura-hachibu* meant a punishment that could practically preclude the chance to survive. Incredible though it may sound, I believe that this explains why even in modern Japan, an act resembling the expulsion of a friend from the group evokes such a strong sense of repulsion and guilt.

One has to behave as a good, consistent, respectable member of the group even to the very end of one's life. This is the modus vivendi for an individual in a group to ensure survival of himself as well as of the group. This aspect of Japanese ethos is superbly described by Marjorie Kagawa-Singer, who made an astonishing observation of two groups of cancer patients, one consisting of 25 Anglo-Americans and the other of 25 Japanese-Americans (second-generation or *nisei*) (Kagawa-Singer 1993).

She noted that a conspicuous difference exists between the two ethnically distinct Americans with respect to their coping behaviors. The Japanese patients frequently denied even objectively established cases of cancer, trying to live to the very end as useful and respected members of the group (family, etc.) as if no cancer were present. The coping behavior of the Anglo-Americans was significantly different from that of the Japanese. However, it is noteworthy that, of both Anglo-Americans and Japanese-Americans, 49 of the 50 cancer patients replied that they were "healthy." This observation is at variance with the image of a human being suggested by rationalist thinkers in the sphere of Western philosophy. It should also be noted that the tactic adopted by the Japanese-Americans in coping with cancer is consistent with RTEO.

The ethos valuing harmony, homogeneity, and efficiency within the group that one commonly sees in rural communities in Japan appears to create an atmosphere that may run counter to, if not altogether block, the implementation of advance directives. First, as previously mentioned, drafting an advance directive might imply that the author is dissatisfied with his current human relationships. And, even when he or she wishes to have the family do something specific during the terminal stages of the illness, it would suffice to tell them the request, provided the matter is simple. Yet, on the other hand, a traditional custom involves the composition of a short poem [*tanka, haiku*] by the dying and sometimes the drafting of advance directives to communicate one's wishes for funeral arrangements.

Physicians Are Reluctant Communicators

As described above, physicians often find it psychologically unbearable to disclose the truth to patients with incurable cancer. Naturally, sometimes it is imperative to impart accurate information to ensure the patient's cooperation in a procedure such as a mastectomy. However, it is still not accepted medical practice to inform a patient of the incurable nature of a disease simply for the purpose of giving the patient a chance to write an advance directive, unless the patient so requests specifically.

A 50-year-old internist found that one of his clients had developed a polyp in the sigmoid colon. A biopsy revealed adenocarcinoma and a CT scan showed that metastatic lesions had already spread throughout the liver. The physician told the patient's family the diagnosis and expected clinical course, but his explanation to the patient remained vague. On one occasion, the patient brought up the subject of the diagnosis but did not insist that he should be informed of the definite diagnosis. His clinical course rapidly deteriorated, and the physician's visits to the patient became increasingly short and infrequent. The patient, however, remained calm to the end, always expressing his hope to get well. When he died, his family found in his diary that he had clearly known the diagnosis and hopelessness of his disease.

COMMENT. Although this case may appear somewhat incomprehensible to those accustomed to straightforward expression, it describes a behavior that is relatively common among Japanese patients, particularly in rural areas. First, the physician found it difficult to maintain a relationship with the patient, probably because of his sense of guilt. Second, the patient behaved as if he had no knowledge of his imminent death to the end. Why did he play the role of a hopeful patient? Being a tender husband and father, he probably thought that had he shown a sign of his knowing the truth, his family and his friends would have been embarrassed; they would not have known how to face him or talk to him. Revealing to his family and friends that he knew the truth would have made him an alien or *mura-hachibu*.

Review of the Literature

The issue of advance directives is a touchy one in Japan, where RTEO prevails in both urban and rural areas. Japanese loyalty to a group accompanies both a drive to expel any agent disturbing the homogeneity of the group and a compassionate desire not to harm its members.

When the first survey of the use of advance directives targeting physicians, nurses, patients, and residents was conducted a decade ago in a rural community (population 60,000) in Nagano, it ignited various emotional reactions (Ohi 1989). The question was phrased in this way: "If you were to learn that you had an incurable disease, would you like to convey your wishes to your family or doctor in an advance directive communicating the treatment strategy?" Although the respondents found it very difficult to choose with only a yes or no option, a majority (60–80%) in each of the four groups replied that they would.

However, when the health workers were asked about the advisability of implementing a system at the hospital in which patients write advance directives related to truthful disclosure and the use of cardiopulmonary resuscitation, nearly 70 percent of physicians were opposed to the idea, while 60 percent of nurses agreed.

The pros and cons of the issue could be summarized as follows: those in opposition stated that implementing a system of advance directives would (1) make patients unnecessarily concerned, eliciting reactions such as "Might I have a bad disease like incurable cancer?" (2) impair the fiduciary relation between the physician and the patient, and (3) fail to reflect the true state of the constantly changing human mind. Those who agreed gave reasons such as (1) the patient has a right to know the truth and to choose a therapy, and (2) advance directives will reveal the intention of the patient, thereby giving health workers an opportunity to honor his or her wishes.

Currently, at least two factors in Japan are at work to facilitate the use of advance directives: First, there has been some shift in ethical orientation from RTEO to ATEO as a result of economic affluence lasting for a half century as well as a loosening of the group ethos. Isolated in an urban environment, an individual must become autonomous in order to survive. Second, an increasing number of therapeutic alternatives, none of which, however, has a decisive edge, inevitably will allow the patient a wider range of options and opportunities to communicate more actively with physicians.

Although nonverbal communication [*ishin-denshin*] was cherished in traditional Japanese culture, Kai et al. clearly demonstrated that nonverbal communication was not feasible between patients and physicians (Kai et al. 1993). They assessed patient-physician communication about terminal care in Japan by examining the accuracy of physicians' estimation of their patients' preferences as regards (1) information about diagnosis and prognosis, (2) the place of death, and (3) the therapeutic strategy at the terminal stage (life prolongation versus pain control), and conducted a questionnaire survey on inpatients (n = 201) in three hospitals; two in rural areas (Nagano and Okinawa) and one in an urban area (Tokyo). Simultaneously they asked physicians (n = 40) in charge of the patients to estimate their attitudes.

Approximately 80 percent of the patients preferred to have candid information about diagnosis and prognosis, regardless of the nature of their disease. The physicians were correct in their estimates in only about half the cases. About one-sixth of their guesses were wrong, while about one-third failed to make any estimate at all. Thus, the overall correct estimation rate (CER) was 42 57, and 62 percent in Nagano, Okinawa, and Tokyo, respectively.

Whereas 70 percent of the patients wished to meet their death at home, the physicians estimated this fact correctly in less than half of the cases. The physicians frequently could not make any estimate (CER 21%, 36%, and 40%, respectively).

Two-thirds of the patients preferred pain control over life prolongation. Again, CER remained in the neighborhood of 50 percent (CER 49%, 49%, and 64%, respectively). The concordance between patients' preferences and physicians' estimates was not far from a figure expected by chance alone. These findings indicate that the physicians had practically no knowledge of their patients' preferences and strongly suggest absence of effective communication between patients and physicians concerning terminal care. This situation inevitably enhances physicians' effort toward prolongation of patients' life at the expense of quality of life and in part accounts for expansion of medical expenditure during the least effective stage of therapy.

It is still rare in Japan to encounter documented examples of advance directives (*ribingu wiru* or living will in Japanese terms). Two such cases were reported this year by a surgeon writer still active in his practice (Kuroyanagi 1994).

1. A 56-year-old man with small-cell carcinoma of the lung (stage IV) articulated the following advance directive: "I have learned from my wife that I have lung cancer and that, although therapeutic efforts including the administration of anti-cancer medication are to be continued, I have little time to live. However, at the end of my life when treatment becomes ineffective and meaningless, I wish to decline all therapeutic endeavor by executing my 'living will' as follows:

> a. "When metastases to the brain or bone are found at the end of my disease course, I request that further treatment be discontinued and decline the implementation of cardiopulmonary resuscitation;
>
> b. "In order to make my death as painless and peaceful as possible, I condone the use of narcotics that might be excessive, causing a premature termination of my life;
>
> c. "This living will was drafted while I was lucid. I hereby declare my will and intention."

2. One of the physician's former classmates died of liver cancer. He left a living will with the intention of protecting the physician from the possible charge of having assisted in euthanasia:

> a. "I will not authorize treatment like radiation, artificial respiration, artificial heart, oxygen inhalation, anticancer agents, etc., or any means that might unduly prolong my life;
>
> b. "I decline the administration of ordinary painkillers and request the use of morphine to reduce pain and hasten death. I request the execution of the foregoing with due deference and leave this advance directive as evidence.

In summary, RTEO, which appears to prevail in Japan, may be regarded as both an outcome of the traditional Japanese way of living for generations and the survival strategy molding the Japanese mentality. It stresses mutual empathy, which is more or less discordant with a clear and straightforward expression of an individual mind such as advance directives. However, with the advance of medical technology, we are witnessing artificial prolongation of life that is more often than not of reduced quality. With this realization, the number of people who wish to rely on advance directives is gradually on the rise.

References

Kagawa-Singer, M. 1993. "Redefining Health: Living with Cancer." *Social Science and Medicine* 37:295–304.

Kai, I., et al. 1993. "Communication between Patients and Physicians about Terminal Care: A Survey in Japan." *Social Science and Medicine* 36:1151–59.

Kuroyanagi, Y. 1994. *Songenshi o Kangaeru* (On Dignified Death). Tokyo: Iwanami Shoten.

Lebra, T. Sugiyama. 1976. *Social Relativism as the Japanese Ethos: A Postulate, in Japanese Patterns of Behavior.* Honolulu: University of Hawaii Press.

Ministry of Health and Welfare. 1993. *Makkiiro nikansuru Kokumin no Ishikichosato Kentokai* (Report of the Committee Studying the Attitude of the Japanese toward Terminal Care). Tokyo: Koseisho.

Ohi, G. 1989. *Shumatsuki Iryo: Jibun no shio torimodosu tameni*(Terminal Care: To Regain One's Own Death). Tokyo: Kobundo.

Ohi, G., and T. Y. Chiu. 1995. Unpublished data.

8

Death, Dying, and Advance Directives in Japan

Sociocultural and Legal Points of View

Rihito Kimura, J.D.

Introduction: The Traditional and Cultural Acceptance of Death

Human death and dying are sociocultural events and processes of human persons embedded in particular historical contexts and environments. The end of human life should be understood by society not only in terms of medical criteria but also as a cultural phenomenon. At present, a majority of Japanese feel that modern biomedical and medicotechnological innovations affecting human life and death have effected a change in our common understanding of the process of death and dying. Historically, death was a natural event, and the criteria for death—cessation of heart beat and respiration—was unquestioned. This is no longer the case because the new Organ Transplantation Law (effective October 16, 1997) permits harvesting organs from those who had declared in advance their acceptance of brain-death criteria and their willingness to donate organs in a written document when they were alive.

An individual's death should be a personal and private matter as well as a familial, communal, and social one. It has been so regarded for many thousands of years in Japanese society and culture. It is well understood that our traditional sociocultural understanding of human life admits the natural process of death as a positive event marking of the end of life. The ideas expressed in Zen-Buddhist phrases such as "accept death as it is" and "life-death as one phenomenon" have been a key motif totally integrated in our traditional understanding of life (Fujii 1991).

Indeed, even the intentional ending of one's life has been regarded as positive, if it was intended for some noble cause within a particular historical context that justified the action. For example, *jyunshi* (self-immolation) and *seppuku* (disembowelment—the same as *harakiri*) are methods of sacrificing one's life for the greater benefit of one's feudal lord or emperor, and in some cases for family and friends. This emphasis on readiness for self-sacrifice, of course, also has its negative side. The expression "education for death" still causes negative sentiment and resentment among some Japanese as a result of strong encouragement in Japan during World War II to wage a "sacred, just war." By this it was meant that all Japanese people needed to be ready to sacrifice their own lives with glory for the honor and victory of the God-Nation of the Japanese Empire. This ideology was initiated by the Japanese military government and its ultra-nationalistic leaders of the time. For the Japanese citizenry, life and death were totally in the hands of a militaristic national authority (Pinguet 1993).

In both war and peace, however, it is certain that we Japanese value communal goals as more important than mere biological life and have a tendency to sacrifice our individual lives for larger ideals. In our cultural tradition, death is given special concern and recognition as an event. Many heroic and unique Japanese figures have appeared in historical documents, usually expressing their last word in the form of a *jisei.* A jisei is a kind of poem composed on the occasion of one's death consisting of 31 syllables (Hoffmann 1986). Although death itself is abhorred, it is understood and accepted as a natural part of the life process. In this sense, a Jisei could be interpreted as a traditional cultural expression of a dying person, almost a "living will," according to Japanese folk study expert Tetsuo Yamaori (Yamaori 1994). However, in my understanding, a Jisei is by no means a legal document or an "advance directive" expressing one's wishes when end-of-life decisions need to be made.

Recent Trends in Views about Dying in Japan

These traditional sociocultural elements of perceiving death as an acceptable process have been vanishing as the Japanese have applied modern biomedical technologies more frequently in well-equipped hospital settings. However, the involvement of family members in the process of dying and particularly in the event of death itself continues in a variety of ways. The Japanese situation in regard to dying patients is becoming much similar to that found in advanced hospital settings in many countries of the world rather than different. Now, in Japan, a majority of people end their lives in the hospital, surrounded by high-technology machines, apparatuses, and equipment. However, in a recent survey published by the *Yomiuri Shimbun* on June 15, 1991, half the respondents said they would prefer to die at home.

There has been a tradition of not explaining to terminally ill people the true nature of their condition, on the grounds that this is the kindest way to proceed (Kimura 1991a). However, views about this matter are changing. In the same nationwide opinion poll published by *Yomiuri Shimbun,* 65 percent of the participants said that if they were terminally ill they would like to be given full diagnostic information about their condition. However, only 22 percent of the people questioned said they themselves would definitely be prepared to disclose such information to a member of their family. The same survey indicated that 78 percent of the respondents considered palliative care desirable, even though it might shorten life; 16 percent thought life should be sustained as long as possible, regardless of the pain that patients might be suffering.

The National Matsudo Hospital is one of the few hospitals in Japan with a palliative care unit. The use of morphine has significantly reduced pain levels for a high proportion of the patients in this establishment (MHWJ 1995). However, until very recently, methods of pain control were not well developed in the Japanese medical service system. For example, my father was hospitalized with lung cancer 20 years ago. Although he suffered very severe pain, he was never told the result of the diagnosis. Even the easing of his pain through the administration of morphine was restricted to a particular time sequence, and often his pleas for an injection were rejected on the grounds that the proper time had not yet arrived. This was the reason he sincerely expressed his final wish to die peacefully at that very moment; tragically, however, he suffered tremendously with this unbearable pain until his death (Kimura 1987).

One of very few surveys exploring cancer pain, conducted by Dr. K. Mizuguchi of Chiba University in 1987, revealed that 68.9 percent of end-stage cancer patients experience pain and 8.7 percent of them die without having that pain relieved (Mizuguchi 1987). Mizuguchi has also gathered some interesting comments indicating less understanding of and interest in the use of pain control among physicians than is desirable. These physicians seem to fear that their use of such measures may create a narcotic addict or possibly shorten a patient's life.

Japan has a very rigid Narcotics Control Law (Law 14, March 17, 1953) that functions effectively, but according to this survey the medical use of narcotics is extremely limited. Such a rigid and complicated system of justifying the use of narcotics has forced many cancer patients with treatable pain to suffer, compared with other advanced countries. The situation is changing only slowly (Takeda and Uki 1994).

A special task force on terminal care, set up by the Ministry of Health and Welfare, issued a report in 1989 that encouraged the disclosure of diagnostic information to patients, provided that consideration was given to patients' life histories, personalities, relationships with family members, and other factors. The use of drugs for pain control was favored. The report also dealt with various additional matters such as spiritual requirements and the care of family members. The idea that people should not have to accept without question the authority of doctors is gaining ground in Japan.

Unfortunately there are still too few trained people to cope with the many problems associated with dying. Therefore, responsibility for the care of the dying should be shared among health professionals as well as those in other fields. Changes in the mentalities of both health care providers and patients, including a recognition that medical systems and institutions are not immutable, are sorely needed.

Efforts have been made by some volunteers and hospitals in Tokyo, Osaka, and elsewhere to improve the care of the dying. There are signs of public approval for such work; since April 1990, the government has increasingly approved the provision of financial support for palliative care through the national health insurance system (Kimura 1991a).

Advance Directives as a Nonlegal Document in Japan

In the context of terminal care in Japan, the notion of "advance directives" has never been regarded as a legally endorsed expression of the patient's intention, whatever the form of particular documents. For example, various kinds of documented advance directives issued by several voluntary organizations have no legally binding force on the medical provider.

It is true that the number of members of the Japanese Euthanasia Society, established in 1976 and recently renamed the Japan Society for Dying with Dignity (JSDD), is increasing. It is also notable that the JSDD makes available a very general form called the "Dying with Dignity Declaration (Living Will)," which seeks to prevent the provision of futile medical treatment. However, the number of living will cardholders is very small, and the JSDD's "Dying with Dignity Declaration" has never been legally recognized during the 22 years of its existence (JSDD 1990/1992).

Sociocultural Aspects

Several factors particular to Japanese culture and society may serve to explain this situation. Traditionally, the physician-patient relationship in Japan has been based on the patient's complete and unquestioning trust of the physician such that the physician acts to make health care decisions on behalf of the patient.

To further complicate matters, although patients' families are informed of the incurable nature of the disease affecting their family member, patients themselves usually are not told of terminal diagnoses. Therefore, the patients often do not have the information necessary to articulate health care preferences in advance, should they wish to do so. A mixture of Shinto, Confucian, and Buddhist beliefs wherein death should not be hastened to avoid disturbing the harmony of the universe also muddle the issue, as does a commonly held view that life and one's body are to be regarded as gifts from one's parents to be treated with traditional filial piety.

The traditional Japanese mentality of *amae,* which is a sense of interdependence, turns the focus away from the individual and toward the family or socially related group (Doi 1971). This almost certainly plays a role in limiting the appeal of the notion of advance directives.

The authority given to the family in making decisions about organ donation is illustrative of the major role the family plays in medical decision making. Some people express their uneasiness about having documents relating to the end of life. They think that this serious event of ending one's life should be dealt with in a more harmonious way, such as a "tacit agreement" or *Ishin-denshin* (heart-to-heart communication without words) among the patient, family members, and attending physician (Lebra 1976).

Dr. Gen Ohi, in his book *Terminal Care,* discussed the difficulties he encountered in conducting a survey on death and dying issues in rural Japan. He commented that the majority of the participants were uneasy about the concept of a documented expression (Ohi 1988).

There is a particularly strong concern among medical providers and their patients that a complicated legal intervention such as an advance directive would be inconsonant with life-and-death issues. This mentality is one of the most important sociocultural factors that mitigate against advance directives, even though some people acknowledge that these documents will become increasingly necessary in the future.

Do-Not-Resuscitate (DNR) orders provide an example of another kind of advance directive in Japan. According to recent data compiled in 1994, 96.7 percent of those surveyed answered that, depending on the situation, a DNR order was necessary. The idea of "dying with dignity" was cited as the main reason for having a DNR order. The unique finding of this survey is that 84.9 percent agreed that the patient's wishes are not indispensable. In other words, a patient's physician and family members would be granted the authority to make a decision. More specifically, 68.4 percent agreed to have a decision made by the attending physician, perhaps after consultation with other relevant physicians. This finding clearly shows the strong medical and professional orientation that impacts the decision to make a DNR order in Japan (Arai et al. 1994).

Legal Aspects

Unlike the codes of Germany and several states in the United States, the Criminal Code of Japan (Law No. 45, April 24, 1907) has provisions related to assisted suicide (*Jisatsu Hojyo*), murder by request (*Shokutaku Satsujin*), and murder with consent (*Doi Satsujin*). They are classified as criminal offenses as follows. Article 202 (Participation in suicide): A person who instigates or assists another to commit suicide or kills another at the request or with the consent of the latter shall be punished with penal servitude or imprisonment for not less than six months nor more than seven years. This article has provided an enormously powerful justification for physicians to prolong life as long as possible. Physicians are considered to be experts in the care of patients and therefore are usually permitted to ignore the patient's desire to be treated in a way that allows the natural ending of life. Instead of respecting such wishes, many physicians favor the provision of aggressive medical intervention to prolong life. For example, when my mother-in-law's 85-year-old mother was dying of colon cancer and suffering severe pain, my mother-in-law suggested to the attending physician that aggressive intervention be forgone. However, this suggestion was simply rejected by the physician, who stated, "My professional ethics cannot accept such a proposal."

However, if the physician him- or herself determines on the basis of medical judgment that additional treatment would be futile, the physician is able to end the treatment. This is considered a justifiable act, according to article 35 of the Criminal Code of Japan, which provides that "No person shall be punished for an act done under law or ordinance or in the course of legitimate business." When considered in this context of Japanese Criminal Law, the reason for and aim of efforts to legalize advance directives may be properly understood as very important steps.

There are several legal opinions regarding a patient's wish or autonomy to end his or her life peacefully and to reject treatment in the process of terminal care. The situation surrounding terminal care in Japan is gradually changing. However, I think that, particularly in our country with its article 202 (described above), the legal difference between the phrases "agree and act based on patient's rejection of treatment" and "assisting committing suicide" should be recognized. If we strictly apply article 202 to both situations, the person who acted will be prosecuted. However, in the particular clinical context of end-stage illness, the former case should be understood as a justifiable "omission" (*Fusakui,* which is a legal term similar to *Unterlassung* in German) because of the counterbenefits of relieving severe pain and honoring the patient's own intention to reject treatment.

Some Unique Elements in Japanese Advance Directives

As I mentioned before, in Japan advanced directives are not legally binding documents. Rather, an advance directive is merely a private document expressing a person's wishes for future medical treatment and care at the end of life (JMA 1992). However, there have been some efforts among concerned individuals and organizations to make an "advanced directive document" similar to the type that has been developed in some countries in Europe and the United States.

I will discuss three different types of advance directives: (1) *Songenshi no Sengensho* (Declaration Document of Death with Dignity–Living Will), which is provided by the Japan Society for Dying with Dignity; (2) *Shumatsuki Sengensho* (Declaration for the End of Life Stage), which is provided by the Citizen's Group in Thinking of the End-of-Life Stage; and (3) "Living Will: Proposal by Kyoto Women's University."

Since 1976 the Japan Society for Dying with Dignity has made available a very general form that enables individuals to declare their desire to avoid futile medical treatment. The "Dying with Dignity Declaration" requests that medical technology not be used to artificially prolong life in irreversible or incurable situations, asks that effective pain-reduction methods be used even though they may hasten death, and permits the withdrawing of life-sustaining technologies in the case of a persistent vegetative state of several months' duration (see book appendix).

As of October 1997, no legal mechanism exists to honor this declaration or any other advance directive in Japanese society. However, public awareness of the death with dignity movement is rapidly increasing, and as of June 1997 the number of memberships in the Japan Society for Dying with Dignity stood at 83,273.

Another organization, called the "Citizen's Group in Thinking of Terminal Care" has become very active during the past five years. They issued another type of advance directive, which attempted to simplify matters by providing a place for a check mark in front of each statement. There are some unique elements in this document that address "Truth Telling," "Vegetative State," and "Brain-Death Situations." For example, sentence No. 1 says, "Please tell my family members as things actually are but don't tell me the truth clearly," while No. 2 states, "I do not want to be connected continuously to a life sustaining machine when I became PVS [Persistent Vegetative State]," and No. 4 offers a choice of "Brain-dead status as death or not." An opportunity to express one's wishes in terms of organ donation was also provided in the following sentences. Finally, this document has a place expressly designed for the designation of a surrogate decision maker, to be signed by the person who made the statement. This means that the statement has combined the characteristics of a "Living Will" and a "Durable Power of Attorney" in one document. Of course, similar to the JSDD's Living Will declaration, such a document is not legally binding in any way and need not be respected by the physician in charge. Naturally, however, these expressions of patient preference might have some influence, depending on the individual opinion of the physician (see appendix no. 4).

The Student Bioethics Study Group at Kyoto Women's University proposed a unique advance directive model document, written from the perspective of a pregnant woman. Statement II.B.a says that, if a guardian for the unborn baby had previously been designated, the document specifying this should be retracted and the best medical treatment for continuation of pregnancy and delivery should be performed. This proposal also has statements that request the forgoing of life-sustaining technologies in the event of the onset of PVS and attempts to address the situation in which a mental disability would make a decision impossible. The statement says that in the case of an incurable disease in which death is imminent, hydration, nutrition, and cleaning of the body should be provided, however, the mere prolongation of the dying process through the use of life-sustaining machines should be avoided.

This proposed living will has suggested having the names of two physicians listed as witnesses to this document, as well as choices of physicians for making a diagnosis of PVS (see book appendix).

Case Discussion

In addition to the efforts of the JSDD and other recent interest groups focusing on issues in death and dying, and the validity of the explicit expression of individual intent in advance directive documents, there are three important cases that serve to reflect the Japanese situation concerning advance directives and the experience of an extremely painful terminal stage of life due to chronic disease.

Rejection of the Suit Claiming Legal Validity of a Living Will

There is only one legal case relating to the legal validity of a living will that should be mentioned here. In 1980, Mr. Tobita, who was then the chairman of the Edogawa Machine Metal Industrial Cooperatives and a board member of the JSDD, filed an action in the Tokyo District Court. He asked for a confirmation of the validity (*Feststellungsklage*) of an individual person's intention of "dying with dignity." He, as the plaintiff, quoted articles 13 and 25 of the Japanese Constitution, which endorse the "pursuit of happiness" and the "right to live." Mr. Tobita insisted that the opportunity to experience pleasure, displeasure, pain, and nonpain has been guaranteed to all Japanese citizens by this fundamental constitutional law and that, thus, a person has a right to choose a way of death according to his or her individual intention.

For this reason he claimed that the state should confirm "the person's intention to express his or her wishes precisely as written in a document such as a living will, when the person is competent, not to suffer in death unnecessarily, and to reject futile treatment." The Tokyo District Court decided on February 17, 1982, that this case could not be accepted for ruling in the court as it was not concrete and could not be included in the category of "all kinds of legal conflicts" delineated by the Court Law, article 3, section 1. Also, the court claimed that this case lacked the legally necessary conditions to be dealt with as a suit in the court. The court concluded that this case must be turned down (*Zurückweisung*), by applying article 202 of the Civil Procedure Code (Tokyo District Court 1982).

This example of case No. 1 shows that such a suit that seeks the confirmation of the validity of personal choice in dying cannot be accepted by the court. This idea of dying with dignity according to an individual's value of life might be possible only through the legislation of laws supporting living wills in Japan.

Questions about advance directives were raised in a concrete legal case in which a patient was dying painfully due to an incurable disease. The following two cases involve "oral directives," one made by the patient and the other by a close family member who sought the termination of treatment and an end to suffering through active euthanasia, performed by the patient's son in the first case and by the physician in charge in the latter case.

Legal Criteria for Active Euthanasia in Japan

One of the most important Japanese legal precedents relating to the issue of death and dying has never been applied since it was set in 1962. The case is usually cited as the "Nagoya High Court Decision of 1962." In this case, a son killed his terminally ill father, was charged with "ascendant homicide," and was subsequently prosecuted. In the Japanese legal system, ascendant homicide, or the killing of one's lineal ascendant or a lineal ascendant of one's spouse, is a more serious crime than ordinary homicide. The punishment for ascendant homicide carries a sentence of death or penal servitude for life, while the sentence for murder can be as little as three years. The standard sentence for cases of assisted suicide is six months to seven years. The particulars of the Nagoya case are as follows: the father, a farmer and head of a household, became completely paralyzed. Because of his very severe pain and suffering, exacerbated by frequent occurrences of hiccups, the father repeatedly expressed his wish to die, saying, "Please let me die, please let me go. I want to go to the other world."

The physician informed the family that the farmer's situation was worsening and that his death would probably occur within ten days. The man's son, a kind person, thought that his last filial duty required him to save his father from his severe pain and suffering by killing him, based on his father's verbally articulated "directive." The son prepared milk mixed with an agricultural pesticide to which he had ready access. The glass was given to the man by his wife who did not know its poisonous content, and the man died.

In reaching its judgment, the court identified the following six conditions that must be fulfilled before one is legally permitted to end a suffering patient's life.

> First, the patient's situation should be regarded as incurable with no hope of recovery, and death should be imminent;
> Second, the patient must be suffering from unbearable and severe pain that cannot be relieved;
> Third, the act of killing should be undertaken with the intention of alleviating the patient's pain;
> Fourth, the act should be done only if the patient him- or herself makes an explicit request;
> Fifth, the euthanasia should be carried out by a physician, although if that is not possible, special situations shall be admitted for receiving some other person's assistance, and
> Sixth, the euthanasia must carried out using ethically acceptable methods (Nagoya High Court 1962).

In this case, the Nagoya High Court ruled that, although the first four criteria had been met, the final two conditions had not. The son was sentenced to four years' imprisonment with three years suspended. As mentioned earlier, the Japanese Criminal Code (JCC) provides for severe punishment, such as capital punishment or life imprisonment, for ascendant homicide; however, in this case, the court believed that the son's desire to honor his filial duty and to follow his father's spoken "directives" was evident and warranted a lesser sentence.

In the light of medical and technological advances, the ramifications of the Nagoya High Court decision have changed in many ways. Conditions once considered fatal can now be treated effectively or even cured. Better methods of pain control have been developed, and new centers for palliative care have been developed (Kimura 1991a).

The interpretation of the Nagoya criteria has been very strict. In the 33 years since the Nagoya High Court decision, there have been only four cases brought before the court wherein a family member acted to end the life of a patient suffering grave pain. All of these cases were prosecuted as criminal cases, and none were found to be in accordance with the six requirements laid out by the Nagoya High Court, but the defendants all received lesser sentences: (1) Homicide case of a wife suffering from a chronic disease of the autonomic nervous system, severe hip gout, and tuberculosis (Kagoshima District Court Decision 1975); defendant was sentenced to one-year imprisonment suspended for two years on the criminal charge of "murder with consent." (2) Homicide case of a mother suffering from a cerebral hemorrhage (Kobe District Court 1975); defendant was sentenced to three years' imprisonment suspended for four years on the criminal charge of "homicide." (3) Homicide case of a wife with painful stomach cancer (Osaka District Court Decision 1977); defendant was sentenced to one-year imprisonment suspended for two years on the criminal charge of "murder with consent." (4) Homicide case of a wife having severe pain due to sarcoma (Kochi District Court Decision 1990); defendant was sentenced to three years' imprisonment suspended for one year on the criminal charge of "murder with consent."

Although the Nagoya High Court ruling established the legal criteria for active euthanasia and specifically confirmed the importance of the individual wish of the patient to have his or her life terminated, all three district courts seem reluctant to apply these conditions fully. An explanation for this phenomenon may be the court's unwillingness to accept the concept of active euthanasia.

On April 4, 1973, in another case of ascendant homicide relevant to case No. 1 as presented above, there was a drastic change in this reluctant attitude. In this case, the Supreme Court ruled that article 200 of the Japanese Criminal Code, which entails a heavy criminal charge in cases of ascendant homicide, is an illegal and unfair clause contrary to the equal treatment clause of the Japanese Constitution. "If the sentence is extremely heavy and if there is no justifiable ground for it, this discriminatory provision is very much unreasonable to be applied. Therefore, it is against article 14, section 1 of the Japanese Constitution and it is invalid." This ruling indicates a positive change in the established legal values of the Criminal Code, based on a cultural ethos that is significantly influenced by a Confucian ideology of filial piety. In the enforcement of new and more contemporary official phrasing and modification of the Criminal Code of Japan, article 200 was completely eliminated on June 1, 1995.

A Physician's Active Ending of a Patient's Life by Family Request

The most recent case in which a physician actively ended the life of a patient happened in 1991 at Tokai University Hospital. The case attracted great media attention because it involved a physician who ended the life of a patient based on the request of a family member. According to the physician, the patient's son asked the physician to alleviate his father's suffering. However, when questioned later, the son stated that he had not meant the ending of his father's life. At the time of the alleged request, the patient was hospitalized with an incurable and terminal condition and was already comatose when the physician administered an injection of potassium chloride. Due to the family's denial that they had asked for help to end the patient's life, the physician was accused of murder and dismissed from the hospital. On March 28, 1995, the Yokohama District Court sentenced the physician to two years' imprisonment with a stay of execution of two additional years. This ruling is significant for its clear statement of the principle of individual autonomy based on the patient's own intention and its establishment of a limit on a physician's immunity for failing to treat those patients whose treatment is deemed medically futile. According to this ruling, when making a decision to withhold a treatment, it is clearly necessary to have a confirmed statement of the patient's intention to stop treatment. The decision goes on to note that, although there is at present a general lack of these kinds of clear patient statements, in the future there will be widespread acceptance of living wills among the public. The presence of a patient's advance expression of his or her wishes could serve as a verification that the physician indeed made a judgment by taking into account the patient's own wishes when decisions to withhold treatment are made.

Moreover, if the patient has communicated openly enough with family members about his or her view of life, character, and values, the family will be able to make a conjectural decision to end his or her life in a natural way (without aggressive overtreatment). By endorsing the family's ability to guess a patient's wishes, this ruling has set a sort of standard for allowing indirect euthanasia provided that the physician considers it to be an appropriate medical procedure for terminal care in the clinical context. In such cases, the withdrawal of treatment could be justified. However, in the case of positive or direct euthanasia, the ruling does not endorse familial decision making based on the presumed wishes of the patient. The following four points should be taken into account in making the decision: (1) the patient is suffering with intolerable, severe physical pain caused by disease, (2) the patient's death is imminent, (3) there is no possible medical treatment that can ease the pain, and (4) the patient has clearly agreed to the shortening of his or her life (Yokohama District Court 1995).

Although this is not a case focusing only on a patient's advance directive, public opinion is rather supportive of the defendant physician in recognizing the family member's oral "directive" to ease the life of the dying patient. As the involvement of family members in making decisions on behalf of the patient is generally accepted behavior, the inter-relationship with patient, family, and physician is very important in our Japanese social context and human relations (Kimura 1991c).

However, one must be very careful in making any sort of surrogate decision for a family member, even though the process of dying is regarded not as an individual event but as a family event in the Japanese culture.

Family Role in Medical Decision Making

It is not clear whether the situation would be different in the Tokai Hospital Case if the family declared that they had asked the physician to assist in the euthanasia of their father. If this were the case, the first through third, fifth, and sixth conditions of the Nagoya High Court criteria for permissible euthanasia would have been fulfilled, although it is not clear if the patient or only his family made the request for death.

The traditional importance and authority of the family in medical decision making is illuminated by the fact that they, and not the patient, are informed of a terminal diagnosis. The family's role has been discussed in the process of the debate about brain-death criteria and organ transplantation. The draft of legislation and additional guidelines issued by the Inter-party Council on Brain Death and Transplantation in December 1993 cited a number of situations in which the family may *sontaku,* or make a guess as to some other person's mind to allow the pronouncement of brain death and permit organ donation even in the absence of any clear expression of wishes in that regard by the deceased. Even the idea of *sontaku* was not embodied in the final legislation. The scope of family authority in medical decision making is highlighted again by the fact that consent from the family is required concurrently to consent from a potential donor when the individual's desire to donate organs is expressed according to the new Organ Transplantation Law of 1997.

Cases of comatose and terminally ill patients are rarely brought to the court, as these problems are usually regarded as medical and clinical cases to be confined to the authority of the medical profession. A very strong sense of the rights associated with professional discretion is confirmed in many legal cases. In Japan, those in the field of medicine want to practice medicine and conduct research without intervention from any other profession, such as law, religion, or economics.

Traditionally, the paternalistic behavior of physicians has been accepted without question. The recommendations regarding medical treatment made by physicians on behalf of comatose or terminally ill patients are accepted unquestionably by the family members of these patients. The traditional practice of not explaining to terminally ill people the nature of their illness, on the grounds that this is the kindest course of action, often results in surrogate decision making by the family on behalf of the patient, as mentioned before. Some gradual movement toward truthfulness toward the patient is underway, and the notion of informed consent has been widely publicized in clinical settings (Morikawa 1994).

Review of the Literature

There have been several important and influential books and documents published in recent years, among them a book by Professor Koichi Bai, an official report of the Japanese Medical Association's Bioethics Council, and the final report of the Special Committee on Death and Medical Services of the Japan Science Council.

Professor Koichi Bai's Book

One of the most important Japanese books in this area was written by Koichi Bai, *Seimei Iji Chiryo no Hori to Rinri* (Legal Reasoning and the Ethics of Life-Sustaining Therapy; 1990). Even though the book focuses mainly on the analysis of cases and the situation in the United States concerning treatment at the end of life, section 4, entitled "Terminal Care and Law," does comment on relevant issues in Japan. Professor Bai points out several elements in the process of making the decision to forgo a patient's treatment: first, a confirmation of the patient's real wishes ; second, the importance of informed consent; third, an assessment of the patient's competency; fourth, continued treatment for the prolongation of life if the patient's intent is not clear; fifth, a respect for a patient's wish to change hospitals due to a difference in values between the physician and patient; and sixth, the necessity of care and the continuation of minimum treatment even if life-sustaining technology is terminated. Professor Bai's book is unique in its legal analysis and overview of the implications for advance directives in Japan (Bai 1990). Other resource books are mentioned in the Japanese section of the annotated bibliography at the end of this volume.

An Official Report of the Japanese Medical Association's Bioethics Council

The title of the report issued by the Japanese Medical Association's Bioethics Council on March 18, 1992, is "How a Physician Should Handle the Treatment of Terminal Patients in the Final Stage" (JMA 1992). An official statement in 1978 by the JMA stated, "When a doctor is held responsible for disconnecting a life-prolonging device, the existence of a living will is significant as a mitigating factor only, and nothing more." After 14 years, the JMA changed its position, saying, "Even without the force of law, the attending physician will not be held responsible for a patient's death as a result of withdrawal of life-prolonging treatment." This did not state that the physician should follow any advance directive document prepared by a patient or presented by a family member on behalf of the patient. But this sentence implies an acceptance of the patient's wish not to have life-prolonging treatment, and an assertion that the physician will not be blamed for carrying out whatever action is in accordance with those wishes. It goes even further in affirming the patient's wishes, stating that "still, even if the patient does not have a signed document, a clear and unequivocal verbal statement expressing his /her wishes should be respected," and "In cases where the patient is unable to express his/her wishes, the question arises as to the extent to which family or friends may act on the patient's behalf. In principle, however, it is the patient's wishes [not those of others] that should be adhered to. In cases where there is reliable testimony from friends or family with respect to the patient's wishes, such testimony may be taken as an accurate reflection of the patient's wishes [and treatment undertaken accordingly]."

However, the following statement is problematic: "On the basis of connections with the Civil Code, for anyone over the age of 15, some declaration written by that person is, in essence, required. Further, in cases where the person is deemed to possess the capacity to make a decision, there may be no objection to the decisions of a person under the age of 15." The relevant Civil Code Article 961 states, "Persons who have attained the age of 15 are entitled to write a will."

These statements may appear acceptable and practical in a clinical setting. However, I think the underlying message is one of avoidance of a clearly documented legal framework to which physicians must adhere. The intention seems to have been to retain, in the tradition of paternalism, medical professional hegemony in order to exclude legal control and legislation of living will laws, which are seen as a source of complications.

The Japan Science Council's Final Report on Death with Dignity

The Japan Science Council's final report on Death with Dignity was most recently issued on May 26, 1994. This report caused a heated debate among professionals already in the midst of the ongoing Tokai University Hospital case mentioned above. The JSC is a sort of house of representatives sponsored by the Japanese government that consists of various eminent scholars elected by national academic societies in the fields of humanities, social sciences, natural sciences, medical sciences, and so on. In this report, the words "death with dignity" mean a withdrawal of life-prolonging treatment. The report confirms that in the terminal stage, the patient's wishes should be respected based on the patient's autonomous choice. The importance of the patient's intention is particularly stressed. The treatment plan, according to this report, should be based on "advance directives such as living wills," thus respecting the patient's own choice for deciding when to withdraw life-prolonging treatment, including hydration and nutrition (JSC 1994).

However, the report concludes by stating, "We have to consider seriously whether we need to have legislation endorsing living wills or not." This report points out the possible risk of abuse and the difficulties in applying such a law. In conclusion, this report articulates that the withdrawal of life-prolonging treatment could be justifiable under specified conditions and states that appropriate and cautious application of this law to actual cases should be performed.

Once again we are faced with a repeated unwillingness to legalize advance directives, and an avoidance of legal support in this kind of discussion. In addition, public policy debates regarding how life-and-death decisions should be handled in medical and clinical settings have been neglected (Kimura 1994).

Conclusion

There is a widening gap between the position of medical professionals and the lay public on issues in terminal care. The general public is relatively positive in their support of the actions of the accused physician at Tokai University; however, the society of medical professionals has a very negative view of such actions in the case of terminally ill patients. It is almost impossible to legalize living wills in Japan. If any advance directives are to be developed in Japan, they will need to be based on a familial type of directive. It might be possible for individual family members to make different decisions. However, the individual family member's idea should be shared with another family member; otherwise, the individual wish cannot be respected and followed. It might be called a Family Unit Advance Directive. This type of advance directive might have a more practical effect for future family preparation for life-and-death issues.

For many years, issues relating to death have not been openly discussed in Japan, as it is considered a "taboo" topic (Kimura 1991c). However, in considering the reality of advanced medical technology and its impact on medical decision making, an opinion poll conducted by the Ministry of Health and Welfare in 1993 revealed that around 80 percent of all Japanese citizens are concerned about the issues relating to death with dignity, euthanasia, and terminal care. Conferences, research efforts, and educational programs focusing on death and dying are now very popular. Dr. Alfons Deeken's pioneering educational program at Sophia University on preparing for death had its thirteenth anniversary in 1995. International dialogue and joint research programs on death and dying issues are taking place between various institutions around the world, such as the Bioethics Project of Advanced Research Center for Human Sciences at Waseda University and the Kennedy Institute of Ethics at Georgetown University (Waseda University 1992). In working on this Volkswagen Project and comparing advance directives in Germany, the United States, and Japan, we have learned a great deal about cultural differences and similarities (Olick et al. 1966).

Finally, I will briefly discuss a survey I conducted at Waseda University with 473 students in a bioethics class. Approximately 70 percent of students responded no to the statement "I want to live as long as possible if I am permanently unconscious," and 77 percent wanted their own values to govern treatment decisions. Approximately 87 percent responded yes to the statement "I want to be without pain," while around 87 percent of students expressed a desire to have a comfortable dying process (appendix 2, p. 206).

One might speculate that some of these data might elicit similar responses from students of other countries. We now share common values relating to issues such as the ability to understand the limits of life and death, the capability to alleviate pain and to foster a comfortable dying process, and the right to govern treatment decisions based on our own values. This commonality of values illustrates the enormous importance that advance directives have among the younger generation in Japan.

Appendix 1

Japan Society for Death with Dignity

A Draft of Legislation by JSDD: Official Translation by JSDD

A draft of the bill of special measures in the medical treatment of terminally ill individuals

Article One (Purpose)

Every human being has the right to decide whether to accept or refuse measures to maintain one's own life. In accordance with this right, the purpose of this law is to provide procedures for stopping life prolonging measures for patients who are terminally and incurably ill and have declared they do not want excessive life prolonging treatment.

Article Two (Definition)

The patient must be deemed by medical authorities to be terminally and incurably ill where life prolonging treatment would merely prolong the time of death. Excessive life prolonging measures mean treatment from which a patient shows no signs of improving, but which only serves to prolong the time of death. This does not include treatment to lessen pain.

Article Three (Declaration by an Individual to Refuse Excessive Life Prolonging Measures)

An individual older than fifteen, possessing the ability to express intent, can indicate in advance a desire to refuse excessive life prolonging measures in the event he/she should become terminally and incurably ill, in any of the following ways.

(1) An individual, while of sound mind, can indicate on a written form his/her desire in advance to refuse excessive life prolonging measures should that individual become terminally and incurably ill. This form must be dated and carry the individual's address and name in handwriting as well as his/her personal stamp. At least two others must bear witness by signing and putting their personal stamps on the above form to verify that the above individual did indeed sign in normal consciousness.

(2) If due to illness or other reasons, an individual is not able to sign the form, at least two doctors must sign and put their personal stamps on the form where the individual's signature would go. Furthermore, the form must be dated, in order to verify that these doctors were present when the individual indicated his/her desire and that this request was made while the individual was of sound mind.

[Subpoint 1 omitted]

2. Article Number 964 of the civil code applies to the witnesses described in (1) above.

3. The format of the written form to be used, mentioned in the first item of (1) above, is shown in a separate table.

Article Four (Withdrawal of Form by an Individual)

In order for an individual to change his/her mind about the written form mentioned in item 1 of the previous article, he/she must either destroy the form, or write in his/her own handwriting a request for the form to be withdrawn, with the date and the individual's signature.

Article Five (Measures for Individuals Who Do Not Possess the Ability to Decide)

The individual's right to decide, as provided in article one, cannot be taken on by others. However, in cases where an individual does not possess the ability to decide, the courts may be asked to decide for the individual.

Article Six (Verification that an Individual Is Terminally and Incurably Ill)

At least two doctors need to verify that an individual is terminally and incurably ill. The doctors carrying out the verification must sign and put their personal stamps on the form certifying that an individual is terminally and incurably ill. This does not include the patient's doctor who will either decide to not start life prolonging measures or who will decide to stop them.

Article Seven (Doctors Not Legally Accountable for Carrying Out Request)

The doctors who have decided to not start or to stop excessive life prolonging measures, in accordance with the regulations or law, are not to be held legally accountable under the penal and civil codes.

Article Eight (Duty of Keeping the Form)

The forms mentioned in articles three, four, and six must be kept by the doctor who decided to not start or to stop the life-prolonging measures of an individual for a period of five years.

Article Nine (Relation to Life Insurance Policies)

An individual's refusal of excessive life prolonging measures must not be interpreted as suicide in life insurance policies.

Article Ten (Punishment)

Those who destroy or hide the form in article four, four, or six falsify facts, or sign as a witness knowing the facts are false, or forge or adulterate the form, are punishable by imprisonment for a term no greater than ~ years or a fine no greater than ~ yen.

APPENDIX 2

Survey for Waseda University Students (SHS)

Bioethics: Prof. Rihito Kimura

R. Kielstein and H. M. Sass. 1993. "Using Stories to Assess Values." *Kennedy Institute of Ethics Journal* 3 (3): 322–23.

WHICH VALUES AND WISHES SHALL GOVERN YOUR TREATMENT? . . . Others might not make the correct proxy decisions when deciding for you. Therefore you should let them know about your preferences and give them directions. Tell them which values and wishes you would prefer to govern the last days and hours of your life story.

PRESENT SELF-ASSESSMENT	FUTURE SELF-DETERMINATION
1. Yes, very important	A. Yes, very important
2. Important	B. Important
3. Not important	C. Depending on situation
4. I cannot decide	D. I cannot decide
5. No	E. No

1. I want to live as long as possible:		
—if I am permanently unconscious	1,2,3,4,5	A,B,C,D,E
—if I am mentally incompetent	1,2,3,4,5	A,B,C,D,E
—if I am terminally ill	1,2,3,4,5	A,B,C,D,E
2. I want to be without pain.	1,2,3,4,5	A,B,C,D,E
3. I do not want to be dependent.	1,2,3,4,5	A,B,C,D,E
4. I do not want to die in the hospital.	1,2,3,4,5	A,B,C,D,E
5. I want a comfortable dying process.	1,2,3,4,5	A,B,C,D,E

6. I do not want to be left alone.	1,2,3,4,5	A,B,C,D,E
7. I do not want to be a burden.	1,2,3,4,5	A,B,C,D,E
8. I want my values to govern treatment.	1,2,3,4,5	A,B,C,D,E

If you intend this to be a legally binding document, please sign it and have it witnessed according to the laws of your state. If you change your story, comments, or directives, do so in writing by dating and signing those changes. It is always a good idea to review stories, comments, and directives from time to time and to sign and date them again, even if you do not change anything, as this would indicate your repeated commitment to previous statements.

If you wish, please include comments on these and other stories, wishes, or preferences on additional pages.

Signed ______________________________ Date ________________

Witnessed ____________________________ Date ________________

References

Arai, Tatsuru, et al. 1994. "Shumatsuki kanjyani taisuru DNR wa doarubekika" (What Should be Done to Terminal Care Patient Relating to DNR?). *Journal Masui (Anastesia)* 43 (4): 600–611.

Bai, Koichi. 1990. *Seimei Iji Chiryo no Hori to Rinri* (Legal Reasoning and Ethics of Life-Sustaining Therapy). Tokyo: Yuhikaku.

Doi, Takeo. 1971. *Amae no Kozo* (Anatomy of Dependence). Tokyo: Kobundo.

Fujii, Masao. 1991. "Gendai no Shi to Bukkyosha" (Contemporary Death and Buddhists). In *Bukkyo no Ningengaku* (Anthropology of Buddhism), ed. Z. Ishigami, 234–48. Tokyo: Suzuki Shuppan.

Hoffman, Yoel. 1986. *Japanese Death Poems*. Tokyo: Charles E. Tuttles.

Japan Medical Association (JMA). 1992. *Makki Iro ninozomu Ishino arikata* (How Physicians Should Handle the Treatment of Terminal Patients in the Final Stage). Tokyo: Japan Medical Association.

Japan Science Council (JSC). 1994. *Shi to Iryo Tokubetsuiinkai Hokoku-Songenshi ni tsuite* (Report of Special Committee on Death and Medical Services—On Dying with Dignity). Tokyo: Japan Science Council.

Japan Society for Dying with Dignity (JSDD). 1990/1992. "The Development of the Movement for Dying with Dignity in Japan," Part 1. Tokyo: Japan Society for Dying with Dignity.

Kimura, Rihito. 1987. *Inochi o Kangaeru* (Thinking of Life). Tokyo: Nippon Hyoron Sha.

Kimura, Rihito. 1991a. "The Right to be Informed: An Aspect of Dignity." *World Health Forum* 12:391–92.

Kimura, Rihito. 1991b. "Fiduciary Relationship and Medical Profession: A Japanese Point of View." In *Ethics, Trust, and the Professions,* ed. Edmund Pellegrino, R. M. Veatch, and J. P. Langan. Washington, D.C.: Georgetown University Press.

Kimura, Rihito. 1991c. "Japan's Dilemma with the Definition of Death." *Kennedy Institute of Ethics Journal* 1 (2): 123–31.

Kimura, Rihito. 1994. "Bioethics and Japanese Health Care." *Washington-Japan Journal* 2 (4): 1–7.

Kobe District Court, Showa 50 nen. October 29, 1975, no. 484.

Kochi District Court, Heisei 2 nen (Wa). September 17, 1990, no. 94.

Lebra, T. S. 1976. *Japanese Patterns of Behavior.* Honolulu: University Press of Hawaii.

Ministry of Health and Welfare of Japan (MHWJ). 1995. *Kosei Hakusho* (*Annual Report on Health and Welfare*). Tokyo: Gyosei.

Mizuguchi, Kiminobu. 1987. *"Shumatsukiiryo no Genkyo"* (Present Situation of Terminal Medical Services). *Nippon Iji Shinpo* (Japan Medical Journal) no. 3290, 14–18.

Morikawa, Isao. 1994. "Patients' Rights in Japan: Progress and Resistance." *Kennedy Institute of Ethics Journal* 4 (4): 337–43.

Nagoya High Court, Showa 37 nen (U). December 22, 1962, no. 496.

Ohi, Gen. 1988, *Shumatsuki Iryo* (Terminal Care). Tokyo: Kobundo.

Olick, Robert S., Rihito Kimura, et al. 1996. "Advance Care Planning and the ALS Patient: A Cross-cultural perspective on Advance Directives." In *Annual Review of Law and Ethics,* ed. B. Sharon Byrd, Joachim Hruschka, and Jan C. Joerden. Berlin: Duncker & Humblot, 529–51.

Osaka District Court, Showa 52 nen (Wa). November 30, 1977, no. 3083.

Pinguet, Maurice. 1993. *Voluntary Death in Japan.* Cambridge: Polity Press.

Takeda, F., and J. Uki. 1994. "Recent Progress in Cancer Pain Management and Palliative Care in Japan." *Annals of the Academy of Medicine* 23 (2): 296–99.

Tokyo District Court, Showa 55 nen (Wa). February 17, 1982, no. 2812.

Waseda University (Center for Advanced Study of Human Sciences). 1992. *Kanjyanitotte Iryo towa nanika* (The Meaning of Medical Service for Patients). Bioethics Project, Waseda University.

Yamaori, Tetsuo. 1994, *Omukae no Toki: Nipponjin no Shiseikan* (When Time Comes: Japanese View of Death and Life). Tokyo: Shodensha.

Yokohama District Court, Heisei 4 nen (Wa). March 28, 1995, no. 1172.

9

A Differing Perspective on Advance Directives

Tomoaki Tsuchida, Ph.D.

Introduction

In recent decades, the Japanese have also been wrestling with biomedical challenges. Advances in medicine have raised questions among the Japanese about traditional understandings of human life and the proper ways of living and dying. The Japanese have begun to consider the need for advance directives and actually have put them into effect in certain limited areas, such as the provision of options about the treatment of cancer.

This limited utilization of advance directives is not just a result of slowness or "underdevelopment" in terms of human rights among the Japanese. Certainly, however, the Japanese in general have yet to catch up with American and European counterparts in terms of being aware of and respecting individual human rights. In addition to the issue of rights, there are some basic differences in the Japanese concept of human life and death and in their view of "nature," and so on, which contribute to somewhat different attitudes among the Japanese toward advance directives. The traditional views, which used to furnish Japanese society with a remarkably high contextuality, are now more or less fragmented, and some have been consigned to oblivion. Modern Western values and behavior patterns have been adopted and juxtaposed with traditional Japanese concepts and values. Japanese society retains some traditional views of life and death, including continued adherence to the sense of the naturalness of the dying process, and resists quick changes. Advance directives will certainly facilitate a more individualized way of coping with illnesses and matters of life and death, protecting personal dignity toward the end of one's life and thereby promoting a society of reasonable, mature persons; directives will also help eliminate merely inhuman or wasteful medical practices. What seems to be demanding our attention is the basic horizon of contemporary medicine in which advance directives are called for and contrived. Is this horizon truly humane or "ethical," or at least is it in harmony with the coherence and continuity of a cultural tradition on which "common people" depend for the attainment of a personally meaningful life and for the integrity of their life and death? In this chapter I attempt to clarify what lies behind this slowness or hesitation to implement advance directives in Japan.

A Preliminary Analysis of the Japanese Ethos

Is the Matter of Life and Death beyond One's Own Control?

In general, it is still considered social anathema for a Japanese citizen to act individually without regard to the viewpoints of the family (or community, if one lives in a rural area), or to disregard the traditional ethos. This ethos, traditionally handed down from generation to generation, is what matters to the Japanese people in general, even if it has not yet been rationally reflected upon or formulated into a code of ethics. As a people, they would prefer to act as "together-beings," in accordance with the traditional ethos, which places priority on communal well-being.

It is not surprising, then, to find among the Japanese a universal attitude of dependency, *o-makase* (or *amae,* as Dr. Takeo Doi formulated in his very popular book *Anatomy of Dependence*). This attitude, *omakase,* entails entrusting one's care to one's family and physician, assuming that they would certainly give the patient the most beneficial or appropriate care. The patient would, thus, defer to his or her family and the physician in charge for a decision about continuing or forgoing treatment, a matter that is very likely to affect his or her life and death. Telling the truth to the patient him- or herself is still not practiced at the majority of medical institutions; rather, the patient's family are typically the only ones told the truth about the illness. Then the family members get together, share the news, consult the physician, and finally come to a decision or, alternately, leave the decision up to the physician.

No doubt this attitude has been tied to, and is responsible for, rampant paternalism on the part of physicians and the medical establishment, as well as indecision and dependency on the part of patients. In conjunction with this, there has not been much discussion of the adequacy of, and proper ways of defining the role of, surrogate decision makers. However, the so-called discretion of the physician has been challenged in several court cases, such as in a case involving the failure on the part of a physician to tell the truth about a diagnosis of cancer, which led to the patient's untimely and painful death, and in a case in which a doctor improperly used an antitumor agent under a clinical testing program without written consent from the patient or from her husband. People are increasingly better-informed and more alert to doctors' ways of giving or withholding information.

Yet, in the traditional context this attitude of entrusting vital decisions to others (family and/or physician) is interwoven with the Japanese view of the nature of human beings. As has been pointed out by philosophers (such as Tetsuro Watsuji 1934, 1961/1935), psychiatrists (such as Bin Kimura 1984, 1988), and others, the Japanese concept of human being is embodied in the German word *Mitsein,* for example, that humans are human insofar as they live together with fellow humans and that one's life and death as a human renders one part of the whole community of humans. Life and death are not wholly private acts but rather concern the entire community of which one is a member.[1]

Although this notion of community, reflected in the attitudes of rural villages or old townships, has been steadily disintegrating in the wake of the industrialization and urbanization into which Japanese were abruptly thrust in the middle of the last century, still it is fair to say that it is far stronger, in actuality and in sentiment, than in Western nations. An ordinary Japanese person would, primarily and ultimately, think of his or her own family as the source of meaning in his or her life, his or her raison d'être. This tendency has been steady and even increasing among the Japanese, as every recent poll shows. It is natural, then, that many people think of the family as the primary agent of the life-and-death decision-making process.

The Japanese have traditionally held first the family, and then the community, as the locus of their religious life. The family was also the social unit for religion during the last four centuries. Religious traditions including Buddhism and Confucianism (the first tending toward a more personal self-transcendence, and the latter placing more emphasis on society and nation) did modify and influence this basic focus on family to a certain extent, but on the whole the movement toward individual and personal atonement and salvation in the ultimate Real was mitigated and "domesticated." One should always keep in mind that in Japan there never was one single, united national church, except during several decades in modern times [1868–1945] when state Shintoism was forced upon the people. In other words, there has never been one institutionalized religious authority to set moral codes, to judge people's state of faith, and so forth.

Kunio Yanagita (1875–1962), pioneer of Japanese folklore studies, has suggested that for ordinary Japanese, for example, for the vast majority of the people, one's identity and meaning of life are closely tied up with belief in ancestors' spirits. One is born and grows up with the help of parents and ancestors; one sometimes reincarnates one of his or her ancestors, thereby becoming an ancestor; and finally, by shedding off individuality and merging with other ancestors in the course of a generation or so, one will become the spirit of an ancestor. As the spirit of an ancestor, one will always be concerned about the welfare of the offspring.

Yanagita summarized the Japanese view of death in one of his important and influential works, *About Our Ancestors* (1988/1945, section 64), by way of attempting to answer the question of why the Japanese were not so afraid of dying, or were less fearful of death, than people of other cultures. He came to the following conclusions: (1) Most Japanese thought that after death one's spirit would remain close to the living sphere of his or her offspring and would thus never wander very far away from one's descendants (although some, under Buddhist influence, would insist that they would be reborn in Buddha's paradise, in hell, or in a different mode of life); (2) they believed that there has been frequent intercourse between our corporeal world and the world of the spirit, not limited to the occasions of quarterly festivals for the ancestor and that one could invite the spirit on one's initiative or the spirit could visit the living of its own accord; (3) they believed that the most serious wishes of the dying would eventually be realized after one's death; and (4) they held that one could continue one's mission in one's next or future rebirth.

These characteristics have been more or less affirmed by other scholars and can be considered basic tenets in the Japanese view of dying. A Japanese individual envisions his or her life and death in view of the continuity and solidarity between the dead and the living, and therefore his or her life is not just his or her own personal affair.

Complicating medical decision making today is the changing face of the institution of family. Since the end of World War II in particular, patriarchal authority has eroded a great deal. When the family was clearly the basic unit in society and patriarchal power was taken for granted, difficult decisions were left with the father of the family. Today, however, the locus of authority may not rest with the husband or father. Each family has to make their decisions together by sharing their views about grave decisions. Thus, final authority is wanting; people feel at a loss without recourse to a consensus that not only the family of the patient but also the general community can accept.

The Notion of Symbiosis of All Living Beings

In conjunction with this belief that one's life and death must be viewed in the context of one's family, there is another strain of thought continuously forming an undercurrent in Japanese tradition: a prescientific notion of the symbiosis of all beings. This view, originally an animistic worldview, is based on the conviction that each living being is endowed with spirit and is interrelated and interdependent with all other beings, each with its own place in the world. This belief was much endorsed and supported by the Buddhist thesis of interdependent co-arising (Sanskrit: *pratityasamutpada*). It is now receiving new attention because of a dominant Japanese biological view (proposed by Kinji Imanishi [1990] and others) that each living being has its own habitat and that, in contradiction to the natural selection theory, beings survive without exterminating others.

Desire for Natural Death

As modern medicine intervenes increasingly and more vitally in the final days of human life, it has reached the extent of excluding or devaluing the individual wishes and the worldviews of the patient and his or her family. In response, a new cult among the elderly in Japan has come into being. Those who would identify themselves as members of this group share a desire to die without much suffering either for the dying person or the family and to spare whoever may be concerned about the patient or the elderly person anticipating the approaching day. A fairly recent phenomenon has been observed in Japanese religious behavior: many more pilgrimages have been made to those Buddhist temples that are believed to be efficacious in procuring a sudden death. This desire to die quickly is based in part on the Japanese ethos that it is not proper to trouble others too much, especially about one's own physical care, and in part on the traditional view of nature, which we will examine below. It is a view that is in line with the recent remarkable increase in the membership at the Society for Death with Dignity, one very well-known citizen's group promoting the proliferation of living wills and urging the medical profession to honor them.

On the whole, these efforts represent minor phenomena in Japanese society. The Society for Death with Dignity has grown rapidly to more than one hundred thousand members, but clearly the majority remain undecided about the issue. Many people seem to think that the decision of whether to envision one's final days and to request or reject a specific medical treatment belongs not to the dying but to the surviving family members.

Leave It to What Nature Provides

It is apparent to even the most casual observer that the Japanese prize nature and naturalness in their aesthetic tradition. These people have inherited a keen awareness that nature provides as well as takes back what and who we are. The word for nature, *shizen,* was adopted in the latter half of the nineteenth century to translate the Western term "nature," by which was meant the nonartificial, undomesticated state of nonhuman beings. However, the original meaning of the word *shizen* was a force that transcends human control and follows its own course of changes or processes. It thus sometimes came to mean "that's the way it happens" (as far as humans can see). This idea still lingers in the minds of many, making it hard for the Japanese to objectify quantitatively or to freely process nature as material or natural resources. Implicit still in many folk customs and festivals is an animistic reverence, as mentioned above, to the vital force that is found in all living beings, including plants.

In connection with this idea, the concept of "allotted life" (*jomyo*) or "fate" is alive in the minds of many traditionalists. It affirms the attitude of resignation or heroic acceptance of even great suffering as a perspective that is more humane than trying to live on beyond one's lot, or beyond what "common sense" finds to be within the scope of medical possibility.

In light of the Japanese family-community orientation and the notion of "nature" as transcending each person's control, one can see that the Japanese have not yet totally resigned themselves to the authority of modern medicine when it comes to life or death issues. Humane approaches by the family and physicians toward fatal illnesses and death are more desirable than die-hard medical technology. People tend to feel that they are helpless in the face of tremendously specialized modern medicine and are hardly in a position to determine what is in the best interests of the patient or exactly how the family is concerned. Most of us, after all, have trouble coming to grips with, or putting our faith in, medical technology. The level of comfort with the idea of medicalizing one's life and death (or for that matter, with the suggestion to legalize them) is still low among the Japanese. Thus, to a typical Japanese person, the idea of dying medically, such as, say, in Dr. Kevorkian's old van, is still remote.

To the Japanese, death is too solemn a moment to be reduced by any rational considerations to a biomedical phenomenon, let alone to a resource for other beneficent objectives, such as donation of organs for transplant. Death must be embraced in toto, not only rationally but also emotionally and spiritually. This is an important point to consider when it comes to advance directives. There is resistance to the idea of letting doctors, or any scientists, technologically preside over the death of a human being, particularly because the death of a human is different from the death of other living beings. A human being is essentially a being insofar as he or she communicates with other human beings. Therefore, his or her death is not entirely an individual biological affair, but rather a communal concern, and especially a most important matter for the family. The experience of parting is a process for the dying and his or her family to go through over a certain length of time, especially if the patient suffers a sudden accident entailing brain death.

Universal Health Care Coverage

With regard to the actual availability of health care, all Japanese residents are covered by national health insurance, so an individual does not have to worry about basic health care. He or she can expect to be taken care of by the social institution at least, if not by their own family, which most people prefer. This health care setup insulates the individual from the difficult decisions he or she may face upon suffering the misfortune of an incurable chronic disease, an acute grave illness, or a terminal illness. One is free, at least in terms of basic medicine, from financial concern about who will pay for medical treatment.

An Illustration: The Case of Brain-Death Criteria

One of the major difficulties in instituting advance directives can be illustrated through the ongoing argument over the brain-death issue.

Brain death as a standard by which to determine when human death has occurred has been discussed for more than twenty years; legislators in the Japanese Diet finally considered this issue in 1997.[2] Until questions about the validity of the brain-death standard can be clarified, organ transplantation has been suspended with the exception of more than one hundred cases of live liver-section transplants between family members and numerous cases of kidney transplants from a living family member or from the cardiac dead. In response to the current prohibition of organ transplantation, many an individual has gone abroad to seek an organ transplant.

On December 10, 1993, the Ministry of Health and Welfare announced that when a law is passed in the parliament allowing the brain-death standard and the taking of organs from brain-dead bodies, it will enact a supplementary special provision to the current health insurance system to cover the cost (estimated at 100,000 to 200,000 yen per day) incurred during the period between brain death and removal of organs. National insurance would also cover the cost until cardiac death after brain death in a case where the organs are not to be donated and the brain-death standard is not employed. This provision purports to eliminate one of the objections to organ transplantation but also indicates the prevailing attitude of indecisiveness about brain death.

In light of the impending enactment of a law concerning brain death and organ transplants, on January 11, 1994, the Ministry of Health and Welfare submitted guidelines for the procedure of organ transplantation from a brain-dead donor to the Interparty Conference on Organ Transplant (which has been discussing the legalization of organ transplantation and brain death). The gist of the proposal for a new law includes the following: the irreversible cessation of brain functions, as examined and determined according to the ministry's Takeuchi criteria (1985) will be regarded as death, and, in the absence of written consent from the brain-dead donor, the surviving family can give consent to organ donation by guessing the wishes of the deceased. This consent shall be written in the presence of an attorney, free of any pressure from physicians. The guidelines give six justifiable reasons by which the survivors can consent to donation:

1. The donor used to speak positively about organ transplant.
2. He or she was inquiring about a donor card.
3. He or she was positive about giving organs and tissues (like giving blood often and registering with an eyebank, etc.), even though the organ(s) requested for an actual donation is not the one he or she was considering giving.
4. He or she had a wish to contribute to medicine and medical science.
5. He or she wanted part of his or her body to live on.
6. He or she did not speak specifically about organ transplantation, but judging from his or her words and behavior, the family can conjecture that he or she had somehow expressed a wish to donate his or her organs.

The guidelines obviously set out to promote organ transplantation. The potentially most controversial is the sixth point, which could allow family members' subjective impression or empathy to be the ground for consenting to donation. The composition of an ethics committee whose purpose would be to represent the potential donor, and the restriction of institutions permitted to remove organs for the purpose of donation to only a handful, must also be debated. Because societal recognition and the development of a transplant coordinator are only beginning to grow, physicians in charge (including emergency-room doctors) are faced with the difficult question of how to take the initiative in asking the bereaved about the possibility of organ donation.

In addition to all these problems, this proposal does not take into account the possible differences of opinion among the surviving family members, according to whether their loved one has suffered brain death or cardiac death. Considering the Japanese viewpoint, this is rather a crucial point that deserves careful consideration.

An Analysis of the Situation

The number of people who see brain death as the death of a human being has steadily but slowly increased over the years. According to a recent survey, 53.6 percent agree that a brain-dead person is dead, which is 20 points up from 10 years ago; 70 percent support the promotion of heart and liver transplants; and 60 percent are in favor of legalizing organ transplants (*Yomiuri Shimbun,* Jan. 13, 1994). Whether we view this increasing support for the brain-death standard as an encouraging sign or not, the slow increase is very intriguing and demands that we take a good look at the complexity of the situation. It might be beneficial to ponder the significance of our findings, for although this is a Japanese case, one could surmise that many other non-Western traditional societies are faced with similar problems.

For one thing, it is clear that we have yet to institute a law regulating the method of determining human death or to establish a framework within which organ transplantation should be handled. Legislation will come about in the not-too-distant future, probably allowing for both brain and cardiac standards of determining death.

In addition, technical frameworks that will ensure fair distribution of organs need to be developed. Also, ethics committee and institutional review boards will have to be run so as to be accountable to public critical review, a requirement being prepared for through the training of transplant coordinators and efforts by ethics committees to study better ways of conducting ethics.

The least articulated and most difficult factor lies, it seems, in the cultural and traditional ethos of the people. Think, for example, about advance directives concerning brain death and organ transplants. At the moment, there is no nationwide system such as the completion of donor cards for expressing, recognizing, and honoring one's wishes. Although the general public is becoming aware of the possibility of drafting advance directives, it is not yet a well-developed option (some 40 thousand people are registered at the present). One factor that may explain such reluctance to actually create one's own advance directive is that the national ethos is not ready for the idea of prescribing the way one's dead body should be handled due to a traditional belief that such a matter is out of one's discretion.

One survey recently conducted among physicians seems to reflect the sentiment of the general public concerning this point. To the question of whether patients think it proper to donate their own organs, 38.3 percent of doctors (general practitioners) said they would donate, whereas 38.5 percent responded that they would leave the decision to their family. Those who responded "No" for various reasons or for no reason at all totaled 6.4 percent, and 12.8 percent were undecided (*Nikkei Medical* 1985).

Another study (conducted by Tomio Kinoshita, Professor Emeritus in Social Psychology, Kyoto University, and others) indicates that, while the majority of the 960 citizens questioned in the Osaka area had correct knowledge about brain death, 55 percent said that it is hard for them to give up on a brain-dead but warm-blooded patient. Two-thirds or 65 percent of the respondents said that, once diagnosed as brain dead, they would understand it as death as far as they themselves were concerned, but only 41 percent agreed to the same proposition if the person involved was a loved one. Likewise, although only 33 percent indicated that they would hope for an organ transplant for themselves, 61 percent would want it for a loved one. Two-thirds of the inquirers thought that there could be both brain and cardiac criteria for death. Very few agreed to the idea of using dead bodies as resources, such as for the sale of organs (*Kyoto Shimbun,* Dec. 21, 1993). It is then easy to see that the Japanese are reticent to accept advance directives. Possibly, that may explain why the Ministry of Health and Welfare committee of specialists who wrote up the proposal described above included an ambiguous clause (the sixth point).

It is the family to whom people turn for crucial decisions, especially those concerning life and death. One recalls the clause in the final report that the Consultation Committee on Biomedical Ethics submitted to its governing body, the Japan Medical Association, in January 1988, and that was accepted as the official view of the association on brain-death issues: the actual moment of death (using brain-death criteria) will be determined with respect for, and with the consent of, the patient him- or herself or the family. The inclusion of the family's wishes in determining the moment of brain death seems to compromise the objectivity of the physicians' findings, but the aim of such inclusion was to honor the wishes of the bereaved in regard to a possible removal of organs and the turning off of life-support machines (Kato 1986). In conjunction with these findings, the following facts should also be considered: Most kidney transplants are performed between blood relatives, and transplantation from the dead accounts for only 26 percent. Very few of these donors (20 of approximately 1,100 dead donors through the end of 1991) had expressed their desire, in the form of a donor card or otherwise, to donate an organ postmortem. A number of live liver section transplants have been performed since November 1989, but the majority of the transplants have been between family members.

Conclusion

A coherent system of ethics prevailed in the premodern period, drawn mainly from Confucian and Buddhist ethical teachings that were contextual with the feudal social structure and based primarily on premodern economic life. The onslaught of modern Western values, embedded in technoscientific culture and society, ranged from the material view of the human body to a belief in the autonomy of individuals. This invasion of ideas has jolted the Japanese tremendously, breaking into pieces a public code of ethics and fragmenting a traditional ethos that had previously instructed the common people how to cope properly with birth, aging, illnesses, and death as respectable Japanese and as good ancestors-to-be.

Today, advanced medical technoscience has forced us to face the need to determine, in the name of individual rights and autonomy, the kind of medicine we desire or can afford. This advanced technological force, backed by the capitalist principles of free enterprise and cost-benefit analysis and counterbalanced by socialized medicine in differing degrees from one developed country to another, of course promises us much in the way of lessening or obscuring our pain and suffering. But modern medicine thus almost enslaves us by forcing us to acquiesce to its positivist outlook on life and on being in general, often depriving us of the *shizen* sense of nature, of which we are part and partaker. Medicine is becoming the modern affluent society's obsession and appears to further biologize and atomize people by segmenting their bodies and minds.

Advance directives are a necessary part of this type of medicine and the society that enables it to flourish. Advance directives have to be implemented in Japanese society, too, although it will take a long time before we come to see these instruments as effective and meaningful. Proponents of advance directives will have to find a way to incorporate the role of the family, even though the shape of the family itself is undergoing significant changes.

One final comment: What has been said above may not be peculiar to the Japanese but may be rather common among non-Western peoples. There are important factors other than mere economics that must be considered if people living in the North are willing to reflect on the significance of advance directives in a global health care context.

Notes

1. The Japanese word *awai* and its collateral words (such as *aida, baai*) are quite indicative of their ethos. (*Awai* and *aida* come from the root *afu* [to meet], which signifies space/time between two beings and, further, relatedness and relationship.) The word for humans, *ningen* (although composed of two Chinese characters, human and between/among, thereby signifying earthly human world in Chinese, the word lost this meaning in Japanese), individual or collective, involves a concept of human being as *Mitsein.* In the traditional conception, a being was not so much determined by natural law as by its participatory interaction with other beings (humans foremost, of course, but also other beings). A life's acts are conditioned by the milieu and physiological conditions, other beings' response and reaction, yet they would as such reverberate through the world, be remembered, and mold the (especially human) world into a certain (although historically developing) shape. The world of beings is closely interwoven, and no single being can claim to its being apart from other beings. A human being's raison d'être cannot solely draw upon the cerebral cortex or a collection of "rights," which modern civilization has accorded him and her. Nor is it sound in the Japanese ethos to think of a human death only in terms of brain death that technology judges, and then the brain-dead form is disposed of. The loss of *awai* in between life and death, the living and the dying, creates a profound warp in a Japanese conception of life, at least to some, not a few, people.

2. A long-awaited law was finally passed by the Diet in June 1997, after three years of delay and involving considerable changes. It permits brain death as the definition of the death of a person only when (1) the person has left his or her will in writing that he or she accepts brain death as a definition of death and is willing to donate his or her organs and (2) when the family also endorses his or her will thus written. If either condition is lacking, the law does not define brain death as death and prohibits the harvesting of organs. The law became effective as of October 16, 1997.

References

Doi, Takeo. 1973. *The Anatomy of Dependence.* Translated by John Bester. Tokyo: Kodansha International. Originally published as *Amae no kozo*. Tokyo: Kobundo, 1972.

Imanishi, Kinji. 1990. *Shizengaku no tenkai* (The Development of Natural History). Tokyo: Kodansha.

Nihon Ishikai Zasshi (Journal of the Japanese Medical Association). 1985. Vol. 94, no. 11.

Kato, Ichiro, Takeuchi Kazuo, Ota Kazuo, and Nimi Ikufumi. 1986. *Noshi, zoki ishoku to jinken* (Brain Death, Organ Transplants, and Human Rights). Tokyo: Yuhikaku.

Kimura, Bin. 1984. *Jiko, aida, jikan* (Self, Between, Time). Tokyo: Kobundo.

———. 1988. *Aida* (Between). Tokyo: Kobundo.

Koseisho Noshi kenkyu-han (Ministry of Health and Welfare Study Group on Brain Death). 1985. *Noshi no hantei shishin oyobi hantei kijun* (Guidelines for Judging Brain Death and Its Criteria; so-called Takeuchi Criteria). Tokyo: Ministry of Health and Welfare.

Watsuji, Tetsuro. 1934. *Ningen no gaku toshiteno rinrigaku* (Ethics as Study of Man). Tokyo: Iwanami Shoten.

———. 1961. *Climate and Culture: A Philosophical Study.* Translated by Geoffrey Bownas. New York: Greenwood Press. Originally published as *Fudo*. Tokyo: Iwanami Shoten, 1935.

Yanagita, Kunio. 1988. *About Our Ancestors: The Japanese Family System.* Translated by Fanny H. Mayer and Ishiwara Yasuyo. New York: Greenwood Press. Originally published as *Senzo no hanashi.* Tokyo: Chikuma Shobo, 1946.

Appendix

Model Forms of Medical Directives and Advance Care Documents

Overview

Hans-Martin Sass

Given different degrees and methods of imposing a person's own values, wishes, and visions on future medical treatment before and during the process of dying, different models have been developed. The first type is the classical form of a living will, which provides an opportunity to reject in advance certain life-sustaining intervention (in some cases termed extraordinary means). More recently, the basic concept of a living will has been expanded to encompass those forms that establish value histories and other narrative information that requires one to translate general convictions into the paradigm of a specific scenario. Another burgeoning type of advance document is the disease-specific advance directive, which is often part of a specific long-term care plan for chronic disease. Naturally, each form of advance care document has its own advantages and disadvantages. There are increasing interdisciplinary bioethical and clinical efforts to improve the validity, accessibility, prevalence, and actual use of these instruments.

1. *The Living Will Model.* Living will forms that are short and use terminology such as "no futile treatment" or "no artificial means" are difficult to translate into specific clinical scenarios. In addition, they do not give detailed or significant insight into the person's reasoning for rejecting or requesting life-prolonging or other interventions; some religious forms, however, use religious language that may shed light on the person's fundamental beliefs that may underlie such decisions. Rejectionist living will forms have been enacted in most states of the United States; most of them include the possibility of designating a proxy. The Choice in Dying form (No. 1) and the form in the hymnbook of the Bavarian Lutheran Church (No. 3) represent classical models for a nondetailed living will in nonreligious and religious forms, respectively. It has been argued that extended and detailed forms may hurt more than help in extending the prospective patient's values into the yet-unknown scenarios of dementia, preterminal, and terminal situations. In particular, forms drafted primarily for legal purposes in liability cases are rarely informative for specific clinical situations and therefore of no help in clinical decision making.

2. *The Proxy Model.* The durable power of attorney for a trusted family member, friend, or other representative is a model that, instead of voicing preferences or directing others in yet-unclear future scenarios, designates another person to make decisions when the time is ripe and the circumstances are clear. The proxy model probably is the model of choice if the designated person (1) knows the person, his or her values, wishes, and attitudes well, and (2) has good judgment, communication skills, and adequate knowledge to assess complex medical situations. The proxy model, in written or oral form or assumed by the family or

a family member or friend, seems to be accepted nearly everywhere except in cases of the most conservative paternalistic attitudes of physicians. The representative's personal authority, without which a proxy's legal mandate may be undercut, is indispensible. Cultural and familial specifics determine whether or not a respected family member or the family as a whole best meets the requirements to be a good proxy. Representatives who are available to make decisions at the right time need not confront the theoretical and practical problems associated with advance risk assessment for future unknown situations. Powers and duties of the proxy can be broad, unspecified, or spelled out in detail. Traditional proxy models name one or two designates and in many cases a substitute, whereas some exclude certain persons by name whom others might likely be considered to be the natural or logical representatives. But as the directions in living wills can be either general or differentiated and specific, proxy forms can specify which individuals shall serve in which capacity and in regard to which problems or conflicts (No. 8). Therefore, they can be extended to include eventually the recommendation or even the request to the designated proxy to seek advice from other designees as "value experts" or special "medical experts." A value expert can be another trusted friend, the pastor of the congregation, a priest, or philosopher; a medical expert can be a specialist who already knows the patient or to whom the patient will entrust complicated technical or clinical decision making. Upgraded in such a way by subproxies, the proxy model can become as efficient for detailed clinical decision making as the instructional medical directive but without the shortcomings that are sometimes associated with inflexibility of instructions and directives.

3. *The Value History Model.* Value statements and lists of treatment preferences, on the other hand, are more direct and more personal than proxy representation ever can be (Nos. 9-11). The risks associated with value statements are that (1) they might be too general to be translated into a specific clinical situation and (2) their interpretation requires a high degree of experience in differential ethics and clinical hermeneutics, for which health care providers have not yet been educated and trained. Treatment preferences, if given without a situational context, are often difficult to interpret. On the other hand, if presented within a specific clinical context, they might be too inflexible to allow for treating the patient in his or her best interest, as this interest might be defined by other statements of the patient or voiced by the proxy.

4. *The Medical Instruction Model.* Instructional medical directives, which give health care providers specific and strict directives for specific situations, focus on details of intervention and nonintervention (Nos. 5–6). For laypersons, it is very difficult to envision clearly the technical as well as ethical parameters of such future medical situations. Detailed and treatment-specific medical instruc-

tions and directives carry a high risk to those who execute them. There seem to be four scenarios in which detailed instructional directives are better than general and vague ones: (a) if individuals are very determined and are strong-willed, know the issues or have received sufficient professional support, and do not want to burden others with major decisions; (b) where religious or philosophical convictions can be directly translated into a very specific action, such as the pregnancy clause in the Kyoto Women's University form (No. 13); (c) if certain chronic diseases are present, the likelihood and the detailed parameters of which can well be predicted, such as in the case of patients with amyotrophic lateral sclerosis (No. 15), or if specific future medical situations and the options are spelled out very clearly and have been discussed and explained by a medical expert (No. 12).

5. *The combination model.* Various forms combine the instruments of designated representative, value statements, and directives for treatment (Nos. 16-18). Combination forms try to prevent the disadvantages of the more basic forms. As advance directives may, for good reason, differ from person to person and from culture to culture, there cannot be one uniform instrument that is applicable to and appropriate for everyone. Courts and state legislators should accept and welcome different forms and approaches whose purposes are to express valid wishes and preferences for future treatment and to share values that shall govern treatment. But complex forms require complex instructions that explain how to reconcile conflicts between the proxy section and the directive or value section; those conflicts can be reduced by using simpler forms or by presenting possible solutions to such conflicts within the instrument itself.

On the one hand, the establishment of valid advance medical care documents primarily presents a challenge to lay and expert attitudes in the medical field, whereas matters of administration, regulation, and legal actions and parameters seem to be secondary. On the other hand, the role of law in ensuring the validity of advance care documents in the clinical encounter and in alleviating concerns about legal liability that often incline physicians toward overtreatment should not be underestimated. Bioethical and interdisciplinary work at the crossroads of medical, legal, cultural, and personal responsibility and decision making at the end of life have just begun but are expanding rapidly. The following samples, representing different approaches to reasoning, validation, clear expression, and flexibility toward unknown future scenarios, are not recipes to choose from but, rather, are raw materials for further debate and interdisciplinary research.

1. Euthanasia Educational Council: A Classical Living Will

[This form, originally developed by the Euthanasia Educational Council in 1974, resembles the major feature of a living will: a refusal of "extraordinary medical means" that extend life at its end under certain conditions. Most living wills also include the nomination of a designated proxy. The Euthanasia Educational Council later changed its name to Society for the Right to Die, now Choice in Dying, 200 Varick Street, New York, N.Y. 10014. In the United States, most states have legislated state-specific advance directive forms based on this model.]

Living Will and Health Care Proxy

To my family, my physician, my lawyer, my clergy; to any medical faculty in whose care I happen to be; to any individual who may become responsible for my health, welfare, or affairs:

Death is as much a reality as birth, growth, maturity, and old age; it is the one certainty of life. If the time comes when I, ________________________, can no longer take part in decisions for my own future, let this statement stand as an expression of my wishes, while I am still of sound mind.

If the situation should arise in which there is no reasonable expectation of my recovery from physical or mental disability, I request that I be allowed to die and not be kept alive by artificial means or "heroic measures." I do not fear death itself as much as the indignities of deterioration, dependence, and hopeless pain. I, therefore, ask that medication be mercifully administered to me to alleviate suffering even though this may hasten the moment of death.

This request is made after careful consideration. I hope you who care for me will feel morally bound to follow its mandate. I recognize that this appears to place a heavy responsibility on you, but it is with the intention of relieving you of such responsibility and of placing it on myself in accordance with my strong convictions, that this statement is made.

Signed ________________________

Dated ________________________

Witness ________________________

Witness ________________________

Copies of this request have been given to ________________________

____

____

____

2. County Council for Senior Citizens, Böblingen, Germany: A German Senior Citizens' Group Model of a Living Will

[This form was developed by the County Council for Senior Citizens in Böblingen, Germany (Kreisseniorenrat beim Kreissozialamt Böblingen, Parkstrasse 16, 71034 Böblingen); it was translated by Deborah Vester, Esq. The Kreisseniorenrat office provides an information hotline and individual counseling for those seeking assistance with drafting advance directives. A footnote on the pamphlet reads: "The advance directive on the reverse side of this document is also available as a pocket-sized card. Upon request, we can laminate this card for you. Please fill out and sign the enclosed card and send it to the Kreissozialamt (County Social Welfare Office), Geschäftsstelle des Kreisseniorenrates (Office of the County Council for Senior Citizens). We can also help you fill out the information (Landratsamt [State Administration Office], Room 170, Tel. 07031/663-234). Your information will not be electronically documented."]

Living Will

Last name _______________ First name _______________

Date of birth _____________ Place of birth ____________

City ____________________ Street ___________________

Should I become incapacitated to the extent that I am no longer capable of making decisions or judgments, I refuse to accept any type of treatment that would result only in prolonging the dying process or my suffering. I want my life to end in peace and dignity.

The following persons and/or physician of my choice must be consulted before any decisions are made with respect to further necessary measures or treatment:

Last name ________________ First name _______________

Address ________________

Signature ________________

The persons above confirm with their signature that they have knowledge of my advance directive and that I have signed this last disposition in full possession of my faculties and on my own free will.

Place ______________________ Date __________________

Signature __________________

3. Bavarian Lutheran Church: A Christian Patient's Request

[This form was developed and is distributed by the Bavarian Lutheran Church (Landeskirchenrat der Evangelisch-Lutherischen Kirche in Baveria, Box 200751, 80007 Munich, Germany). It is reprinted in the official hymnbook of the Lutheran churches in the German states of Bavaria and Thuringia; see *Evangelisches Kirchengesangbuch: Ausgabe für die Evangelisch-Lutherischen Kirchen in Bayern und Thüringen* (Munich: Verlag Evangelischer Pressedienst o.J.), pp. 1486–87).]

A Christian Request

I believe that my time is in God's hands. As long as there is a realistic chance of sustaining my life under tolerable conditions, I expect medical and nursing care to the extent of all appropriate measures. In any case, I expect sufficient treatment of pain. If possible, I would like to remain in my familiar surroundings. In the event that I,

____________________ ____________________

Name Date of birth

am no longer capable of setting forth or expressing my will due to illness, accident, or other circumstances, I hereby declare that I refuse active aid in dying; however, I also do not want my life to be prolonged at all costs. Therefore, I request that no life-sustaining measures be applied which will only prevent me from dying in peace. In such a situation I request Christian support. Should a court be required to order the appointment of a welfare officer as my legal representative who is to be responsible for me and my affairs, I request that

__________________ Name __________________ Date of birth

__________________ Address __________________ Telephone

be appointed. Before a court order, the treating physicians are to be released from their physician-patient privilege with respect to my legal representative and are obligated to discuss all necessary measures with the aforementioned in my place.

________________ Signature ______________________ Place, date

COMMENT

The possibilities created by modern medicine have contributed to the prolonging of life, even when there is no chance of returning to a state of tolerable living. At the same time, there is a clear appeal for the shortening of life. This is where the Christian advance directive comes into play. It is an attempt to achieve a compromise between a senseless prolongation of the dying process and an irresponsible shortening of life.

The advance directive—an advance declaration of an individual's will:

Whenever a physician has to make a medical decision with regard to a patient who is unconscious or no longer capable of declaring his or her own will, the physician is required to establish the alleged will of the patient.

For this reason, it makes sense for a person to prepare an advance directive in "days of good health" which will later help the physician make a responsible decision.

Legally, an advance directive serves as an indication of a patient's alleged will. Of course, the final decision to be made lies in the hands of the physician.

Person of trust and Christian support: A person of trust should be named in the advance directive. This person has the role of supporting the patient and discussing with the physician the necessary measures to be taken.

The church has an obligation to patients and their family members to offer them Christian support through pastoral care. All attempts must be made to ensure "death in peace."

WHAT SHOULD ONE DO?

1. The patient should locate a person of trust as soon as possible.

2. The patient should discuss and fill out the advance directive together with the person of trust.

3. Under certain circumstances, subsequent additions might be necessary. These additions can be notarized if need be.

4. The advance directive belongs with the patient's identification papers. The person of trust retains a copy of the directive. For legal reasons, the person of trust is referred to in the directive as the "legal representative."

5. Should the case of patient incapacity described above occur, the person of trust is to contact the physician or vice versa. The physician can be assured of the validity of the person of trust's role as "legal representative" of the patient where the advance directive corresponds to the copy presented by the person of trust.

4. Japan Society for Dying with Dignity: To My Family, Friends, and Medical Attendants

[This is the official translation of the Dying with Dignity Declaration, drafted in 1979 for its members.]

To My Family, My Friends, and My Medical Attendants

In preparation of a time when I might face an incurable illness and death is near, I declare that my wishes are as follows:

This declaration is made by me at a time when I am of sound mind. Therefore, this is effective and in full force unless I revoke or withdraw this declaration in writing while I am mentally sound.

1. I request that medical technology should not be used to artificially prolong my life if modern medicine concludes that my disease is an irreversible or incurable one and my life is certified to be terminal.

2. I request, however, that effective pain reduction should be fully achieved by any method, such as from the use of narcotics, etc., even though such treatment may shorten my life.

3. I request that all life-sustaining procedures be withdrawn if I lie for several months in a condition known as a "persistent vegetative state."

I express my heartfelt thanks to all those concerned who will faithfully realize my requests. I further declare that I hereby absolve these people from any civil liability arising from any actions taken in response to and in fulfillment of the terms of this declaration.

Signature ______________________ Date_________________

5. Japanese Citizens' Association for Thinking about the Terminal Stage Medical Directive

[This form of a detailed medical directive was developed by the Citizens' Association for Thinking about the Terminal Stage [Shuumatsuki o Kangaeru Shimin no Kai]; it was translated by Rihito Kimura.]

Terminal Stage Declaration

In my mentally and physically sound situation and with my voluntary intention, I express the following wishes and declare them to my family members and medical providers in preparing for my terminal stage and death. I expect that this declaration will be honored as my final intention by my family members and physicians unless I abandon it or I make documents to retract my statement.

1. If the diagnosis was made that death is inevitable due to my disease, then the name of the disease, its character, and how long I will be able to live with dignity as a human being should be mentioned as suggested in the following:

   1. Please let me know the information in its entirety without hiding anything.

   2. Please tell my family members how it stands, but not me.

   3. I can't decide whether or not I would like to know now. As my ideas will possibly change in the future, I would like to reserve the expression of my wishes at this moment.

2. When my death becomes imminent, I go into an irreversible coma, or enter a persistent vegetative state:

   1. I reject life-prolonging measures, application of resuscitation techniques, and hooking up or continuing the use of life-sustaining apparatus.

   2. Please prolong my life up to last moment by applying high-technology medical treatment and life-sustaining measures.

3. When all other alternative treatments become meaningless, and the only option is to accept the natural course of the disease:

   1. I want to die in my own home. I accept only that medical and nursing care that is possible at home.

   2. I want to die in this hospital.

   3. Other choice _____________

4. If I become brain-dead:

   1. I recognize that this is my death.

   2. I do not recognize this as my death.

3. I agree to donate my organs.
4. I do not want to donate my organs.
5. Other additional wishes: ____________

To observe a faithful fulfillment of the above declaration, I hereby nominate the following person(s) as my proxy for making medical decisions, including prolongation of life, continuation or withdrawal of life-sustaining machines, etc.

Name ____________________ Relationship to me ________________
Telephone __________________ Address ______________________

The result and responsibility of the actions in accordance with the above declaration totally rest with me.

Signature____________________
Year ________ Month _________ Date ________ Birth date ______________
Address ________________________________ Telephone ________________

COMMENT

Please mark X in each square according to your wish and sign with your seal stamped on this document. Our association keeps this document on file with a registered number and will mail back two copies, one to be kept by you and the other to be delivered to your proxy. If it becomes necessary, this document should be shown to the attending physician by the person himself or herself, or by the proxy. If consideration to the stated preferences is not given or the wishes are disregarded, please let us know your registered number and name, together with the name and address of the attending physician. Our association would then seek the understanding of the attending physician.

6. Rabbinal Assembly of Conservative Judaism's Committee on Jewish Law and Standards Model of a Living Will

[This document was prepared by Rabbi Avram Reisner and is one of two living wills that were accepted by the R. A. Committee on Jewish Law and Standards in 1991. See *United Synagogue Review* 44 (2): 22-23. It is written in religious language and expresses specific religious visions, beliefs, and hopes. In contrast to the simple and nonspecific model of the Bavarian-Lutheran Church, this form is very specific and detailed in its medical instruction.]

Introduction and Comment

In our social and medical circumstances, it is increasingly clear that provision should be made for our medical treatment in the last stages of life. As we are called upon to undertake such provision, we should be guided not only, nor preeminently, by legislators and lawyers, but by our commitment to Judaism, by Jewish law and ethics. To that end, "Instructions for the Valley of the Shadow" has been constructed to serve as a halakhically proper medical directive (or living will).

This document must be signed in the presence of witnesses, and the signature of the designated representative(s) should be solicited wherever possible. It is further suggested that the document be dated and the signature notarized, and that the document be reviewed periodically. Whether this document and these procedures will be recognized in every local jurisdiction remains to be seen. Consultation with a lawyer familiar with local regulations is advisable.

As we undertake to instruct our care in advance against a time of need, may God grant us health and wisdom, and may we be blessed further never to see such need.

Instructions for the Valley of the Shadow: A Medical Directive (Living Will)

Name ____________________________

I live and I die by God's will. That fact is as clear to me as the sun at noonday and as the stars on a moonless night. It is my wish in all things to live in a manner that graces God's image, to carry out God's instructions and, when all that is to be said has been said, and all that is to be done has been done, to quit this life upon God's call.

To that end, I set out the following guidelines toward my treatment should I be taken seriously ill and be unable to express my wishes at that time.

It is my wish and instruction that all prudent medical treatment should be extended to me with the aim of effecting my recovery. Should that be deemed impossible, all nutrition, hydration, medication and necessary surgical procedures should be continued where these are understood to be effective measures for extending my life.

Medical knowledge, however, may find itself at a loss as to which form of treatment is best for me, or whether a given treatment will be helpful or harmful. In such circumstances, I call upon my designated representative, in consultation with my physician and in accordance with these guidelines, to choose a course of action that protects me from unnecessary pain and degradation while pursuing the goal of life.

Specifically, I would instruct as follows (choose one):

1. Surgery:

   ( ) I would consent to reasonable surgery as proposed by my physicians to effect my comfort.

   ( ) All surgery carries an implicit risk through anesthesia, the introduction of infection and through trauma to the body. I do not consent to such risk save in pursuit of the immediate and overriding demands of extending my life and of freedom from unbearable pain.

2. Amputation:

   ( ) I am prepared to lose a limb if in the best medical judgment of my physicians this is necessary to prolong my life.

   ( ) There may come a time when my condition is such that there is no reasonable expectation of my recovery and when my physicians feel that my life is threatened by infection, and that the most effective defense lies in amputation of the affected limb. I find the notion of amputation in such a circumstance unbearable and am convinced that I will not survive the loss of a limb in such a weakened state. I prefer all other treatments to fight the infection, save where the limb has already been substantially severed.

Nasogastric Feeding:

   ( ) I will accept the maintenance of nutrition and hydration through a nasogastric tube. I understand that that may at some point require restraint so that I not dislodge the tubes.

   ( ) I find reliance on nutrition forcibly provided through tubes emplaced in my nose to be abhorrent. I fear the pain and the risk of aspiration. I prefer to feed myself. Where that is not possible, let arrangements be made so that I may be fed orally or provided nutrition and hydration intravenously or in other ways acceptable to me.

4. Surgically Emplaced Feeding Tubes:

   ( ) I will accept the maintenance of nutrition and hydration through surgically emplaced feeding tubes. I understand the risks involved in this type of surgery.

( ) I find reliance on nutrition provided through tubes emplaced surgically in my stomach or intestines to be abhorrent. I fear the risks of surgery and aspiration. I prefer to feed myself. Where that is not possible, let arrangements be made so that I may be fed orally or provided nutrition and hydration intravenously or in other ways acceptable to me.

5. Aggressive Chemotherapy:

( ) I wish above all to live. To that end, I would undertake any regimen, however difficult, which stands a reasonable chance of helping me.

( ) Aggressive chemotherapy can be most debilitating and destructive. While I desire to fight my disease with all the tools at my command, I do not wish to undertake treatments which are futile, untested or unlikely to offer meaningful, measurable results.

6. Diagnostic Tests:

( ) I wish to have available all possible information concerning my condition. I consent to diagnostic tests as ordered by my physician.

( ) I wish to be cured or, where that is not possible, to extend my life. I do not wish simply to know the etiology or ramifications of my illness. Let me not be poked and prodded save in the specific interest of treatment.

7. Knowledge of My Condition:

( ) I wish to know all relevant facts of my condition. With knowledge, I shall better be able to find comfort.

( ) I do not wish to know all the details of my condition. I fear that such knowledge will diminish my will to live and will cast a shadow over the time left to me.

8. Mechanical Life Support:

( ) I consider that as long as I breathe, even with the aid of life support equipment, and my brain is still active, my God-given life has not yet been called back. These technologies should therefore be maintained. I recognize, however, that if the total absence of brain activity can be verified, I may be considered dead despite mechanically induced respiration and heartbeat.

( ) I consider mechanical means of life support to be impediments to my death at God's behest, even though they may prolong biological function, if they cannot contribute to my recovery or return to unaided functioning. Therefore, I instruct that they be forgone or withdrawn when my physician and designated representative jointly conclude that they offer no reasonable chance of return to unaided functioning.

9. Cardiopulmonary Resuscitation:

( ) Should my cardiopulmonary system fail for any reason, in every case I would like the utmost done in my behalf.

( ) If my heart has stopped beating and my condition is such that there is no reasonable expectation of my recovery, I would consider cardiopulmonary resuscitation (CPR) to be contrary to God's will, and therefore ask that my body not be subjected to such handling. In such a case, I would consider a Do Not Resuscitate order to be in order.

10. Pain Relief:

( ) I trust that all possible pain relief will be provided to me, save that I do not wish to accept significant risk that my death will be hastened thereby. I will accept considerable periods of sedation to avoid pain.

( ) I trust that all possible pain relief will be provided to me, save that I do not wish my death to be hastened thereby. If I remain alert, however, I am prepared to accept a reasonable amount of pain in order to maintain my awareness.

11. Hospital or Home Care:

( ) I prefer to be supported by the best medical technology. To that end, if my death is not sudden, I expect that it will occur in the confines of a hospital.

( ) To the extent that it is practicable and not an undue hardship upon my family, I would prefer to die at home or in a congenial supportive care facility rather than a hospital. When hospital care is no longer able with confidence to effect my recovery, I would prefer such comfort-oriented care, with the clear understanding that all palliative and essential medical care will be continued.

12. Organ Donation:

( ) When I die, I hereby empower my representative to effect the donation of any or all of my vital organs for the purpose of transplant only. The rest of my remains should then be buried in a Jewish cemetery in accordance with local Jewish custom.

13. Autopsy:

( ) I understand that governmental authorities may require an autopsy in certain circumstances. If such an autopsy is performed, I ask that it be conducted with all possible respect and that all of my body parts subsequently be buried in a Jewish cemetery in accordance with local Jewish custom.

Should I be incapacitated, I name as my representative to make medical decisions in accordance with these directives, along with my physicians, my ________________, currently residing at ____________________________.

( ) I have obtained his/her consent to serve in this capacity.
Should s/he be unavailable to serve in this capacity, I designate in his/her stead ________________, currently residing at ____________________________.

( ) I have obtained his/her consent to serve in this capacity.

I would prefer, if possible, that these matters be reviewed with my rabbi,

________________.

Nothing in this directive should be construed, God forbid, as a wish to die; only as a wish to live in accordance with God's desires. Should this directive be unclear in any way, it is my wish that a rabbi be consulted and that s/he consider my situation in light of the guidance offered by the Rabbinical Assembly (3080 Broadway, New York, N.Y. 10027) in the Committee on Jewish Law and Standards responsum of December 1990, "A Halakhic Ethic of Care for the Terminally Ill," *Conservative Judiasm Magazine* 43, no. 3 (spring 1991).

As God is my rock and my fortress and my deliverer, so may God be my refuge, my shield and my salvation, forever.

Being of sound mind, I hereby affix my name to the above declaration.

Signed ________________________
Signature of designated representative ________________________
Signature of alternative representative ________________________

Witness ________________________
Witness ________________________

Notary's Seal

Dated: ________________________
Reaffirmed: ____________________
Reaffirmed: ____________________

7. OMEGA Friendship Contract

[OMEGA is an incorporated association of concerned citizens in Germany. The Friendship Contract (*Freundschaftsvertrag*) was translated by Deborah Vester, Esq.]

Friendship Contract

____

Last name First name

____

Address

hereinafter "friend," and

____

Last name First name

____

Address

hereinafter "friendship recipient,"
have entered into the following contract ("friendship contract") effective as of today. The parties are obligated according to the best of their knowledge and good will to meet their obligations under this agreement and uphold this agreement with respect to third parties using their best efforts. They agree to undertake all action necessary to ensure the effectiveness of this contract.

1. Purpose of this Contract

This contract seeks to regulate the support relationship between an ill patient (friendship recipient) and a person of his choice (friend). The friend becomes the support and companion of the ill patient; he represents him with respect to third parties (physicians, nurses, institutions, etc.) to the extent that the friendship recipient desires this or himself is no longer capable of asserting his rights.

2. Obligations of the Friend

The aforementioned friend is obligated

- To maintain complete confidentiality with respect to all information relating to the friendship recipient to the extent that the information in question is not necessary for carrying out the purpose of this contract;
- To be available at all times within the constraints of his professional and other personal obligations;

- To refrain from taking long trips, vacations, etc., apart from the times which are to be agreed upon with the friendship recipient at three-month intervals as well as other absences resulting from professional or other personal obligations. All absences resulting from professional and other personal obligations are to be reported without delay to the friendship recipient;
- To be able to be reached within reason (telephone number, address, etc.);
- To comply with the required measures of support pursuant to the conception and methodology of the Association for Aid and Accompaniment in Dying (Vereinigung für Sterbebeistand und Sterbebegleitung) "OMEGA—Living with Dying" as well as to the extent determined by the friendship recipient and the best efforts of the friend himself;
- To cooperate with persons and institutions as agreed upon with the friendship recipient.

3. Rights of the Friendship Recipient

The friendship contract does not terminate any rights of the friendship recipient. The friendship recipient remains free to establish similar relationships with other persons. Nonetheless, the friend should be informed as best as possible about such relationships so that no conflicts arise in the event of illness.

4. Effectiveness against Third Parties

The parties to this contract agree that upon presentation of this contract the hospital or any medical/health care personnel is required to consult the friend in all matters and decisions for which the friendship recipient has expressly provided as well as in the event of the total or partial unconsciousness or hearing or speech impairment of the friendship recipient, even in the absence of the express will of the latter. The friendship recipient requires all persons involved in any way in his illness, life, or state of dying to cooperate closely with the aforementioned friend and to support him in the friendship recipient's dying process according to their best efforts.

5. Disclosure Rights of the Friend

The aforementioned friend has the right to demand and receive all information that is necessary for fulfilling the purpose of this contract. The friendship recipient expressly grants the friend the right to ask the recipient himself, all personnel involved in the recipient's treatment, as well as other important persons any questions which have a bearing on the recipient's express or alleged will.

6. Termination of the Contract

Apart from the death of either contracting party, this contract can be canceled or terminated by the express will of the friendship recipient or upon the expiration of a period of three weeks as stipulated by the friend or upon the closing of a new friendship contract (with a new friend).

7. Witnesses to the Contract

The two parties bearing witness to this contract confirm with their signatures below that the parties to the contract are in full possession of their faculties and were capable of entering into the contract at the time of its formation.

8. Legal Consequences

This contract creates no effective legal consequences upon the death of a contracting party or any other termination of the contractual relationship. However, the contracting parties may enter into ancillary agreements (e.g., testamentary powers of representation). Such agreements must be in writing. They may be included in this instrument as an additional agreement (10).

9. Deposit

This contract is deposited with an attorney or the witnesses to the contract.

10. Additional Agreements

____

Signature of the friendship recipient

____________________	____________________
Place	Date

____

Signature of the friend

____________________	____________________
Place	Date

Witnesses to the contract

Last name	First name	Address
Signature		Place, date
Last name	First name	Address
Signature		Place, date

8. A Detailed Form for Designating a Proxy

[This form provides for the designation of more than one proxy or, in addition to the main designee, for additional proxies for specific value-related, clinical, financial, or legal issues, where the designator might want to authorize trusted friends with specific professional expertise in addition to or in support of a prime agent. See Hans-Martin Sass, Frederick O. Bonkovsky, Akira Akabayashi, Rita Kielstein, and Robert S. Olick, "Advance Health Care Documents in Multicultural Perspectives," *Jahrbuch für Recht und Ethik* (Annual Review of Law and Ethics) 4 (1996): 492–93.]

A Detailed Form for Designating a Proxy

1. I hereby designate: Name ______________________________
Address ______________________ City ____________________
Telephone and fax ____________________ as my health care representative (proxy) to make any and all health care decisions for me, including decisions to accept or refuse any treatment, service, or procedure used to diagnose or treat my physical or mental condition, including decisions to provide, withhold, or withdraw life-sustaining measures.

2. If the person I have designated above is unable, unwilling, or unavailable to act as my health care representative, I hereby designate the following person(s) to act as my health care representative, in the following order: 1. __________, 2.__________, 3.__________.

3. If none of the above mentioned persons is able, willing, or available to act as my proxy, I direct that [specify one]: (a) the medical team which has primary responsibility, (b) the physician who has primary responsibility, or (c) an ethics committee of the institution responsible make decisions based on my value profile and list of treatment preferences.

4. I do not wish that the following person(s) be involved in making health care decisions for me: 1. ______________, 2. ______________.

5. I recommend / request that my health care representative seeks advice/and follows advice/in specific medical issues from __________,

- seeks advice/and follows advice in specific religious or ethical issues from ________,
- seeks advice/and follows advice in legal matters from ____________,
- seeks advice/and follows advice in financial matters from __________.

6. If a conflict arises between my health care representative (proxy), those friends and experts I have mentioned under (5) and/or the medical team or physician having primary responsibility, and if their interpretation of my value profile and medical directives varies, I hereby direct that the final authority for decision making is [I specify one]: (a) my health care representative, (b) my family, (c) the phy-

sician who has primary responsibility, (d) the medical team which has primary responsibility, (e) the friend or expert I have mentioned in (5) in his/her field, (f) an ethics committee, (g) a religious advisor of the ________ religion, (h) other: ________________________.

My signature______________ My proxy's signature________________ Date __________
My signature______________ My proxy's signature________________ Redated_________

9. The Value History Form

[This value history form was developed and tested by David Doukas and Laurence McCullough. See D. Doukas and L. McCullough, "The Values History: The Evaluation of the Patient's Values and Advance Directives," *Journal of Family Practice* 32 (1991): 151–53). Primarily a model to establish a patient's values, this form nevertheless is combined with a section allowing for medical directives regarding specific interventions.]

The Value History

Patient Name ____

This Values History serves as a set of my specific value-based directives for various medical interventions. It is to be used in health care circumstances when I may be unable to voice my preferences. These directives shall be made a part of the medical record and used as supplementary to my Living Will.

Values Section

There are several values important in decisions about terminal treatment and care. This section of the Values History invites you to identify your most important values.

BASIC LIFE VALUES

Perhaps the most basic values in this context concern length of life versus quality of life. Which of the following two statements is the most important to you?

____1. I want to live as long as possible, regardless of the quality of life that I experience.

____2. I want to preserve a good quality of life, even if this means that I may not live as long.

QUALITY OF LIFE VALUES

Many values help to define the quality of life that we want to live. The following list contains some that appear to be the most common. Review this list (and feel free to either elaborate on it or add to it) and circle those values that are important to your definition of quality of life.

1. I want to maintain my capacity to think clearly.
2. I want to feel safe and secure.
3. I want to avoid unnecessary pain and suffering.
4. I want to be treated with respect.
5. I want to be treated with dignity when I can no longer speak for myself.
6. I do not want to be an unnecessary burden on my family.

7. I want to be able to make my own decisions.

8. I want to experience a comfortable dying process.

9. I want to be with my loved ones before I die.

10. I want to leave good memories of me to my loved ones.

11. I want to be treated in accord with my religious beliefs and traditions.

12. I want respect shown for my body after I die.

13. I want to help others by making a contribution to medical education and research.

14. Other values or clarification of values above:

Directives Section

Some directives involve simple yes/no decisions. Others provide for the choice of a trial of intervention.

Initials/Date

1. I want to undergo cardiopulmonary resuscitation.

_____Yes

_____No

2. I want to be placed on a ventilator.

_____Yes

_____TRIAL for the period of _________

_____trial to determine effectiveness using reasonable medical judgment

_____No

Why?

3. I want to have an endotracheal tube used in order to perform items 1 and 2.

_____Yes

_____TRIAL for the period of _________

_____trial to determine effectiveness using reasonable medical judgment

_____No

Why?

4. I want to have total parenteral nutrition administered for my nutrition.

_____Yes

_____TRIAL for the period of _________

_____TRIAL to determine effectiveness using reasonable medical judgment

_____No

Why?

5. I want to have intravenous medication and hydration administered; regardless of my decision, I understand that intravenous hydration to alleviate discomfort

or pain medication will not be withheld from me if I so request them.

_____Yes

_____TRIAL for the period of _________

_____TRIAL to determine effectiveness using reasonable medical judgment

_____No

Why?

6. I want to have all medications used for the treatment of my illness continued; regardless of my decision, I understand that pain medication will continue to be administered, including narcotic medications.

_____Yes

_____TRIAL for the period of _________

_____TRIAL to determine effectiveness using reasonable medical judgment

_____No

Why?

7. I want to have nasogastric, gastrostomy, or other enteral feeding tubes introduced and administered for my nutrition.

_____Yes

_____TRIAL for the period of _________

_____TRIAL to determine effectiveness using reasonable medical judgment

_____No

Why?

8. I want to be placed on a dialysis machine.

_____Yes

_____TRIAL for the period of _________

_____TRIAL to determine effectiveness using reasonable medical judgment

_____No

Why?

9. I want to have an autopsy done to determine the cause(s) of my death.

_____Yes

_____ No

Why?

10. I want to be admitted to the Intensive Care Unit.

_____Yes

_____ No

Why?

11. [For patients in long-term care facilities who experience a life-threatening change in health status] I want 911 called in case of a medical emergency.

_____Yes

_____ No

Why?

12. Other Directives

I consent to these directives after receiving honest disclosure of their implications, risks, and benefits by my physician, free from constraints and being of sound mind.

______________________________ ______________

Signature Date

______________________________ ______________

Witness Date

______________________________ ______________

Witness Date

13. Proxy Negation

I request that the following persons *not* be allowed to make decisions on my behalf in the event of my disability or incapacity: ______________________________

______________________________ ______________

Signature Date

______________________________ ______________

Witness Date

______________________________ ______________

Witness Date

14. Organ Donation [Specific state version inserted here]
15. Durable Power of Attorney [Specific state version inserted here]

10. A Narrative Model

[This story-based narrative model was first developed and tested in 1993 by Rita Kielstein and Hans-Martin Sass as an alternative to inflexible rejectionist medical directives. See Hans-Martin Sass and Rita Kielstein, *Wertanamnese und Betreuungsverfügung,* 3d ed. (Bochum: Zentrum für medizinische Ethik, 1995). For an earlier version, see R. Kielstein and H. M. Sass, "Using Stories to Assess Values and Establish Medical Directives," *Kennedy Institute of Ethics Journal* 3 (1993): 303–25.]

A Narrative Method to Initiate Value Statements and Treatment Preferences
Stories for Self-evaluation and Self-determination

INTRODUCTION

It is neither easy nor pleasant for healthy people to discuss values and preferences that shall govern one's health care decisions in future situations of pain, suffering, illness, and dying. Here are five stories of patients at the end of their lives. As these stories of disease, suffering, and dying are as different as the patients' life stories are, they might help you to reflect on risks and challenges in making value statements and giving directives in advance for future situations. But our medical history is part of our personal history. The stories of our last days will one day become a part of the stories of our own lives. Our own future stories may be full of rich and enjoyable events, but there will also be dark hours of weakness, harm, pain, and reduced physical and mental mobility. Early on we should reflect on those personal values, wishes, and preferences that we expect to guide our medical treatment decisions. To make advance assessments and to reflect on directives prior to acute situations not only strengthens our capacity for self-evaluation and self-determination in situations of dementia, coma, severe pain, agony, and dying, but also will increase our health risk competence and improve attitudes in good and preventive health risk management.

If we have valid advance directives that reflect our values and that are treatment-specific, then others—proxies, family and friends, physicians and nurses—will have advice, guidance, or directives to care for us in our best interest. While these five stories challenge you to recollect and to reaffirm those values that are essential for you, an introductory part asks you to reflect on your own experiences with disease, dying, and the hospital setting.

You might want to discuss these stories and your comments with family and friends, as you share many values with them or want their contribution to your reflections and their comment on values they do not share with you. It is also advisable to share your comments and preferences with your physician as there might be medical terms or interventions you do not fully understand. You definitely want to discuss your thoughts with the person you want to act as your health care representative or proxy for situations in which you might not be able to speak for yourself.

From time to time, after new insights and experiences, you should review the stories and change comments or directives. We strongly suggest that you familiarize yourself with the medical language used in Advance Directives and to discuss these or other stories with a health care professional you trust before you give specific directives for future medical treatment.

RECOLLECTIONS

Stories of fatal disease, suffering, and dying are catalysts for the recollection of one's own often unpleasant and agonizing experiences. Many of us have our own stories to tell, stories that have already become a part of our own life histories. What are your stories? What has become a part of your life story?

1. Have you been in the hospital? Why? How long?
2. Has your own suffering or illnesses of loved ones or friends become a part of your own history and influenced your understanding of disease and pain?
3. Have you been a witness to death and dying? What were your reactions and impressions? What still moves you?

Story 1: Who Shall Decide? How Should It Be Decided?

Mr. B. is 79 years old and dependent on others. His eyesight and hearing have diminished. He seems to have lost all interest in life. At times he is very confused and does not even recognize others. He has pain in his legs and can only walk short distances, because of poor blood supply to his legs, which is caused by previous smoking. Blood vessel surgery might improve his mobility and reduce pain, thus improving his quality of life. Mr. B. does not understand the situation nor can he make his preferences clear; he does not have an "advance directive," nor has he named a proxy. One daughter and the physician favor surgery while the other daughter is opposed.

1. If you were in Mr. B.'s situation, unable to decide for yourself, who should decide for you, your son or daughter, both together, your spouse or friend, your physician, who else? Give names and addresses:
2. How closely should physicians follow advance directives?
3. How would you have wished to be treated?
4. Rewrite the story the way you would like it to end!

Story 2: Dying of Incurable Cancer?

Mrs. M., 38 years old, had her left breast removed five years ago because she had breast cancer. Now she has increasing pain in her lower back; her physicians have diagnosed metastatic bone cancer. They recommend chemotherapeutic treatment to reduce pain and to prevent or to slow down the development of more metastatic cancer. Mrs. M. undergoes chemotherapy with uncomfortable side effects. Her pain increases and is not treated adequately. The physicians do not tell her the "full truth," that chemotherapy will not cure her cancer but might prolong her life. Mrs. M. dies in the hospital eight months after the bone cancer was detected; she did not die at home as she had wished. Without chemotherapy she might have died a few months earlier.

1. How would you have wished to be treated?
2. Would you want your physicians to fully inform you about your condition, even if it is terminal?
3. Would you want intensive and aggressive pain treatment, even if it might reduce your mental alertness?
4. Rewrite the story you would like it to end!

Story 3: A Sudden Brain Damage

Ms. A., 55 years old, suffers from stroke in her office, a result of many years of inconsistent hypertension control. An accumulated blood clot in the brain tissue cannot be removed surgically without major additional brain damage but may disappear in part or totally over a period of several months. At this point it is unpredictable which neurological damages will remain. They can vary from partial or total paresis to partial or total loss of cognition, speech, memory, or thinking.

1. Which neurological defects do you think would allow you to continue a life worth living?
2. Which neurological defects would you think are so severe that you would not want to continue living and therefore refuse all medical treatment, including treatment of infections and minor injuries, while at the same time continue to accept treatment against pain, restlessness, angst, and also foods and liquids?
3. Which damages would be so severe that you would want to have palliative treatment and hydration only, so that you would be allowed to die as soon as your body allows you to die?
4. Rewrite the story the way you would like it to end!

Story 4: Losing the Will to Live

Mrs. S., 80 years old, is alert and competent but suffers from heart pain and arthritis, in addition to her often painful and incurable intestine inflammation. Her two sons are living in another state. Since her husband died two years ago, she has lost the will to live. She told her family physician about her plans to commit suicide and asked that her decision be respected. Now, she calls the doctor and tells him that she has taken the necessary pills and wants to die in peace and not be revived or put into the hospital. A few hours later, the doctor makes a house call. No one opens the door, and a neighbor lets him into Mrs. S.'s apartment. They find her lying on the couch unconscious and a note on the table reading, "Please, let me die!" The doctor follows her wishes. A court did not hold him responsible for not saving her life.

1. Can you imagine that you would act like Mrs. S. in similar situations?
2. Would you want your doctor to give you detailed information on how to commit suicide or even assist you in doing so?
3. How do you evaluate the doctor's reaction in moral and in legal terms?
4. Rewrite the story the way you would like it to end!

Story 5: A Severe Accident and Deep Coma

Mr. W., 26 years old, survives a motorcycle accident with severe fractures of the cranium, of the hip and the right leg. His spleen and his right kidney are injured and have to be surgically removed; two days later the right leg becomes seriously infected and has to be taken off from the knee downward. Now, after four months, Mr. W. still is unconscious. The statistical evidence that he will awake from his coma is very low. He depends on artificial nutrition and on a mechanical ventilator.

1. Would you want artificial nutrition and ventilation, if after some time the probability that you will regain your consciousness will be less than 1:10/ 1:100?
2. What arguments support your decision?
3. What are the mental or physical handicaps that might cause you to wish to be dead rather than alive?
4. Rewrite the story the way you would like it to end!

11. A Situational Medical Directive

[This model was developed and tested by Linda L. Emanuel and Ezekiel J. Emanuel to provide a forum for the expression of more situation-specific preferences and directives. The situational approach can be combined with proxy designation as well as with personal and value statements but stands on its own as a method for specifying treatment directives for classical situations in the care of the incompetent. See L. L. Emanuel and E. J. Emanuel, "The Medical Directive: A New Comprehensive Advance Care Document," *Journal of the American Medical Association* 261 (June 9, 1989): 3288–93; the following revised and extended version is from Fred H. Cate and Barbara A. Gill, "The Patient Self-determination Act: Implementation Issues and Opportunities" (Northwestern University: Annenberg Washington Program, 1991), appendix F: 59–62.]

THE MEDICAL DIRECTIVE: AN INTRODUCTION

As part of a person's right to self determination every adult has the freedom to accept or refuse any recommended medical treatment. This is relatively easy when people are well and can communicate. Unfortunately, during severe illness, people are often unable to communicate their wishes at the very time that many critical decisions about medical interventions need to be made.

The Medical Directive states a person's wishes for or against types of medical interventions in several key sitations, so that the person's wishes can be respected even when he or she cannot communicate.

A Medical Directive only comes into effect if a person becomes incompetent, or unable to make decisions or to express his or her wishes. It can be changed at any time up until then. Decisions not involving incompetence should be discussed directly with the physician.

The Medical Directive also allows for appointing someone to make medical decisions for a person should he or she become unable to make his or her own; this is a proxy or durable power of attorney. The Medical Directive also allows for a statement of wishes concerning organ donation.

A copy of the completed Medical Directive should be given to a person's regular physician and to his or her family or friend to ensure that it is available when necessary.

Medical Directives should be seen not only as legal protection for personal rights but also as a guide to a person's physician. Discussion of Medical Directives with the physician can help in making plans for health care that suit a person's values.

* * *

A person's wishes usually reflect personal, philosophical, and religious views, so people may wish to discuss the issues with his or her family, friends, and religious mentor as well.

Before recording a personal statement in the Medical Directive it may be helpful to consider the following question. What kind of medical condition, if any, would make life hard enough that attempts to prolong life would be undesirable? Some may say none. For others the answer may be intractable pain. For other people the limit may be permanent dependence on others, or irreversible mental damage, or inability to exchange affection.

Under such circumstances as these the goal of medical treatment may be to secure comfort only, or it may be to use ordinary treatments while avoiding heroic ones, or to use treatments that offer improved function (palliation), or to use all appropriate interventions to prolong life independent of quality. These points may help to clarify a person's thoughts and wishes.

DURABLE POWER OF ATTORNEY

I understand that my wishes expressed in these four cases may not cover all possible aspects of my care if I become incompetent. I also may be undecided about whether I want a particular treatment or not. Consequently there may be a need for someone to accept or refuse medical interventions for me in consultation with my physicians. I authorize:

____

____

as my proxy(s) to make the decision for me whenever my wishes expressed in this document are insufficient or undecided.

Should there be any disagreement between the wishes I have indicated in this document and the decisions favored by my above named proxy(s), I wish my proxy(s) to have authority over my medical directive /I wish my medical directive to have authority over my proxy(s). (Please delete as necessary.)

Should there be any disagreement between the wishes of my proxies,

____

shall have final authority.

ORGAN DONATION

I hereby make this anatomical gift to take effect upon my death.

I give: _____ my body; _____ any needed organs or parts; _____ the following organs or parts ______________________________

to the following person or institution; _____ the physician in attendance at my death; _____ the hospital in which I die; _____ the following named physician, hospital, storage bank or other medical institution ________________________;

for the following purposes: _____ any purpose authorized by law; _____ transplantation; _____ therapy; _____ research; _____ medical education.

MY PERSONAL STATEMENT (use another page if necessary.)

____

____

____

Signed __________________________ Date __________

Witness __________________________ Date __________

Witness __________________________ Date __________

MY MEDICAL DIRECTIVE

This Medical Directive expresses, and shall stand for, my wishes regarding medical treatments in the event that illness should make me unable to comunicate them directly. I make this Directive, being 18 years or more of age, of sound mind and appreciating the consequences of my decisions.

SITUATION (A)

If I am in a coma or in a persistent vegetative state, and in the opinion of my physician and several consultants have no known hope of regaining awareness and higher mental functions no matter what is done, then my wishes regarding use of the following, if considered medically reasonable, would be:

SITUATION (B)

If I am in a coma, and I have a small likelihood of recovering fully, a slightly larger likelihood of surviving with permanent brain damage, and a much larger likelihood of dying, then my wishes regarding the use of the following, if considered medically reasonable, would be:

SITUATION (C)

If I have brain damage or some brain disease which cannot be reversed and which makes me unable to recognize people, or to speak understandably, *and I also have a terminal illness,* such as incurable cancer which will likely be the cause of my death, then my wishes regarding use of the following, if considered medically reasonable, would be:

SITUATION (D)

If I have brain damage or some brain disease which cannot be reversed and which makes me unable to recognize people, or to speak understandably, *but I have no terminal illness,* and I can live in this condition for a long time, then my wishes regarding use of the following, if considered medically reasonable, would be:

	SITUATION (A)				SITUATION (B)				SITUATION (C)				SITUATION (D)			
	I WANT	I DO NOT WANT	I AM UNDECIDED	I WANT A TRIAL: IF NO CLEAR IMPROVEMENT STOP TREATMENT	I WANT	I DO NOT WANT	I AM UNDECIDED	I WANT A TRIAL: IF NO CLEAR IMPROVEMENT STOP TREATMENT	I WANT	I DO NOT WANT	I AM UNDECIDED	I WANT A TRIAL: IF NO CLEAR IMPROVEMENT STOP TREATMENT	I WANT	I DO NOT WANT	I AM UNDECIDED	I WANT A TRIAL: IF NO CLEAR IMPROVEMENT STOP TREATMENT
1) **CARDIOPULMONARY RESUSCITATION—** if on the point of dying the use of drugs and electric shock to start the heart beating, and artificial breathing.																
2) **MECHANICAL BREATHING—** breathing by a machine.																
3) **ARTIFICIAL NUTRITION AND HYDRATION—** nutrition and fluid given through a tube in the veins, nose, or stomach.																
4) **MAJOR SURGERY—** such as removing the gall bladder or part of the intestines.																
5) **KIDNEY DIALYSIS—** cleaning the blood by machine or by fluid passed through the belly.																
6) **CHEMOTHERAPY—** drugs to fight cancer.																
7) **MINOR SURGERY—** such as removing some tissue from an infected toe.																
8) **INVASIVE DIAGNOSTIC TESTS—** such as using a flexible tube to look into the stomach.																
9) **BLOOD OR BLOOD PRODUCTS—**																
10) **ANTIBIOTICS—** drugs to fight infection.																
11) **SIMPLE DIAGNOSTIC TESTS—** such as blood tests or x-rays.																
12) **PAIN MEDICATIONS, EVEN IF THEY DULL CONSCIOUSNESS AND INDIRECTLY SHORTEN MY LIFE—**																

The Medical Directive.

12. Kyoto Women's University: A Medical Directive Containing a Pregnancy Clause

[This living will form was drafted by Kyoto Women's University students for use by women. It is interesting, as it addresses the rare instances of letting a comatose pregnant woman die or extending her life for the sole purpose of saving the unborn child. The form was translated by Rihito Kimura.]

A Living Will for Women

I. IN THE CASE OF VEGETATIVE STATE

1. If I lapse into a vegetative state and if two physicians diagnose it to be impossible for me to regain consciousness, I would like to ask my physician in charge or the attending physician not to use life-sustaining machines. If the machine is already in use, please withdraw the use of the machine and do not use it again. As this discontinuation of life-sustaining treatment is based on my rejection of medical treatment, it is not necessary for physicians to have my informed consent in this case.

2. However, please continue to provide hydration, nutrition, and cleansing of my body.

II. IN THE CASE THAT RATIONAL AND MENTAL JUDGMENT BECOME IMPOSSIBLE

1. If two physicians diagnose that my disease is incurable and that death is imminent, please do not institute treatment to prolong my life merely to extend my moment of death. In such a case, it is not necessary to have my informed consent.

2. However, please continue to provide hydration, nutrition, and the cleansing of my body.

3. If I express my feeling of pain, please try to do the best possible to alleviate the symptoms in giving palliative care.

In regard to the following alternatives, I express my intentions by making X marks.

a. In the event that I enter into a vegetative state, the physician who diagnoses that it is medically impossible for me to regain consciousness will be:

1. Any physician

2. The physician-in-charge or the attending physician at that time

3. I would like to nominate the following physician, who has agreed to fulfill my living will (one or two physicians):

Physician's Name and Address______________________________________

____

Physician's Name and Address____

____

____

III. IF I AM PREGNANT WHEN THIS LIVING WILL COMES INTO EFFECT

1. If consultation among family members has determined that a guardian of the baby shall be appointed, I retract this living will statement and request that treatment be the best possible for my pregnancy and delivery.
2. Please accept this living will as effective.

To draft this document, while I have my normal intellectual and mental capacities to make a judgment, I have asked the physician about those items referred to above that relate to medical items. I received a full explanation, which I understood and to which I consented. I then made an autonomous judgment in deciding to make this living will. Hereafter, whenever I want to change any intention stated in this document, I can do so, reserving my freedom to retract or change any individual condition of any clause, or to write an alternative statement of this document.

Signature____

13. Japanese Hospice Society: A Hospice Patient's Directives

[This form, drafted in 1994 by the Japanese Hospice Society as a Living Will for dying patients in hospice care, was translated by Rihito Kimura.]

I have been informed of and understand the purpose behind the hospice living will after reading the explanation that accompanies the membership agreement of the society. I request the following of my family and of those who would be involved in the delivery of my medical services and care when I am faced with a terminal condition caused by incurable disease.

I hope to be admitted to hospice (a palliative care unit), which focuses on the relief of my generalized pain, or, if this is impossible, I hope to be granted a similar sort of terminal care to complete my life in a natural and dignified manner without merely prolonging my life in order to receive medical examinations and aggressive treatment.

I will, in addition to the signing of this document, draft in my own words and in a concrete manner the way in which I want to spend the final stage of my life (see below). (If additional pages are necessary, please attach them to this document.)

I, being of sound mind, hereby confirm the validity of this request. In signing this document, I clearly state that the responsibility for all of the events that may be caused in executing this request rests solely with me.

Name (signature)______________________________ Seal

Year_______ Month _______ Date______________

Date of birth _____________ (male, female) (please circle)

I have included for your information the following statement concerning my request noted on the previous page of "My Living Will." I describe here my thoughts that, though frank and accurate now, might change in the future. Please use these statements in determining the proper course of my actual hospice care or similar type of terminal care. I will circle each applicable statement and include a statement of my own reasons for choosing it.

I. Issues relating to the disclosure of the name, condition, treatment choice, and prognosis of the disease that I have been diagnosed as having (i.e., cancer).

1. I need to have a detailed explanation.

2. I do not want any detailed explanation.

3. I need to have a detailed explanation if the cancer is in an early stage, however I do not want it if the cancer is in an incurable stage.

4. I will let my family make the judgment.

5. I cannot make a decision about this issue.

I will state the reason for choosing the one mentioned above.

II. Issues relating to the name, condition, treatment choice, and prognosis of any kind of disease that I have been diagnosed as having except in the case of cancer.

1. I need to have a detailed explanation.

2. I do not want a detailed explanation.

3. I will let my family make the judgment.

4. I cannot make a decision about this issue.

I will state the reason for choosing the one mentioned above.

III. Issues relating to the situation in which I enter a persistent vegetative state for more than several months.

1. I need my treatment to be continued until the very last moment.

2. I want all life-sustaining machines to be removed.

3. I will let my family make the judgment.

4. I cannot make a decision about this issue.

I will state the reason for choosing the one mentioned above.

IV. Issues relating to the situation in which I am judged to be "brain dead."

1. I will donate necessary organs for organ transplantation.

2. I refuse to donate organs for organ transplantation.

3. I will let my family make the judgment.

4. I cannot make a decision about this issue.

I will state the reasons for choosing the one mentioned above.

V. I do not want to donate organs for organ transplantation; however, I will choose one of the following options.

1. I wish to have a pathological autopsy (to determine the cause of death or for the purpose of researching certain diseases)

2. I wish to be an anatomical gift (for the purpose of anatomical practice on the part of medical students)

3. I wish my eyes to be donated to a cornea bank (to cure a person suffering from diseased corneas).

4. I do not wish to opt for any of the above courses of action (nos. 1–3).

5. I cannot make a decision.

I will state the reason for choosing the one mentioned above.

14. An Advance Directive for the Patient with Amyotrophic Lateral Sclerosis

[This form was written by Robert S. Olick in conjunction with the Volkswagen Foundation Project on "Advance Directives and Durable Powers of Attorney." Portions of this document are adapted from the New Jersey Bioethics Commission. In concept, the disease-specific directive obviates the most serious concerns raised by past experience with advance directives (in particular, living wills), namely, that static written documents, sometimes written remotely in time and before the onset of the patient's illness, may not adequately embody informed decisions and can present serious challenges for those who must faithfully interpret the patient's wishes. Disease-specific directives may be especially useful for patients with chronic, progressive illnesses with a (relatively) predictable clinical course and who retain mental capacities through a substantial period of their illness, such as patients suffering from HIV/AIDS, amyotrophic lateral sclerosis (ALS), multiple sclerosis, or renal disease requiring frequent dialysis. For these patients, advance care planning discussions are more likely to occur within the context of an ongoing, rather than episodic, physician-patient-family relationship that affords all parties ample opportunity to come to understand the patient's illness, its likely course and long-range prognosis, and to appreciate each others' values and perspectives. Thus, the disease-specific directive holds the promise of fostering more informed, less anticipatory planning and offering more explicit guidance for end-of-life decisions. The disease-specific directives for ALS patients reprinted in the pages that follow represent initial efforts to develop such documents. R.S.O.]

Combined Proxy and Instruction Directive

I understand that as a competent adult I have the right to make decisions about my health care. Although patients ordinarily retain mental abilities through most of the course of the illness, there may come a time when I am unable, due to a physical or mental incapacity, to make my own health care decisions. In these circumstances, those caring for me will need direction concerning my care and will turn to someone who knows my values and health care wishes. I understand that those responsible for my care will seek to make health care decisions in accordance with my wishes and best interests. To provide the guidance and authority needed to make decisions on my behalf:

I, ____________, hereby declare and make known my instructions and wishes for my future health care. This advance directive for health care shall take effect in the event I become unable to make my own health care decisions, as determined by the physician who has primary responsibility for my care, and any necessary confirming determinations. I direct that this document become part of my permanent medical records.

[In completing Part I of this document you will designate an individual you trust to act as your legally recognized proxy to make health care decisions for you in the event that you are unable to make decisions for yourself. In completing Part II of this document you will provide instructions concerning your treatment wishes to your proxy, your family, your physicians, and others entrusted with your care and treatment.]

PART I. DESIGNATION OF A HEALTH CARE PROXY

A. I hereby designate:

Name________________________________

Address______________________________ City___________________ State______

Telephone____________________________

as my health care proxy, with durable power of attorney, to make any and all health care decisions for me, including decisions to accept or to refuse any treatment, service or procedure used to diagnose, treat or care for my physical or mental condition and decisions to provide, withhold or withdraw life-sustaining treatments. I direct my health care proxy to make decisions on my behalf in accordance with my wishes as stated in this document, or as otherwise known to him or her. In the event my wishes are not clear, my proxy is authorized to make decisions on my behalf in accordance with what he or she believes to be in my best interests.

B. If the person I designated above is unable, unwilling, or unavailable to act as my health care proxy, I hereby designate the following person(s) to act as my proxy, in the order of priority stated:

1. Name______________________	2. Name______________________
Address______________________	Address______________________
City____________State______	City____________State______
Telephone ___________________	Telephone ___________________

PART II. INSTRUCTION DIRECTIVE

[In Part II you are asked to provide instructions concerning your health care. Before completing your directive, you should discuss these matters with your proxy, family members, your physician, or others who may become responsible for your care.]

C. Statement of Personal Values and Wishes: I understand that ALS is a debilitating disease that will cause me to progressively lose muscle and motor function and become increasingly dependent on others for my medical care and daily living needs. I am also aware that most ALS patients eventually become respiratory-dependent and ultimately die of respiratory failure. To inform those responsible for my care of my specific wishes, I make the following statement of personal views regarding my health care:

Initial ONE of the following statements which best expresses your wishes:

1. _____ I direct that all medically appropriate measures be provided to sustain my life, even if I am dependent on a respirator and am suffering from severe physical and mental disabilities in an advanced stage of ALS.

2. _____ I direct that all medically appropriate measures be provided to sustain my life, even if I am dependent on a respirator and am suffering from severe physical and mental disabilities in an advanced stage of ALS, unless I am unable to communicate meaningfully with my family, physician and others. In this event I direct that the respirator sustaining my life be withdrawn.
3. _____ I believe that being dependent on a respirator and on others for daily living would be an unacceptable quality of life. When my disease reaches the point where I will become dependent on a respirator I direct that it not be started. If respirator support has begun, then I direct that it be discontinued.
4. _____ I recognize that as my disease progresses it will still be possible for me to live for a significant period of time even while dependent on a respirator and on others for my care and daily living needs. I direct that in such circumstances all medically appropriate treatment be provided to sustain my life. However, when my disease progresses to the point where my physician has determined that my condition is terminal, I direct that the respirator support be discontinued.

To me, terminal condition means that my physicians have determined that [fill in the appropriate phrase or write in your own definition]:________________

____

[I will die within a few days/I will die within a few weeks/I have a life expectancy of 6 months or less/I have a life expectancy of 1 year or less.]

D. Pain Relief and Comfort Care: I also direct that at all times I be given all medically appropriate care necessary to make me comfortable and to alleviate pain.

E. Additional Instructions

(In the space below you should provide any additional information about your health care preferences which is important to you and which may help those concerned with your care to implement your wishes. You may wish to direct your health care proxy, family members, or health care providers to consult with others, or may wish to direct that your care be provided by a particular physician, hospital, or home. If you need more space, you should attach an additional statement to this document.)

____

____

PART III. SIGNATURE AND WITNESSES

F. Copies: The original or a copy of this document has been given to my health care proxy and to the following people:

1. Name____________________	2. Name____________________
Address___________________	Address___________________
City____________State_______	City____________State_______
Telephone _________________	Telephone _________________

G. Signature: By writing this advanced directive, I inform those who may become entrusted with my health care of my wishes and intend to ease the burdens of decision making which this responsibility may impose. I have discussed the terms of this designation with my health care proxy and he or she has willingly agreed to accept the responsibility for acting on my behalf in accordance with this directive. I understand the purpose and effect of this document and sign it knowingly, voluntarily and after careful deliberation.

Signed this ____ day of _______, 19___. Signature ______________________________

Address _______________________________

City ___________ State ____.

H. Witnesses: I declare that the person who signed this document, or asked another to sign this document on his or her behalf, did so in my presence, that he or she is personally known to me, and that he or she appears to be of sound mind and free of duress or undue influence. I am 18 years of age or older, and am not designated by this or any other document as the person's health care proxy, nor as an alternate health care proxy.

1. Witness___________________
Address___________________
City___________State______
Signature _________________
Date _____________________

2. Witness___________________
Address___________________
City___________State______
Signature _________________
Date _____________________

15. An Advance Directive Including a Proxy Clause

[This form, developed by Robert M. Veatch in 1976, is one of the first to combine the designation of a trusted proxy agent and information regarding the signee's system of belief with directions on how to proceed in order to determine the moment that the authority to direct and decide should be passed on to the agent. What appears here is a modification of the version appearing in the second edition of Veatch's 1976 book; see Robert M. Veatch, *Death, Dying, and the Biological Revolution* (New Haven: Yale University Press, 1989), pp. 154–55.]

A Model Advance Directive

An advance directive that covers all of these points will not necessarily be complete and unambiguous, but it is likely to be more complete than some of the early model directives. Since the variations are almost infinite, no single model can be definitive. Nevertheless, one such sample, based on one currently signed by the author, will help show how these elements can be combined into a single statement:

DECLARATION made this ______ day of ______, 19 ______. I, ______, being of sound mind, willingly and voluntarily make known my desires that my dying shall not be artificially or in any other way prolonged under the circumstances set forth below, do declare:

If at any time I should have an incurable injury, disease, or illness certified to be a terminal condition by two (2) physicians who have personally examined me, one (1) of whom shall be my attending physician, and the physicians have determined that my death will occur if life-sustaining procedures are not utilized and where the application of life-sustaining procedures would serve only to prolong the dying process, and when such withholding or withdrawal has been approved by __________, I direct that such procedures be withheld or withdrawn, and that I be permitted to die naturally with only the administration of medication or the performance of any medical procedure deemed necessary to provide me with comfort care or to alleviate pain.

Furthermore, if at any time I should have a condition (whether incurable or not) which, in the opinion of __________ (regardless of the opinion of any physician), involves treatment which is ether itself useless or on balance burdensome to me or will sustain life in such a way that it is useless or on balance of no benefit to me or is burdensome to me or others, I direct that any procedures being used to sustain my life or prolong my dying be withheld or withdrawn and that I be permitted to die with only the administration of medication or the performance of any medical procedure deemed necessary to provide me with comfort care or to alleviate pain.

In either circumstance, that is, when continued treatment merely prolongs a terminal condition or is directly or indirectly responsible for grave burden to myself or others, I explicitly instruct that __________ be my agent for the purposes of all medical decisions. I urge him (or her) to refuse any medical procedures which (s)he believes would be useless or on balance burdensome based on my values as (s)he can discern them or based on his (her) own values if (s)he cannot deduce what my position would be. I explicitly instruct him (her) to refuse not only complex procedures such as respirators and dialysis machines, but also simple treatments such as IV's, antibiotics, nasogastric tubes, hyperalimentation, or even oral feeding, if they are no longer appropriate in his (her) judgment. Furthermore, I give him (her) all authority to engage or dismiss the two physicians referred to above (including my attending physician), should I be unable to do so. I expect him (her) to dismiss immediately any physician who fails to comply with his (her) decisions.

Should (s)he want guidance in interpreting what I would have wanted in any particular circumstance, I urge him (her) to consult my own writing. (In doing so, [s]he should note that recently I have expressed concern that some patients who may not want to have treatment stopped, will have it stopped by physicians who are paternalistically trying to do what whey think is best. [S]He should be aware that I have expressed this solely out of concern for the rights of those who want treatment continued. This should not be interpreted to imply that I am one of those people.) Should (s)he want further guidance, I urge him (her) to consult __________, __________, and __________ all of whom hold positions on these subjects which I respect. Should (s)he need medical guidance, I urge him (her) to consult Dr.________ and Dr. ________ whose medical skills and ethical positions I respect. I urge him (her) to transfer me to the medical care of Dr.__________ should that become necessary to have my wishes or his (hers) respected. Should (s)he need legal guidance, I urge him (her) to consult __________.

It is my intention that this document be legally binding as a declaration of my wishes under the law of __________ and all other states having living will or natural death act legislation and that it be seen as expressing my wishes under common law and constitutional law as well as conveying a durable power of attorney in all states.

It is my belief, after studying the matter for many years, that the wishes expressed here are consistent with and based upon principles of Judeo-Christian ethics. In particular, I affirm that while life is precious, it is not the ultimate good. When medical treatments are no longer fitting, when they are useless given the patient's own beliefs and values, or when they are on balance burdensome to the patient or others, then humans should step aside and let nature take its course.

In the absence of my ability to give directions regarding the use of life-sustaining procedures, it is my intention that this declaration shall be honored by my family and physician(s) as the final expression of my legal right to refuse medical or surgical treatment and accept the consequences from such refusal.

I understand the full import of this declaration and I am emotionally and mentally competent to make this declaration.

____

Name

This declarant is personally known to me and I believe him (her) to be of sound mind. I did not sign the declarant's signature above for or at the direction of the declarant. I am at least eighteen (18) years of age and am not related to the declarant by blood or by marriage, entitled to any portion of the estate of the declarant according to the laws of interstate succession of __________ or under a will of the declarant or codicil thereto, or directly financially responsible for declarant's medical care. I am not the declarant's attending physician, an employee of the attending physician, or an employee of the health facility in which the declarant is a patient.

____

Witness

____

Witness

16. A Combination Form: Proxy Designation, Value Statement, and Medical Directives

[This model combines sections of (1) a proxy designation, (2) a value statement, and (3) directives for specific medical situations and interventions; a fourth part (not reprinted here) describes medical "Words I need to know" in lay language. The form was developed by a team of Japanese, German, and American clinicians, bioethicists, and legal experts funded by a grant from the Volkswagen Foundation. See Hans-Martin Sass, Frederick O. Bonkovsky, Akira Akabayashi, Rita Kielstein, and Robert S. Olick, "Advance Health Care Documents in Multicultural Perspectives," *Jahrbuch für Recht und Ethik* [Annual Review of Law and Ethics] 4 (1996): 494–500.]

A Combination Form

____ Name, Date of birth

____ Address

I understand that as a *competent adult* I have the moral and legal right to make decisions about my health care. There may come a time when I am unable, due to physical or mental incapacity, to make informed and competent decisions. In these situations, those caring for me will need advice concerning my care and information about those values, beliefs, and health care wishes which I want to govern my care. *I hereby declare, that the following statements, instructions, directives, and wishes for future health care take effect in the event that I become temporarily or permanently unable to make my own health care decisions.* I wish that those responsible for my care follow these instructions, even though they or others might choose differently for themselves or "normal" or "rational" standard medical practice could suggest or pursue other treatment options. The determination of my incapacity to make competent, informed, and applicable decisions must be made by the physician who has primary responsibility for my care. I direct that this document become part of my permanent medical records.

In Part I of this Directive, I designate a person I trust or my family to be my legal and moral *health care representative* to make health care decisions for me in the event I am unable to make decisions for myself. In Part II I discuss *Values and Preferences which should govern my treatment.* In Part III I discuss more specific *treatment-specific Medical Directives.*

______________________ ______________________

Signature Date

PART I. MY HEALTH CARE REPRESENTATIVE

1. I hereby designate:

Name__________________________________
Address________________________________
City___________________________________
Telephone and Fax_______________________

as my health care representative (proxy) to make any and all health care decisions for me, including decisions to accept or refuse any treatment, service, or procedure used to diagnose or treat my physical or mental condition, including decisions to provide, withhold, or withdraw life-sustaining measures.

2. If the person I have designated above is unable, unwilling, or unavailable to act as my health care representative, I hereby designate the following person(s) to act as my health care representative, in the following order:

1. ______________,
2. ______________,
3. ______________.

3. If none of the above-mentioned persons is able, willing, or available to act as my proxy, I direct that [specify one]: (a) the medical team which has primary responsibility, (b) the physician who has primary responsibility, or (c) an ethics committee of the institution responsible make decisions based on my value profile and list of treatment preferences.

4. I do not wish that the following person(s) be involved in making health care decisions for me:

1. ______________,

5. If a conflict arises between my health care representative (proxy), the medical team or physician having primary responsibility, and their interpretation of my value profile and medical directives, I hereby direct that the final authority for decision making is [I specify one]: (a) my health care representative, (b) my family, (c) the physician who has primary responsibility, (d) the medical team which has primary responsibility, (e) an Ethics Committee, (f) a religious advisor of the __________religion, (g) other: ___________

________________	________________	____________
(my signature)	(my proxy's signature)	(date)
________________	________________	____________
(my signature)	(my proxy's signature)	(re-dated)
________________	________________	____________
(my signature)	(my proxy's signature)	(re-dated)
________________	________________	____________
(my signature)	(my proxy's signature)	(re-dated)

PART II. MY VALUES AND WISHES THAT SHALL GOVERN MY CARE

I want to be treated as a respected person. The visions, values, and beliefs that have formed my attitudes, preferences, and wishes as well as my personal understanding of the quality and meaning of life are to be respected by those who will care for me in situations in which I will be unable to communicate my preferences and directives. I am aware that I might change my preferences and wishes based on future experiences (including mental or physical illness or distress). But as long I have not changed these statements, my health care representative and everyone else shall regard the following statements as the final authoritative and valid expression of my values, preferences, and requests. Being aware of the risk of expressing preferences of future situations I have tried to document how my self-determination for future situations could vary from preferences for actual situations.

PRESENT SELF-ASSESSMENT	FUTURE SELF-DETERMINATION
1. Very important	A. Very important
2. Important	B. Important
3. Not important	C. Depending on situation
4. I cannot decide	D. I cannot decide
5. No	E. No

1. *I want to live as long as possible*	
• if I am in good health	1,2,3,4,5 A,B,C,D,E
• if I am ill but overall recovery is expected	1,2,3,4,5 A,B,C,D,E
• if I am permanently unconscious	1,2,3,4,5 A,B,C,D,E
• if I am mentally incompetent	1,2,3,4,5 A,B,C,D,E
• if I am terminally ill	1,2,3,4,5 A,B,C,D,E
2. *I want to be without pain*	1,2,3,4,5 A,B,C,D,E
• even if clear thinking is compromised	1,2,3,4,5 A,B,C,D,E
• even if I become drowsy or sleepy	1,2,3,4,5 A,B,C,D,E
3. *When time has come, I prefer to die*	
• at home	1,2,3,4,5 A,B,C,D,E
• in the hospital	1,2,3,4,5 A,B,C,D,E
• with loving people around	1,2,3,4,5 A,B,C,D,E
• being left alone	1,2,3,4,5 A,B,C,D,E

4. *I want a comfortable dying process*	1,2,3,4,5 A,B,C,D,E
• even at the cost of heavy sedation	1,2,3,4,5 A,B,C,D,E
• even at the cost of shortening life	1,2,3,4,5 A,B,C,D,E
• even if it means active euthanasia [*]	1,2,3,4,5 A,B,C,D,E
5. *If my prognosis is terminal*	
• I want full disclosure	1,2,3,4,5 A,B,C,D,E
• my proxy must be told	1,2,3,4,5 A,B,C,D,E
• my family must be told	1,2,3,4,5 A,B,C,D,E
• my family physician must be told	1,2,3,4,5 A,B,C,D,E
• _______ must be told	1,2,3,4,5 A,B,C,D,E
6. *I do not want to be a burden*	
• to my family	1,2,3,4,5 A,B,C,D,E
• to the financial resources of my family	1,2,3,4,5 A,B,C,D,E
• to health care professionals	1,2,3,4,5 A,B,C,D,E
• to society	1,2,3,4,5 A,B,C,D,E
7. *I want my values to govern treatment*	1,2,3,4,5 A,B,C,D,E

[* It is important to mention, that it will be very difficult to find responsible and virtuous physicians who will honor requests for euthanasia. Physicians traditionally refuse to assist in suicide or to kill patients, even patients' requests to be killed. They base their refusal primarily on principles of medical ethics but also on laws which might criminalize physician's assisted suicide and active euthanasia.]

______________________	________________
(signature)	(date)
______________________	________________
(signature)	(re-dated)

PART III. MY INSTRUCTIONAL MEDICAL DIRECTIVE

[*Attention:* The following situations and procedures contain complex and complicated medical conditions and interventions. It is therefore strongly recommended to seek professional advice and information about treatment options before expressing preferences or giving directives.]

There are certain mental or physical conditions of suffering and disability in which I do not want to live and rather prefer to be dead. In those situations, I would not want my life to be prolonged by further medical treatment. Life-sustaining measures should not be initiated and if they have been, they should be discontinued. I recognize and hope that such a discontinuation is likely to hasten my death. I am also aware that medical terminology defines situations such as terminal illness, mental incompetence, severe and irreversible illness, even death, in objective technical terms only. I am not a medical expert, but being a competent adult I hereby request that my preferences for treatment be honored. I specifically direct my proxy and those in charge of my care to honor these preferences.

A. INSTRUCTIONS FOR SPECIFIC SITUATIONS

In the following, based on my personal values and wishes, I specify and define the situations in which I request that life-sustaining measures be foregone. I do request that the best possible comfort care be continued and I be medically relieved of pain:

1. *Terminal illness:* I realize that there may come a time when I am diagnosed as having an incurable and irreversible illness, disease, or condition. If this occurs and my attending physician and at least one additional physician who has personally examined me determine that my condition is terminal, I direct that life-sustaining measures that would serve only to artificially prolong my dying be withheld or discontinued. To me, *terminal condition* means that my physicians have determined that [I specify one] (a) I will die within a few days, (b) within a few weeks, (c) within six months, (d) within a year, (e) other.

2. *Incurable and irreversible illness:* There might come a time when I am diagnosed as having an *incurable and irreversible condition* which may not be terminal but causes me to experience severe and progressive physical and mental deterioration and/or the loss of capacities and faculties which I highly value and which are part of my life. Under the following conditions I would rather be dead than continue living and therefore I direct that all life-sustaining measures be withheld or discontinued, but that all comfort care is given to make me feel comfortable and to relieve pain under these circumstances:____________________

3. *Severe physical or mental disabilities:* There might come time when I suffer from severe physical or mental disabilities such as severe and unacceptable pain, incapacity to feel or move the body below the neck, a sudden and severe stroke, mental disabilities which will not allow me any more to recognize friends and loved ones, to understand who I am and where I am, severe and untreatable psychiatric disorders causing paranoia, schizophrenia, or depression. The following situations would cause me to direct that all life-sustaining treatment be withheld or discontinued, but that all care be given necessary to make me comfortable and relieve pain: ____

4. *Multimorbidity:* If I have one or more chronic progressive illnesses (such as severe cardiac arrhythmia, leukemia, rheumatism, progressed diabetes, endstage renal disease, or __________, some associated with blindness or amputation),

which is treated and allows me to continue my life within the limits of this illness, and I incur one or more additional severe mental or physical illnesses or incapacities, then I direct my long term chronic care plan be revised in order to allow for an as comfortable as possible end of my life. I direct that all care be given necessary to make me comfortable and to relieve pain if I am in the following situations:____________________________

5. *Permanent coma:* If there should come a time when I become permanently unconscious, and it is determined by my attending physician and at least one additional physician with appropriate experience who has personally examined me that I have lost my consciousness and my capacity to interact with other people and my surroundings, then I direct that life-sustaining measures be withheld or discontinued. *Permanent unconsciousness* means to me [select any that apply]: that the probability of regaining consciousness is (a) less than 1:10, (b) less than 1:100; I am comatose for (c) more than 10 days, (d) more than 30 days, (e) more than 6 months.

6. *Other situations* [Discuss other situations for which you want to express preferences or directives, based on your actual health risks or illnesses or on situations in which you have seen family members or friends]:________________

B. INSTRUCTIONS FOR SPECIFIC INTERVENTIONS

While I request that best possible comfort care and palliative care be provided, even if there might be only a slight probability that I may feel pain, I direct that the artificial provision of fluids and nutrition, the use of cardiopulmonary resuscitation (CPR), and, where legally acceptable, the use of drugs which will hasten death or result in death (euthanasia) be administered the following way:

1. I reject *artificial nutrition* for the following situations: ________________
2. I reject *artificial hydration* for the following situations: _______________
3. I reject *CPR resuscitation* for the following situations: ________________
4. I reject *major surgery* for the following situations: __________________
5. I request the administration of drugs having the double effect of *hastening my death* for the following situations: _____________________________
6. administration of drugs for the purpose of *ending my life* in the following situations:______________________________

C. INSTRUCTIONS FOR OTHER SITUATIONS

1. *Pregnancy:* If I am pregnant and I am incapacitated to make health care decisions, my statements and directions in this document shall [I specify one]: (a) remain in full force; (b) shall be changed in order to allow my child to be born; (c) shall be changed if a family can be found which will adopt my child. I want the child [I specify one]: (a) not to be born; (b) to be born; (c) to be born only if this can be achieved without discomfort or pain to me.

2. *Change of identity:* I am aware, that under the influence of severe physical or mental disorders or as a result of medication or hospitalization, I might become "another person" than I am now. If that is the case, then I direct that one of the following options be chosen: I want that (a) the values and preferences expressed in this document be followed strictly; (b) my health care representative have the authority to depart from the terms of this medical directive to promote my best interest; (c) only those values and preferences which I will express at that time be authoritative to direct treatment in my best interest.

3. *Death:* I am aware that criteria for declaring death, which previously were based on the cessation of heartbeat and breathing, have been changed in most countries and that physicians now declare a person dead after the irreversible cessation of all functions of the entire brain including the brain stem. I am also aware that the irreversible cessation of the functions of the higher brain (neocortical death) result in permanent loss of consciousness and self-consciousness, and of what is may be called personhood. According to my values and beliefs, I instruct my proxy and the medical experts responsible for my care that I want to be recognized and treated as dead if [I specify one]: (a) my heartbeat and breathing has stopped; (b) my entire brain including the brain stem has irreversibly lost all functions; (c) my higher brain functions have irreversibly been lost and I have become permanently unconscious.

4. *Existing diseases* [you might want to discuss directions for long term care plans for existing disorders, illnesses, and health risks]: __________________

5. *Other* [specify other personal or occupational situations in which your health might be at risk]: ______________________________________

D. MY UNDERSTANDING OF MEDICAL TERMINOLOGY AND OPTIONS

1. The following words and options are clear to me: __________________

2. I have some problems, understanding the following words procedures, and options: ______________________

3. I have discussed this Medical Directive with Dr. ____________________ address ________________, phone ______________, fax ________________

4. Here are Dr. _________'s comments on my state of competence and my understanding of the importance of my treatment preference statements, and any other comments Dr. ______ feels important to make:

___________________________ _______________

(Dr._____'s signature) (date)

___________________________ _______________

(Dr._____'s signature) (re-date)

___________________________ _______________

(Dr._____'s signature) (date)

____________________________	________________
(my signature)	(date)
____________________________	________________
(my signature)	(re-date)
____________________________	________________
(my signature)	(re-date)

17. Advance Health Care Directive: A Flexible Combination Form for Multicultural Use

[This advance health care directive, developed and modified in cooperation with German patients, physicians, nurses, lawyers, and students, is based on a form published in Hans-Martin Sass and Rita Kielstein, *Die Betreuungs-verfügung in der Praxis* (Bochum: Zentrum für Medizinische Ethik, 1996; 3d revised edition, 1997). The model is flexible, as it allows for (1) the modification of the reference to the monotheistic system or its replacement by referring to other religious or metaphysical traditions, (2) the patient's decision to determine content and specifications of letting others know in advance about her/his preferences for medical treatment and care and the preferred mode of identifying and designating proxy decision makers, and (3) use as a form combining and integrating the individual's value history, wishes, and directives for medical treatment and care, and the designation of a proxy by crossing out either one or a combination of these three elements, making it (1) a general value-and-wish statement, (2) a value-based living will, or (3) a durable power of attorney.

The first part affirms basic individual beliefs, values, and expectations; it requests that these and not available clinical technology shall govern treatment decisions; this part should express the individual's assessment of life and death, suffering and dependency, and trust and community within a specific religious or metaphysical tradition. The second part (1) requests care and treatment and (2) describes situations, for which medical treatment resulting in a prolongation of what the individual understands to be a prolongation of suffering only is refused; this part also (3) discusses individual acceptance or refusal of specific interventions on grounds of worldview and belief and (4) discusses medical directives (i.e., palliative care and its extent, and artificial breathing and feeding, reanimation, and specific interventions which might be required due to existing chronic diseases for a limited number of situations (final stages of terminal illness, severe dementia, prolonged coma). The third part designates a proxy and delineates the extent to which the proxy is bound by the specific directives, given in part 2. The fourth part affirms values and wishes, directives and designation, and the acceptance by the proxy and the signature of a witness. A witness is not required under German law, but the authors feel that a witness (preferably a physician, member of the clergy, or public notary under German law) can testify to the legal competence of the signee in case it would be questioned at a later time. The authors remind the prospective signee to seek professional advice before executing an advance directive, to review it periodically, and to cross out those paragraphs that they do not fully understand. Under German law this form would be authoritative even if one of the three parts (in its entirety or in part) is crossed out.

Germany still is a society with strong Christian traditions, but its multiculturality mirrors the diversity of individual and collective values, wishes, and expectations in a global village. Following is a religious (monotheistic) model, which would suit most Jews, Christians, and Muslims. The sentences referring to this signee's system of monotheistic belief are underlined; individuals are encouraged to replace these references with their own (Shinto, Hindu, Buddhist, animistic, environmental, or any philosophical standpoint). As the authors point out in the accompanying information and educational material, the existential challenge of suffering and death is determined by a limited number of situations (suffering and pain, coma, dementia, dependency) and medical responses, but the system of reference in which these challenges are perceived and addressed is individually and culturally different.]

My Life and My Death Are in God's Hands

ADVANCE DIRECTIVE IN HEALTH CARE MATTERS

______________ __________________ (Name, first name, date, and place of birth)

I. MY VALUES, WISHES, AND HOPES

My life and death are in the hand of the Lord. If in a future situation I might not be competent to consent to or refuse medical treatment, then my proxy(ies) and the attending physicians and care givers shall base their decisions and interventions on the wishes, values, and hopes that I have expressed in this document. They shall act in respect of my medical directives and my proxy designation; they shall not base their decisions on clinical availability and feasibility, and not on what others or they for themselves would want to be done in similar situations.

II. DIRECTIVES FOR MEDICAL TREATMENT AND CARE

1. My life is a gift from God. Therefore I expect all prudent medical treatment and care effecting my recovery or the reduction of the effects of chronic or severe illness to support zest and quality of life. It is also my wish to be provided with drugs that are still in the process of development and testing (yes/no); I also accept tissue and organs from others (yes/no) and donated blood (yes/no).

2. But if I would be (a) in the final stages of a terminal illness, (b) severely demented, (c) in a prolonged coma, (d) or in unrelenting and unrelieveable pain, then I request that all life-prolonging intervention be stopped or not initiated, as these would only prevent the natural course of my dying. If one of these situations occurs, I ask for *Christian and* caring support *and nothing be done which would intervene with the will of God who has counted the days of my life*; I also ask for best pain therapy and that I be relieved from all physical and emotional pain and stress. If possible, I would like to live the last days and hours of my life in familiar surroundings.

3. I refuse medication which will directly cause my death. *It is my belief, that life is a gift from God and should not be taken by suicide or assisted suicide.* If, however, the withdrawal of certain interventions or interventions and medication necessary to provide comfort care and pain relief also, as a side effect, cause harm to my body or shorten my life, then let it be, *as this might be the way the Lord has decided to take me away.*

4. *I know that my life is in God's hands, therefore* I request specifically:

A. *Treatment of Pain and Suffering:* I request effective medical treatment of suffering, such as breathlessness, pain, anxiety and fright, restlessness, nausea and vomiting (yes/no)

a. even if treatment makes me sleepy and tired (yes/no),

b. even if strong medication is needed, which might make me lose my awareness such as in anesthesia (yes/no),

c. even if treatment of pain and suffering might indirectly shorten my life (yes/no).

B. *Artificial Breathing and Artificial Nutrition:* I request that artificial breathing support and artificial nutrition and hydration be initiated or continued (yes/no),

a. even if I suffer from unrelenting pain due to ineffective palliative therapy (yes/no),

b. even if I am mentally incapacitated so that I do not know who I am, where I am, or recognize my loved ones and family any more (yes/no),

c. even if I am comatose for more than half a year.

C. *Re-Animation:* When my heart stops beating, I want to be medically re-animated (yes/no),

a. even if I suffer during the last stages of an incurable terminal illness,

b. even if I am mentally incapacitated so that I do not know who I am, where I am, nor recognize my loved ones and family any more (yes/no),

c. even if total dependency and limited capacity to communicate might be expected due to permanent brain injuries (yes/no).

D. *Other Directives and Wishes* (in particular, those related to the continuation or modification of existing chronic conditions such as ALS, AIDS, ESRD, diabetes, progressive neuronal diseases): ________________________________

III. POWER OF ATTORNEY IN HEALTH CARE MATTERS

1. If a situation arises in which due to physical or mental incapacity I will not be able to care for myself or make decisions, I herewith give full power of attorney (paragraph 1896 II of the German Civil Code BGB) to _________(name, first name, date of birth, address, phone and fax) as my legal representative. The person here designated as my proxy in health care matters is familiar with the content of this advance directive and has agreed to serve as my legal representative; therefore the designation of a legal representative by the courts is not necessary.

2. I put my legal representative under the obligation to act and to decide based on my values, wishes, and directives.

3. This power of attorney is also valid and legally binding for proxy decision making and includes the power to handle my accounts, to pay hospitals and nursing homes, to sign contracts on my behalf and to buy or sell real property (yes/no).

4. In the event that the person designated above is not capable or not willing any more to serve as my legal representative, I designate (1) ______________ (name, etc.), (2) one following the other.

5. In case a dispute arises in the interpretation of my wishes, values, and directives among physicians, nurses, my designated proxy, and family members, the final decision shall rest with my legal representative.

6. In the unlikely event that this power of attorney in health care matters is declared invalid by a court, I request that the court designates the above designated proxy(ies) as my legal representative(s) and that courts and proxies fully respect my wishes, values, and directives expressed and given above.

IV. AFFIRMATION AND SIGNATURE

I affirm the above-mentioned wishes, values, and directives as well as the designation of a proxy decision maker in health care matters. I intend to review these commitments and determinations from time to time and to revise them, if they are not in accordance with my wishes and values any more. However, as long as I have not made any changes, this is the last and final expression of my will.

________Date ______________________________________ Name and Signature

Agreement and Acceptance of Proxy in Health Care Matters. I have reviewed the content of this Advance Directive and accept the designation as legal representative.

________ Date __________________________________ Name, signature, and address

Validation by Witness. I confirm that ____________ has signed this advance directive today in my presence and that he (she) has made a free, competent, and self-determined decision in doing so.

________ Date __________________________________ Name, signature, and address

Review and Affirmation. Date of review ___________; changes ____________

_________________________________(Signature)

Bibliography

Compiled by Pat Milnoe McCarrick

Literature from Germany, Japan, and the United States concerned with advance directives and their importance at the end of life has been combined in this bibliography and divided into seven types of documents: bibliographies, collections, governmental papers, organizational statements, court decisions, books, and journal articles and individual chapters in contributed volumes. In some instances, early works or court decisions have been included in the area of death and dying, because of their importance in leading to the development of the advance directive movement around the world.

Document citations and annotations from Germany were selected by Professor Hans-Martin Sass; those from Japan were chosen by Professor Rihito Kimura; and those from the United States were compiled and annotated by Pat Milmoe McCarrick, a reference librarian at the National Reference Center for Bioethics Literature, Kennedy Institute of Ethics, Georgetown University.

Bibliographies

Bernat, Erwin. 1994. *Anfang und Ende des menschlichen Lebens: Eine internationale juristische Bibliographie.* Vienna: Verlag Österreich.

An international bibliography on legal and bioethical issues regarding interventions at the beginning and end of life, including "death as a legal term" (187–202), "suicide" (205–17), and "euthanasia and assisted suicide" (221–89).

Koch, Gerhard. 1984. *Euthanasie und Sterbehilfe: Eine dokumentierte Bibliographie.* Erlangen: Palm & Enke.

An annotated bibliography.

McCarrick, Pat Milmoe. 1992. *Living Wills and Durable Power of Attorney: Advance Directive Legislation and Issues.* Washington, D.C.: National Reference Center for Bioethics Literature.

Part of the Scope Note Series, the paper offers a brief background to the development of advance directives in the United States, a sample generic living will, and citations and annotations to works concerned with both directives and durable power of attorney.

Collections

Advance Directives: A Cross-Cultural Perspective—Patiententestamente in multikultureller Perspektive. 1996. *Jahrbuch für Recht und Recht und Ethik* [Annual Review for Law and Ethics] 4.

The multiauthored articles discuss ethical, cross-cultural, and clinical issues of advance directives and surrogate decision making in reference to the effectiveness and ineffectiveness of national law and regulation and the phenomena and mechanisms of behavior that generate and accompany law and determine its application and development: Hans-Martin Sass, "Klinisch-Ethische Entscheidungskonflikte und die Frage des rechtlichen Regelungbedarfs bei Patientenverfügungen und Stellvertretenden Entscheidungen"; Les Rothenberg et al., "The Relationship of Clinical and Legal Perspectives Regarding Medical Treatment Decision-Making in Four Cultures"; Johannes Gobertus Meran, "Advance Directives and Surrogate Decision Making: Ethical Questions, Legal Response, and Clinical Summary"; Erwin Bernat, "Advance Directives and Surrogate Decision Making in Germany, Japan, and the United States of America: A Comparative Law Analysis"; Hans-Martin Sass, Frederick O. Bonkovsky, Akira Akabayashi, Rita Kielstein, and Robert S. Olick, "Advance Health Care Documents in Multicultural Perspectives"; Robert S. Olick, Rihito Kimura, Jan T. Kielstein, H. Hayashi, Marc Riedl, and Mark Siegler, "Advance Care Planning and the ALS (Amyotrophic Lateral Sclerosis) Patient: A Cross-Cultural Perspective on Advance Directives"; Madison Powers, Carmen Kaminsky, and Motoko Hayashi, "AIDS and Advance Directives: Clinical, Legal and Ethical Perspectives in Japan, Germany and the United States."

"Advance Directives: What Do They Presuppose? How Do They Work?" 1994. *Bioethics* 8 (3): iii–vi, 191–246.

Editors Helga Kuhse and Peter Singer write that they agree that many advance directives are "badly drafted" and think that these documents should not be prepared by patients or by physicians. They prefer that the task be addressed by a governmentally appointed group of consumers, health professionals, lawyers, and philosophers. Articles included in this special issue are Julian Savulescu's "Rational Desires and the Limitation of Life-Sustaining Treatment," and Jim Stone's Advance Directives, "Autonomy and Unintended Death."

Docker, C. G. 1993. *Collected Living Wills.* Edinburgh: Voluntary Euthanasia Society of Scotland.

Noting the worldwide momentum toward living wills, Docker collected examples from 18 different countries on all the continents (except Antarctica), often with proxy directives. He includes addresses for obtaining further information.

Emanuel, Linda, ed. 1993. Advance Directives: Expectations, Experience, and Future Practice. *Journal of Clinical Ethics* 4 (1): 3–81.

Eighteen different articles comment on advance directives, proxies, patient values, the Patient Self-determination Act, incompetent patients, autonomy, and geriatric patients. Divided into sections, the following topics and authors are included in this special issue: Edmund G. Howe, "Editorial: The Vagaries of Patients' and Families' Discussing Advance Directives"; Linda Emanuel, "Research Section: Advance Directives: What Have We Learned So Far?"; Nancy S. Jecker, "Being a Burden on Others"; John Hardwig, "The Problem of Proxies with Interests of Their Own: Toward a Better Theory of Proxy Decisions"; Lawrence J. Schneiderman et al., "Do Physicians' Own Preferences for Life-Sustaining Treatment Influence Their Perceptions of Patients' Preferences?"; Robert A. Pearlman et al., "Insights Pertaining to Patient Assessments of States Worse than Death"; and David Doukas and Daniel W. Gorenflo, "Analyzing the Values History: An Evaluation of Patient Medical Values and Advance Directives."

The section called "Practice" includes: Linda Ganzini et al., "Is the Patient Self-determination Act Appropriate for Elderly Persons Hospitalized for Depression?"; Thomas E. Finucane et al., "Establishing Advance Medical Directives with Demented Patients: A Pilot Study"; Jack P. Freer, "Cases and Discussion Section: Decision Making in an Incapacitated Patient"; Linda Ganzini and Melinda A. Lee, "Authenticity, Autonomy, and Mental Disorders"; and Carl Elliott, "Meaning What You Say."

The issue included further editorials: Carson Strong, "Patients Should Not Always Come First in Treatment Decisions"; Baruch A. Brody, "Hardwig on Proxy Decision Making"; Alisa L. Carse, "Justice within Intimate Spheres"; Harold J. Bursztajn, "From PSDA to PTSD: The Patient Self-determination Act and Post-traumatic Stress Disorder"; Adil E. Shamoo and Dianne N. Irving, "The PSDA and the Depressed Elderly: 'Intermittent Competency' Revisited"; and Jan Marta, "The PSDA and Geriatric Psychiatry: A Cautionary Tale."

Eser, Albin, and Hans-Georg Koch, eds. 1991. *Materialien zur Sterbehilfe: Eine International Dokumentation.* Freiburg im Breisgau: Eigenverlag Max-Planck-Institut.

A well-documented collection from the countries of Germany, Australia, Belgium, France, Greece, Great Britain, Italy, Canada, the Netherlands, Austria, Portugal, Switzerland, Spain, and the United States and Scandinavia. Advance directives and proxy forms from many countries are included and accompanied by informed discussion by legal experts about the different national legal situations.

Howe, Edmund G., ed. 1995. "Substituted Judgment." Special section. *Journal of Clinical Ethics* 6 (1): 14–52.

Howe presents the dilemma faced by surrogate decision makers for incompetent patients, noting that the greatest weight tends to be placed on patients' prior preferences, expressed or inferred. Articles include: Christine Harrison et al., "Should

People Do unto Others as They Would Not Want Done unto Themselves?"; James F. Drane and John L. Coulehan, "The Best-Interest Standard: Surrogate Decision Making and Quality of Life"; Ralph Baergen, "Revising the Substituted Judgment Standard"; John Arthur McClung, "Time and Language in Bioethics: When Patient and Proxy Appear to Disagree"; and Bethany Spielman, "Futility and Bargaining Power."

Japanese Society for Dying with Dignity. 1988. *Ribingu Uiru: Songenshi no Sengensho* (Living Will: A Statement of Death with Dignity). Tokyo: Japanese Society for Dying with Dignity.

A collection of essays on living wills and death and dying in Japan written by various professionals including journalists, lawyers, physicians, and dieticians. The work includes a summary of the international and national context of the living will movement.

Loewy, Erich H., and Richard W. Carlson. 1994. "Talking, Advance Directives, and Medical Practice." *Archives of Internal Medicine* 154 (20).

An editorial by Loewy and Carlson note their reservations concerning advance directive procedures and physicians' failure to talk with patients about values or wishes. Three articles about this situation are included in the issue: Brendan Reilly et al., "Can We Talk?: Inpatient Discussions about Advance Directives in a Community Hospital: Attending Physicians' Attitudes, Their Inpatients' Wishes, and Reported Experience"; R. Sean Morrison et al., "Physician Reluctance to Discuss Advance Directives: An Empiric Investigation of Potential Barriers"; Lawrence J. Markson et al., "Implementing Advance Directives in the Primary Care Setting."

"Responses and Dialogue: Furthering the Dialogue on Advance Directives and the Patient Self-determination Act." 1994. Special issue. *Cambridge Quarterly of Healthcare Ethics* 3 (3).

Various authors in this collection discuss cultural pluralism as it applies to advance directives. Articles include: Miguel Bedolla, "Patient Self-determination Act: A Hispanic Perspective"; Erich H. Loewy, "Advance Directives: A Question of Autonomy"; Melvina McCabe, "Patient Self-determination Act: A Native American (Navajo) Perspective"; Robin Terrell Tucker, "Patient Self-determination Act: An African American Perspective"; and Lawrence P. Ulrich, "The Patient Self-determination Act and Cultural Diversity."

Takagi, Kentaro, ed. 1984. *Gendai no Sei to Shi* (Contemporary Life and Death). Tokyo: Nipponhyoron Sha.

A collection of articles on various aspects in life and death issues, particularly focusing on terminal care, hospice care, right to die, and the bioethical decision-making process.

Government and Organizations

Bundesärztekammer. 1993. Richtlinien der Bundesärztekammer für die ärztliche Sterbebegleitung. *Deutsches Ärzteblatt* 90 (37) C-1628–29.

This official self-regulatory document of the German Chamber of Physicians understands advance directives in oral or written form to be "leads only" [*Anhaltspunkte*] for the physician to determine the presumed actual wishes of the patient. If the patient has named a proxy, the physician is required to take the judgment of the proxy into account when determining the presumed actual wishes of the patient.

Evangelische Kirche in Deutschland, Deutsche Bischofskonferenz. 1989. *Gott ist ein Freund des Lebens.* Herausforderungen und Aufgaben beim Schutz des Lebens. Gütersloh: Mohn.

The Protestant and Catholic churches' joint statement against euthanasia and abortion supports the concept of allowing death with dignity.

Japan Science Council. 1994. *Shi to Iryo Tokubetsuiinkai hokoku: Songenshi nitsuite* (The Report of Special Commission on Death and Medical Service: On Death with Dignity). Tokyo: Japan Science Council.

The report expresses serious concern about death and dying issues in Japan and was the subject of concentrated discussion in the interdisciplinary academic milieu of the Japanese Scholars Congress called the Japanese Science Council. The issue of advance directives and living wills is discussed in the report, but emphasizes that continued open debate is important at least until specific legislation addresses this matter.

Japanese Society for Dying with Dignity. 1992. "The Development of the Movement for Dying with Dignity in Japan," Parts 1 and 2. Tokyo: Japanese Society for Dying with Dignity.

The basic document that delineates the development of the Japanese Society for Dying with Dignity from its establishment to the present time. The society also publishes an English version of the newsletter.

Medical Affairs Division, Health Policy Bureau, Ministry of Health and Welfare. 1985. *Seimei to Rinri nitsuite Kangaeru* (A Consideration on Life and Ethics). Tokyo: Ministry of Health and Welfare.

The Japanese Ministry's consulting body on Life and Ethics that studies bioethical issues relating to reproductive technology, terminal care, organ transplantation, brain death, etc., prepared this report. One of the session reports (section 2, chapter 3) focused on the issues of the living will in the context of terminal care.

Ministry of Health and Welfare. 1995. *Kosei Hakusho* (Annual Report on Health and Welfare). Tokyo: Gyosei.

Chapter 3 of the report discusses issues relating to terminal care and the establishment and payment methods for palliative care (14 palliative care units were operating in Japan in January 1995 at a cost of 33,000 yen per day [U.S. $330]). The ministry quotes the report (1993) of the National Survey on Terminal Care, saying that only 25 percent favored living will laws although 51 percent favored the idea of a living will. A third of those surveyed said that it is not necessary to have such a document. About 80 percent agreed to respect the wishes and intentions of patients in terminal care.

Ministry of Health and Welfare and Japan Medical Association. 1988. *Makki Iryo no Kea* (Care in Terminal Medicine).

An analysis and report of the commission concerned with care relating to terminal medicine established at the ministry. This document was intended to serve as a practical reference manual for terminal care and also contains a brief summary report of U.S. President's Commission for Bioethics concerning the ethics of terminal care. In addition, it includes a Japanese translation of a living will, quoting from the Medical Decision Act (Model Bill).

New Jersey Commission on Legal and Ethical Problems in the Delivery of Health Care. 1991. *New Jersey Advance Directives for Health Care and Declaration of Death Acts.* Trenton, N.J.: New Jersey Bioethics Commission.

The texts of the Advance Directives for Health Care Act and Declaration of Death Act are included along with relevant commentary. Three advance directive forms and a discussion of the brain dead or brain-damaged patient make up the appendix.

Tokyo Metropolitan Government. 1994. *Tokyo-to niokeru Taaminaru kea no arikata nitsuite* (On Terminal Care in the Hospitals of the Tokyo Metropolitan Region).

The report of the Interim Committee on Terminal Care of the Tokyo Metropolitan Government stresses the increasing need for the care of the terminally ill, including AIDS patients, and urges the establishment of specialized research, education, and clinical institutions be recommended to secure humane resources for these patients.

U.S. Omnibus Budget Reconciliation Act of 1990. 1990. Public Law No. 100-508, sec. 4206, 4751.

The Patient Self-determination Act was included in the general budget for the United States. It stated that hospitals and nursing homes receiving federal funds for Medicare and Medicaid patients must inquire about written advance directives and give information about them to all patients at time of admission. The act took effect in December 1991.

U.S. President's Commission for the Study of Ethical Problems in Medicine and Biomedical and Behavioral Research. 1983. *Deciding to Forego Life-Sustaining Treatment: Ethical, Medical, and Legal Issues in Treatment Decisions.* Washington, D.C.: U.S. Goverment Printing Office. (Out-of-print; facsimilies available from National Technical Information Service, Springfield, Va. 22161, doc. no. PB-83236836).

Serving as a reference and resource document since its publication, this extensive study indicates that neither criminal nor civil law precludes the mutual counsel of patient, physician, and family members to make decisions regarding those who are terminally ill.

Court Decisions

Barber/Nejdl v. Superior Court of Los Angeles County. 1983. 147 Cal. App. 3d 1006, 195 Cal. Rptr. 484.

A nurse complained when physicians removed a comatose patient's life-support systems after conferring with the family. The doctors were prosecuted for murder, but the California Court of Appeals dismissed the charges, ruling that they were not required to treat if there was no hope of recovery; the court also said that a spouse could make such a decision if a patient were incompetent, noting that artificial nourishment and hydration were no different from other medical treatment.

Bundesgerichtshof. 1994. *Urteil vom 13. September 1994—1StR 357/94—LG Kempten.* Manuscript. Karlsruhe: BGH.

Contrary to the regulations of the Bundesärztekammer, this first Supreme Court decision holds that the physician has to recognize previously written or oral statements as well as the patient's religious orientation, other personal values, age-related life expectancy, and degree of suffering when determining the presumed wishes of the patient. The Supreme Court stresses that "objective criteria, such as the recognition of an action as 'reasonable' or 'normal' or normally expressing the interests of a reasonable patient, have no self-standing [*eigenständige*] relevance; they may only be used as leads for the determination of the hypothetical individual will." "Objective value concepts" may be used only if the presumed individual wishes of the patient cannot be determined, but with great caution; if there is any doubt, protection of human life shall supersede personal convictions of the physician, family members, or other persons involved.

Cruzan v. Director, Missouri Department of Health, et al. 1990. 110 S. Ct. 2841; Cruzan v. Harmon. 1988. 760 S.W. 2d 410, Mo. banc.

This landmark case was the first considered by the United States Supreme Court concerned with the withdrawal of life support from a patient in a persistent vegetative state. Nancy Cruzan was only 26 years old in 1983 when an automobile accident left her totally incapacitated. In 1987 her parent asked to remove her feeding tubes, but the hospital refused, and then the Missouri courts ruled against the request. The U.S. Supreme Court ruled a competent person could refuse nutrition and hydration, but that a state should require that an incompetent person had made clear such a desire. When the case was returned to the lower courts, the state was dismissed as a party, no appeals followed the court's decision that tubes could be removed, and Ms. Cruzan died shortly afterward at the end of 1990.

In re Quinlan. 1976. 70 N.J. 10, 355 A. 2d 647.

An early case that brought the plight of incompetent patients to the attention of the public, creating interest in the desire to control one's care in the event competence were lost, involved Karen Ann Quinlan. Ms. Quinlan was 21 and had been in a persistent vegetative state, breathing via a respirator, for six months when her family asked the court to discontinue "extraordinary means" of sustaining her. The parents received permission to remove the ventilator; she survived for ten years in the vegetative state, receiving nutrition through a feeding tube.

In the Matter of Selma L. Saunders. 1985. 492 N.Y.S. 2d 510 (Sup. Ct. Nassau County, N.Y., July 16, 1985).

A competent woman who had executed a living will requested that the court determine its validity and effectiveness. Her petition was granted in part and denied in part. The court said that only the state legislature has authority to enact a statute recognizing the validity of living wills, and that the durable power of attorney transfers to another the responsibility for decisions while Ms. Saunders "strives to maintain her own right to self-determination." The court deemed the document to be in the nature of an informed medical consent and the instructions could be fulfilled without additional expensive court proceedings in the course of the natural death process should she become incompetent to continue to express her wishes.

John F. Kennedy Memorial Hospital, Inc. v. Bludworth. 1984. 452 So. 2d 921 Fla.

The Supreme Court of Florida reversed a lower district court decision that held in the case of Francis Landy, a comatose terminally ill patient who had executed a living will, that her guardian did not need to obtain court approval before removing her feeding tube in order for consenting family members, physicians, and the hospital to be relieved of civil and criminal liability. The higher court held that although patients have the right to refuse extraordinary means of artificial support and that living wills are persuasive evidence of intention, the courts still are always open to hear about circumstances caused by disagreement or wrong motives or malpractice that may need judicial intervention.

Rejection of the Claim for Right to Choose Death with Dignity February 17, 1985. Tokyo District Court Decision.

One of the board members of the Japan Society for Dying with Dignity claimed that the right to choose death with dignity is a constitutional right; however, this was rejected as an invalid case because it lacked the concrete legal conflicts normally intrinsic to those cases that are judged by the court. (See Kimura chapter in this volume.)

Superintendent of Belchertown State School v. Saikewicz. 1977. 373 Mass. 728, 370 N.E. 2d 417.

Joseph Saikewicz, a person who had never been competent, was dying when his caretakers asked the court to appoint a guardian to make his health care decisions. The guardian opted for nontreatment, and his decision was upheld by the Massachusetts Supreme Judicial Court based on substituted judgment—the judgment the incompetent would have made if competent, taking into account present and future factors.

Tokai University Hospital Case on Active Euthanasia. 1995. Yokohama District Court Decision, the Third Criminal Section.

This was the first case in which an attending physician was prosecuted and received a sentence of two years' imprisonment. In this court decision, the term *Living Will* was used and the notion of *advance directives* was mentioned officially for the first time in any Japanese court decision. The criminal charge against the physician, which resulted in two years of imprisonment with suspension, was widely accepted as reasonable. This case is presented in Kimura's chapter in this volume.

Books/Special Issues

American Hospital Association. 1991. *Put It in Writing: A Guide to Promoting Advance Directives.* Chicago: AHA Services (P.O. Box 92683, Chicago, Ill. 60675).

Prepared for hospitals, the guide provides information necessary for complying with the U.S. Patient Self-determination Act of 1990 as well as for fulfilling the requirement of the Joint Commission on Accreditation of Healthcare Organizations that all U.S. hospitals have policies and procedures for written advance directives in patient care. It includes a question and answer section, a glossary, sample forms, information about state laws, copies of the AHA's Bill of Rights and Patient's Choice of Treatment Options, a resource list, and a pamphlet prepared for patients.

Amery, Jean. 1976. *Hand an sich legen: Diskurs über den Freitod.* Stuttgart: Klett.

This document is an outspoken and strongly reasoned defense of the freedom to choose one's own death by "laying hands on oneself," a prescription that this famous novelist followed a few years after this essay was written.

Atrott, Hans H. 1990. *Menschenwürdiges und selbstverantwortetes Sterben.* Augsburg: Deutsche Gesellschaft für humanes Sterben.

A for-members-only numbered edition of a "how to" suicide booklet, which, according to informed sources, contains prescriptions and procedures similar to those recommended in Derek Humphry's book *Final Exit* (Eugene, Ore.: Hemlock Society, 1991), which was translated into German in 1992 under the title *In Würde sterben: Praxis Sterbehilfe und Selbsttötung* (Hamburg: Carlsen). This booklet is no longer distributed as a result of the spectacular imprisonment of Mr. Atrott, who was then the president of the German Society for Dying in Dignity, for privately selling lethal doses of cyanide to members of the society.

Atrott, Hans H., and Hermann Pohlmeier, eds. 1990. *Sterbehilfe in der Gegenwart.* Regensburg: Roderer.

A review of cultural and legal approaches to euthanasia and assisted suicide.

Baumann, J., et al. 1986. *Alternativentwurf Sterbehilfe.* Stuttgart, New York: Vandenhoek und Ruprecht.

A proposal by a group of respected legal experts to change the German Penal Code to allow for physician-assisted suicide or the shortening of life on the request of the patient during the final stages of the dying process.

Bernat, Erwin. 1993. "Das Recht an der Grenze zwischen Leben un Tod." In *Ethik und Recht an der Grenze Zwischen Leben und Tod,* ed. Erwin Bernat. Graz: Leykam.

Böckle, Franz. 1979. *Menschenwürdig Sterben.* Theologische Meditationen 52. Zurich: Benziger.

A strong defense of allowing death with dignity by a highly recognized Roman Catholic theologian, former president of the University of Bonn.

Bönisch, Georg, and Hans Leyendecker. 1993. *Das Geschäft mit der Sterbehilfe.* Göttingen: Steidl.

Sensational journalistic report on the selling of deadly doses of killer drugs by Mr. Atrott, the former president of the Deutsche Gesellschaft für Humanes Sterben.

Cantor, Norman L. 1993. *Advance Directives and the Pursuit of Death with Dignity.* Bloomington, Ind.: Indiana University Press.

Cantor outlines legal information about advance directives, suggesting ways to prepare them, guidelines for their implementation, and possible solutions to problems that may arise. He also looks at the moral implications of persons planning future health care long before there is a need. He includes New Jersey's model legislation and sample forms.

Cate, Fred H., and Barbara A. Gill. 1991. *The Patient Self-determination Act: Implementation Issues and Opportunities.* Washington, D.C.: Annenberg Washington Program.

A publication from the Communication Policy Studies Annenberg Program at Northwestern University in Chicago, this book includes a discussion of unresolved issues in the U.S. law in relation to the U.S. Supreme Court decision in the Cruzan case. The appendix provides information sources, a copy of the law, and sample advance directives.

Colen, B. D. 1991. *The Essential Guide to a Living Will.* New York: Prentice Hall.

The author thinks that explicit advance directives are absolutely necessary to ensure the kind of health care one desires, because they provide physicians and family with the patient's competent wishes. He suggests a videotaped directive that would portray the actual patient clearly stating his or her desires.

Deeken, Alfonso. 1986. *Shi eno Jyunbi Kyoiku* (Death Education). Tokyo: Medikaru Frendo Sha.

This three-volume work looks at the philosophical, religious, medical, and psychological aspects of death and dying. One of the first series of books on death education published in Japan.

Doukas, David John, and William Reichel. 1993. *Planning for Uncertainty: A*

Guide to Living Wills and Other Advance Directives for Health Care. Baltimore: Johns Hopkins University Press.

Family physicians Doukas and Reichel use a question-and-answer format to discuss therapies, values, ethical principles, and advance directive choices. They describe the medical consequences of different treatment choices and procedures and include sample documents.

Füllmich, Reiner. 1990. *Der Tod im Krankenhaus und das Selbstbestimmungsrecht des Patienten.* Dissertation, University of Göttingen. Bern: Lang.

A dissertation that discusses the tension between dying in the hospital and patient autonomy.

Hahn, Susanne, and Achim Thoms. 1983. *Sinnvolle Lebensbewahrung—humanes Sterben.* Auseinandersetzung mit dem ärztlichen Bewahrungsauftrag gegenüber menschlichem Leben. Berlin: VEB Verlag der Wissenschaften.

A defense of allowing death with dignity from two academicians writing in the former German Democratic Republic.

Juergens, Andreas, and Detlev Kröger. 1992. *Das neue Betreuungsrecht.* Munich: Beck.

A legal review of the new German Care Law, which gives the mentally incapacitated a stronger role in sharing decisions within a health care setting. The authors recommend the naming of proxy decision makers and the drafting of advance directives for future onset of dementia or for other situations in which there would otherwise be invalid expression of wishes and preferences or no documentation of preference at all.

Kamlah, Wilhelm. 1976. *Meditatio mortis.* Stuttgart: Klett.

Kamlah, Professor of Philosophy at the University of Erlangen, wrote this justification of ending one's own life as an expression of autonomy and self-determination just before his own suicide.

Kielstein, Rita, and Hans-Martin Sass, eds. 1993. *Materialien zur Erstellung von wertanamnestischen Betreuungsverfügungen.* Bochum: Zentrum für Medizinische Ethik.

The authors present and discuss forms for advance directives based on the value histories [*Wertanamnese*] created by Doukas and McCullough, Amato-Grundstein, Emanuel and Emanuel, Gibson, Seghal, and Kielstein and Sass.

King, Nancy M. P. 1991. *Making Sense of Advance Directives.* Boston: Kluwer Academic.

King describes the right-to-die movement and the various proposed laws and legislation.

Koch, Hans-Georg, Johannes-Gobertus Meran, and Hans-Martin Sass. 1994. *Patientenverfügung und stellvertretende Entscheidung in rechtlicher, medizinischer und ethischer Sicht.* Bochum: Zentrum für Medizinische Ethik.

A modified German version of Koch's, Meran's, and Sass's chapters in this volume.

Ohi, Gen. 1990. *Shumatsuki Iryo* (The Terminal Medical Care). Tokyo: Kobundo.

The changing situation of Japanese medical care in the terminal stage is analyzed through the authors' clinical experiences in various regions in Japan, including Okinawa, Nagano, and Tokyo. The authors discuss the ethical implications of communication between patient and physician about terminal care as well as the necessity for Japanese physicians to approach the terminal patient according to each particular patient's needs.

Ohta, Tenrei, ed. 1972. *Anrakushi* (Euthanasia). Tokyo: Kurieitosha.

Two lawyers, T. Uematsu and M. Fukuda, discuss and analyze the legal aspects of euthanasia in this work.

Pichler, Johannes W. 1992. *Internationale Entwicklungen in den Patientenrechten.* Vienna: Bohlau Verlag.

Pichler discusses patients' legal rights in an international perspective.

Saueracker, Luise. 1990. *Die Bedeutung des Patiententestaments in der Bundesrepublik Deutschland aus ethischer, medizinischer und juristischer Sicht.* Frankfurt: Lang.

A dissertation reviewing the ethical, legal, and medical aspects of advance directives in Germany.

Schöllhammer, L. 1993. *Die Rechtsverbindlichkeit des Patiententestaments: Eine Untersuchung aus zivilrechtlicher Sicht.* Berlin: Duncker & Humblot.

The work reviews the civil law aspects of advance directives in Germany before the BGH Supreme Court Decision of 1994.

Stoll, Kathleen D. 1992. *Pregnancy Exclusions in State Living Will and Medical Proxy Statutes.* Washington, D.C.: Center for Women Policy Studies.

The paper looks at state statutes that negate a women's living will or durable power of attorney when she is terminally ill or in a permanent vegetative state and is pregnant. It analyzes pregnancy exclusions in the advance directive laws of 37 states.

Uhlenbruck, Wilhelm. 1992. *Selbstbestimmung im Vorfeld des Sterbens.* Bochum: Zentrum für Medizinische Ethik.

The leading expert's arguments for accepting and promoting advance directives.

Articles

Annas, George J., and Francis H. Miller. 1994. "The Empire of Death: How Culture and Economics Affect Informed Consent in the U.S., the U.K., and Japan." *American Journal of Law and Medicine* 20 (4): 357–94.

A comparative and unique analysis of three different countries that focuses on death and dying issues, including informed consent issues.

Auer, Alfons. 1976. "Das Recht des Menschen auf einen 'natürlichen Tod.'" In

Der Mensch und sein Tod, ed. Johannes Schwartländer. Göttingen: Vandenhoek und Ruprecht, 82–93.

A Roman Catholic theologian's perspective on dying with dignity without the prolongation of life by extraordinary means.

Bai, Koichi. "Amerikaniokeru iwayuru 'Shinu Kenri'? Hanketsu no Doko: Iryo to Saiban no Aidade" (The So-called Right-to-Die Decision in United States: Between Medicine and Court). In *Medicine, Law and Ethics,* ed. Koichi Bai.

The author summarizes legal arguments in the United States by focusing on the cases of Karen Ann Quinlan and Joseph Saikewicz and discussing issues relating to quality of life, autonomy, and medical professional integrity as a justification for proceeding with the treatment of a patient. This article has received much attention in legal and public discussion in Japan, as similar cases could be recognized in the Japanese clinical setting.

Broadwell, Anita W., Eugene V. Boisaubin, J. Kay Dunn, and H. Tristam Engelhardt. 1993. "Advance Directives on Hospital Admission: A Survey of Patient Attitudes." *Southern Medical Journal* 86 (2): 165–68.

The authors surveyed 200 outpatients and found that 18 percent had completed advance directives; only 5 percent of those queried had received information from their physician. Half of those with advance directives had secured the only copy in a safety deposit box.

Brock, Dan W. 1994. "Advance Directives: What Is It Reasonable to Expect from Them?" *Journal of Clinical Ethics* 5 (1): 57–60.

Brock says that it is a very early time in the use and understanding of advance directives; therefore, he thinks enthusiasm should be tempered and more effective usage developed, particularly to improve surrogate decision making for incompetent patients.

Brodeur, Dennis. 1994. "The Saga of Advance Directives." *Issues* 9 (2): 1–5, 8.

Brodeur describes a document drafted by lawyers to address powers of attorney for health care decisions. It contains a list to identify individual wishes, a section to indicate organ donation wishes, and the name of the primary physician. An Oklahoma woman prepared an 18-page advance directive requesting euthanasia, asking that her attorneys use their own desires as criteria for her care. Brodeur notes that she clearly did not wish to live if cogently impaired, but the attorneys continued treatment, backed by the court. Pointing out such weaknesses in the Patient Self-determination Act brings the author to the conclusion that there is a need for communication going beyond the individual to learn about society's concerns.

Brückner, Christian. 1989. "Was leisten Patientenverfügung und Freitoderklärung als Kommunikationsmittel zwischen Unterzeichner und Drittperson?" *Schweizerische Ärztezeitung* 70:1149–58.

A reflection on the validity of advance directives within the Swiss legal and medical culture.

Bundesminister für Justiz. 1992. *Das neue Betreuungsgesetz.* Bonn: Bundesministerium für Justiz.

Informational brochure by the German Federal Ministry of Justice proposing useful language for advance directives and proxy forms.

Bursztajn, Harold J., and Archie Brodsky. 1994. "Clear, Convincing, and Authentic Advance Directives in the Context of Managed Care?" *Journal of Clinical Ethics* 5 (4): 364–66.

The authors raise the issue of cost-driven treatment and say that patients must be free to change their minds in decisions regarding termination of treatment.

Danis, M., J. Garrett, R. Harris, and D. Patrick. 1994. "Stability of Choices about Life-Sustaining Treatments." *Annals of Internal Medicine* 120 (7): 567–73.

Over 2,500 Medicare patients were questioned about living wills and desire for life-sustaining treatment if they became terminally ill. Two years later with an 82 percent follow-up, the authors found that the study group chose to forgo one treatment more than in the earlier study, and that patients who had living wills were less likely to change their wishes. The authors concluded that it is important to review patients' preferences.

Deutsche Bischofskonferenz. 1975. *Das Lebensrecht des Menschen und die Euthanasie.* Hirtenschreiben der Deutschen Bischöfe. Bonn.

Statement by the German Conference of Roman Catholic bishops criticizing calls for physician-assisted suicide and euthanasia but recommending stopping short of doing everything technically possible to prolong suffering life.

Deutsche Bischofskonferenz. 1993. "Die Hospizbewegung: Profil eines hilfreichen Weges im katholischen Verständnis." Bonn: Deutsche Bischofskonferenz.

This article communicates Catholic bishops' support of the hospice movement and the concept of Christian hospices.

Dresser, Rebecca. 1994. "Confronting the 'Near Irrelevance' of Advance Directives." *Journal of Clinical Ethics* 5 (1): 55–56.

Commenting on the Teno et al. study, Dresser notes the failure of advance directives to provide guidance for seriously ill, incompetent patients and says that she is pleased to see state recognition of family members as surrogate decision makers. She urges further study of unjustifiable burdens both to patients and to society.

Elpern, Ellen H., Suzanne B. Yellen, and Laurel A. Burton. 1993. "A Preliminary Investigation of Opinions and Behaviors Regarding Advance Directives for Medical Care." *American Journal of Critical Care* 2 (2): 161–67.

The authors interviewed 46 inpatients and 50 outpatients at a medical center in 1991, finding that most knew of advance directives, but only 52 percent understood the purpose of these documents. Unfamiliarity and procrastination were given as reasons for not having an advance directive, but 65 percent said that they had spoken with relatives or friends about their preferences for treatment; 83 percent said they would be comfortable discussing them with a physician or a nurse.

Emanuel, Linda. 1994. "Appropriate and Inappropriate Use of Advance Directives." *Journal of Clinical Ethics* 5 (4): 357–59.

Commenting on the Wenger and Halpern (1994) article, Emanuel says that "advance directives have defined purposes, require informed consent and are suitable only for some patients." She urges that patients with borderline competence be assessed for their ability to plan in advance.

Emanuel, Linda L., Michael J. Barry, Ezekiel J. Emanuel, and John D. Stoeckle. 1994. "Advance Directives: Can Patients' Stated Treatment Choices Be Used to Infer Unstated Choices?" *Medical Care* 32 (2): 95–105.

By presenting 11 treatment choices in four illness scenarios, the authors learned from their 495 subjects that requests for certain scenarios were strong predictors for how one choice might follow another. A request for major surgery or a declination of antibiotics were found to be the two most predictive preferences, suggesting that advance directives could be potentially useful in unspecified decisions.

Emanuel, Linda L., Marion Danis, Robert A. Pearlman, and Peter A. Singer. 1995. "Advance Care Planning as a Process: Structuring the Discussions in Practice." *Journal of the American Geriatrics Society* 43 (3): 440–46.

The authors present a suggested five-step process: raising the topic and providing information, having a structured discussion, completing and recording a statement, reviewing and updating such a document, and having later decisions match prior wishes.

Emanuel, Linda L., and Ezekiel J. Emanuel. 1993. "Decisions at the End of Life: Guided by Communities of Patients." *Hastings Center Report* 23 (5): 6–14.

The Emanuels write that treatment decisions for incompetent patients without advance directives could be made "according to default guidelines that follow the preferences of the local community of patients." They note limitations inherent in giving prior instructions, and procedural limitations in honoring such documents because they may not be available to those treating the patient. The authors recommend community deliberations to increase respect for autonomy and wider use of dialogue.

Emanuel, Linda L., Ezekiel J. Emanuel, J. D. Stoeckle, L. R. Hummel, and M. J. Barry. 1994. "Advance Directives: Stability of Patients' Treatment Choices." *Archives of Internal Medicine* 154 (2): 209–17.

Studying a group of outpatients and the public in three ongoing interviews, the authors made four possible illness scenarios with the goal of assessing stability. They found a range of stability levels, but patients who were stable at the start generally remained so. They think advance directives can be relied upon one to two years after completion to reflect patient choices.

Eser, Albin. 1976. "Der manipulierte Tod: Möglichkeiten und Grenzen der Sterbehilfe aus rechtlicher Sicht." In *Der Mensch und sein Tod,* ed. Johannes Schwartländer. Göttingen: Vandenhoek und Ruprecht, 61–81.

A legal expert's review of the legal situation in Germany in 1976.

Foytack, Jane, and Daniel J. West. 1994. "Physician Management Guidelines for Advance Directives with Patients." *Omega* 29 (2): 165–75.

The authors offer a model and guidelines about advance directives for physicians to use with patients, identifying variables in the office or inpatient setting, management and clinical factors, and education about such documents. They say that effectiveness depends on the physician's knowledge to guide the patient through treatment and ability to coordinate efforts with other health care providers.

Francis, Leslie Pickering. 1993. "Advance Directives for Voluntary Euthanasia: A Volatile Combination?" *Journal of Medicine & Philosophy* 18 (3): 297–322.

Francis raises what he calls the "most significant doubts" about advance directives along with the "most significant doubts" about voluntary euthanasia if one could request euthanasia in an advance directive. He discusses accuracy, authority (future as opposed to present), uncertainty, finality, and physicians' obligations. He thinks euthanasia guided by an advance directive combined with a current reaffirmation is preferable to euthanasia legislation.

Fukuda, Masaaki. 1975. "A Survey Research of Doctor's Attitudes toward Euthanasia in Boston and in Tokyo." *Osaka University Law Review,* no. 22:19–77.

This is one of the earliest comparative research works on euthanasia issues between United States and Japan that appeared in the English language. It includes many interesting analyses on categorizing the types of euthanasia that may be deemed acceptable.

Ganzini, Linda, Melinda A. Lee, and Ronald T. Heintz. 1994. "The Capacity to Make Decisions in Advance and Borderline Personality Disorder." *Journal of Clinical Ethics* 5 (4): 360–63.

Commenting on the competence of the woman described in the Wenger and Halpern article, the authors think that more research on how decisions are made will help in actual clinical decision making.

Gillick, Muriel R., Katherine Hesse, and Nancy Mazzapica. 1993. "Medical Technology at the End of Life: What Would Physicians and Nurses Want for Themselves?" *Archives of Internal Medicine* 153 (22): 2542–47.

The authors prepared a document modeled on a medical directive that listed 12 treatment interventions. Presented to the full-time nursing and medical staff at a community teaching hospital along with possible illness scenarios, this document allowed the respondents to indicate how they would want to be treated. The authors conclude that physicians and nurses are unlikely to wish aggressive treatment if terminally ill, demented, or in a persistent vegetative state.

Gomibuchi, R. 1991. ["Informed Consent in Orthopaedic Medicine—In Search of Better Relationships between the Doctor and Patient"] (published erratum appears in *Nippon Seikeigeka Gakkai Zasshi* 65 [10], preceding Table of Contents). *Nippon Seikeigeka Gakkai Zasshi* 65 (9): 788–96.

Grodin, Michael A. 1993. "Religious Advance Directives: The Convergence of Law, Religion, Medicine, and Public Health." *American Journal of Public Health* 83 (6): 899–903.

Noting the importance of religion in the lives of many, Grodin says it is not surprising that decisions about death and dying have led to religious advance directives. He analyzes the strengths (expressing religious beliefs and perspectives related to medical practices) and weaknesses (the possibility of removing power from those seeking religious goals) of such documents. He recommends the health care proxy form, which appoints an agent bound to make substituted decisions according to the patient's desires.

Hesse, Katherine A. 1995. "Terminal Care of the Very Old: Changes in the Way We Die." *Archives of Internal Medicine* 155 (14): 1513–18.

The author studied the use of advance directives, limitations of treatment, and medical intervention in patients over 85 years of age who died at one hospital over a five-year period. She found that fewer high-intensity interventions are being used, more attention is paid to comfort, and few receive cardiopulmonary resuscitation. She found that there is little reference to formal advance directives in decision making for these patients.

Hoerster, Norbert. 1989. "Tötungsverbot und Sterbehilfe." In *Medizin und Ethik,* ed. Hans-Martin Sass, 287–95. Stuttgart: Reclam.

A law professor's proposal to change the German Penal Code to allow for physician-assisted suicide on request.

Hoffman, Molly, K. 1994. "Use of Advance Directives: A Social Work Perspective on the Myth Versus the Reality." *Death Studies* 18 (3): 229–41.

Saying that living wills should be called directives to physicians, Hoffman discusses their weaknesses in describing the patient's wishes and urges greater public awareness of the complexities of modern medical care.

Iserson, Kenneth V. 1993. "A Simplified Prehospital Advance Directive Law: Arizona's Approach." *Annals of Emergency Medicine* 22 (11): 1703–10.

Calling the Prehospital Advance Directive the PHAD, Iserson says it allows patients to communicate to emergency medical services their desire not to receive certain procedures. Noting that Arizona is the fourth state in the United States to pass such a law, he praises its simplicity for both providers and patients.

Ishiwata, Ryuji, and Akio Sakai. 1994. "The Physician-Patient Relationship and Medical Ethics in Japan." *Cambridge Quarterly of Health Care Ethics* 3 (1): 60–66.

The unique nature of the Japanese physician-patient relationship is analyzed in reference to cultural and religious aspects. The authors also explore the meaning of *Omakase* (entrusting) in the context of strong paternalism as well as the way in which Buddhism influences the Japanese attitude toward death.

Johnson, Sarah Coate, Mark P. Pfeifer, and Robert McNutt. 1995. "The Discussion about Advance Directives: Patient and Physician Opinions Regarding When and How It Should Be Conducted." *Archives of Internal Medicine* 155 (10): 1025–30.

Indicating that fewer than 10 percent of Americans have advance directives, the authors' queries indicated that patients thought that discussions should occur at an earlier time than physicians did, but that each group agreed that it was the physician's responsibility to open the discussion.

Jonas, Hans. 1984–85. "Das Recht zu sterben." *Scheidewege: Jahresschrift für skeptisches Denken* 14:10–22.

This article presents Jonas's arguments for allowing death with dignity.

Kielstein, Rita. 1994. "Wertanamnese und Patientenverfügung." *Zeitschrift für ärztliche Fortbildung* 88:743–53.

Here, Kielstein presents and discusses a narrative form of an advance directive developed by Kielstein and Sass.

Kielstein, Rita, and Hans-Martin Sass. 1993. "Using Stories to Assess Values and Establish Medical Directives." *Kennedy Institute of Ethics Journal* 3:303–25.

Kimura, Rihito. 1987. "Bioethics as a Prescription for Civic Action: The Japanese Interpretation." *Journal of Medicine and Philosophy* 12 (3): 267–77.

The author looks at traditional and cultural roots of Japanese paternalistic medical service, describing trends in the emergence of patients' rights as well as the bioethics movement in Japan since the 1980s. The Nagoya High Court Case on euthanasia (1962) is quoted with comments in a reference note.

———. 1988. "Bioethical and Sociolegal Aspects of the Elderly in Japan with Special Reference to Life-Sustaining Technologies in Law in East and West." *Waseda University Institute of Comparative Law,* 175–200.

In the social context of Japan's elderly population, Kimura describes the technological problems related to care of the critically and terminally ill aged. He includes issues relating to informed consent and living wills, and goes on to analyze the unique character of the paternalistic physician-patient relationship and the family relationship.

———. 1991. "Death with Dignity: Discussion in Japan." *World Health* 12:391–92. Published by the World Health Organization.

Kimura provides a brief analysis of dying patients in contemporary Japan with a discussion of the problem of lack of communication and changing demands for truth telling and palliative care.

Koch, Hans-Georg. 1991. "Landesbericht Bundesrepublik Deutschland." In *Materialien zur Sterbehilfe,* ed. A. Eser, H. G. Koch, 31–193. Freiburg: Max-Planck-Institut für ausländisches und internationales Strafrecht.

An extended overview of the legal situation in Germany, including review of court decisions and originals of advance directives and durable power of attorney forms.

Koller, Peter. 1993. "Personen, Rechte und Entscheidungen über Leben und Tod." In *Ethik und Recht an der Grenze zwischen Leben und Tod,* ed. Erwin Bernat, 71–95. Graz: Leykam.

This article reviews legal and cultural aspects of self-determination at the end of life.

Kuczewski, Mark G. 1994. "Whose Will Is It, Anyway? A Discussion of Advance Directives, Personal Identity, and Consensus in Medical Ethics." *Bioethics* 8 (1): 27–48.

Kuczewski considers objections that have been raised to the use of advance directives based on the "discontinuity of personal identity." He thinks there is a narrative ongoing concept of a social sense of self and urges discussion of the "values of society and the wishes of the patient."

Lauter, H. 1993. "Tötung ohne Verlangen—Tötung bei unterstelltem Verlangen." *Zeitschrift für ärztliche Fortbildung* 87:46–51.

Discussion of legal and ethical issues involved in the killing on request by physicians.

Lutterotti, Markus von. 1993. "Grenzen ärztlicher Behandlungspflicht und passive Sterbehilfe." *Zeitschrift für medizinische Ethik* 39:3–14.

A noted physician's position against euthanasia and in support of allowing one to die.

Lynn, Joanne, and Joan M. Teno. 1993. "After the Patient Self-determination Act: The Need for Empirical Research on Formal Advance Directives." *Hastings Center Report* 23 (1): 20–24.

The authors look at various studies on the impact of advance directives on patient populations, saying that it is not enough to show usage. Rather, it is necessary to show that decision making and patient outcomes are improved. They urge study of patient preference stability, the effects of directives compared to other methods of decision making for incompetent patients, and reasons why people do or do not choose to have advance directives.

———. 1995. "Death and Dying: Euthanasia and Sustaining Life. III. Advance Directives." In *Encyclopedia of Bioethics,* ed. Warren T. Reich, 572–77. Revised Edition. New York: Simon and Schuster Macmillan.

The authors provide a historical background, describe types of advance directives, discuss considerations in using the documents, their utilization and impact, and possible policy implications. They conclude that decision making for incompetent adults is a perplexing problem; advance directives are limited by "being no better than the counseling that preceded them."

McCrary, S. Van, William L. Allen, and Clarence L. Young. 1993. "Questionable Competency of a Surrogate Decision Maker under a Durable Power of Attorney: Cases and Discussion." *Journal of Clinical Ethics* 4 (2): 166–74.

The designated health care agent in the case study acts in ways contradictory to the patient's desires and in a manner perceived as unusual by the hospital staff. When the patient's condition improves, she names a new decision-making surrogate. The authors note the importance of having a competent surrogate and suggest various ways that legal recourse could insure competency. Commentary by Gail Povar, "Second Guessing the Patient's Trust: Facing the Challenge of the Difficult Surrogate"; Greg A. Sachs, "Improving Advance Directives: More Dialogue, Not More Laws"; and Jonathan D. Moreno, "Health-Care Agents: Decisional Capacity and Legal Compliance." Povar urges anticipatory planning and early physician-patient discussions. Sachs thinks discussion "should and must occur between patients, families, and physicians for advance planning to work. Regardless of the specific clauses built into statutes, if this communication fails, advance directives fail." Moreno stresses the role of the decision maker and says that health staff must not confuse difficult comportment by the agent with his decisions.

Menikoff, J. A., G. R. Sachs, and Mark Siegler. 1992. "Beyond Advance Directives: Health Care Surrogate Laws." *New England Journal of Medicine* 327 (16): 1165–69.

Saying that some values such as the importance of family and the decisions of loved ones are at least as important as "rigid devotion to the goal of patient autonomy," the authors discuss state legislation concerned with surrogate decision making. They think that certain decisions should have a "higher degree of scrutiny," since it would be "inappropriate to defer automatically to surrogate decision makers in the case of all incompetent patients."

Minogue, Brendan, and James E. Reagan. 1994. "Can Complex Legislation Solve Our End-of-Life Problems?" *Cambridge Quarterly of Healthcare Ethics* 3 (1): 115–24.

Minogue and Reagan write that over the last 20 years, a consensus of legal opinion has arisen that holds that the states should minimally interfere with the wishes of patients or surrogates and physicians' decisions about forgoing life-sustaining treatment, but that states can intervene to protect a compelling state interest. They discuss the Ohio law that in their opinion places restrictions that are too complex on all parties involved. The authors recommend that state legislatures consult with hospital ethics committees to draft better laws.

Mower, William R., and Larry J. Baraff. 1993. "Advance Directives: Effect of Type of Directive on Physicians' Therapeutic Decision." *Archives of Internal Medicine* 153 (3): 375–81.

The authors presented patient and advance directive scenarios to medical school faculty in three different surveys. With a therapy-specific advance directive supported by a proxy decision maker and a discussion by the physician with the patient, physicians polled were willing to withhold cardiopulmonary resuscitation. Mower and Baraff say that detailed advance directives, an appointed proxy, and physician-patient discussions are characteristic of the most reliable directives.

Pinch, Winifred J., et al. 1995. "Implementation of the Patient Self-determination Act: A Survey of Nebraska Hospitals." *Research in Nursing and Health* 18 (1): 59–66.

The authors queried 79 hospitals about the role of nurses in advance directive policy and found that they were involved in planning but not implementation. An advocacy role was suggested for nurses to promote patient education.

Pugh, Donna, and Daniel J. West. 1994–1995. "Advance Directives and the Self-determination Act: A Patient's Perspective." *Omega* 30 (4): 249–56.

Patients' ideas on how professionals should be actively involved in meeting their needs, wants, and desires are discussed by the authors, who provide a model for implementing advance directives.

Reinders, M., and Peter A. Singer. 1994. "Which Advance Directive Do Patients Prefer?" *Journal of General Internal Medicine* 9 (1): 49–51.

The study offered two types of advance directives to 128 patients and found that different people preferred different directives. They concluded that a variety of such forms should be made available before one chooses and completes one.

Robinson, Mary K. 1993. "Effects of the Patient Self-determination Act on Patient Knowledge and Behavior." *Journal of Family Practice* 37 (4): 363–68.

Hospital patients were questioned about advance directives. The study results indicate that although awareness increased, the number of patients who acted on this awareness to prepare advance directives for themselves did not increase.

Rubin, Susan M., William M. Strull, Michael F. Fialkow, Sarah J. Weiss, and Bernard Lo. 1994. "Increasing the Completion of Durable Power of Attorney for Health Care: A Randomized, Controlled Trial." *Journal of the American Medical Association* 271 (3): 209–12. "Increasing Completion of Advance Directives: Letters." *Journal of the American Medical Association* 271 (24): 1907–1908.

The authors sent information and a form about the durable power of attorney to a group of patients older that 65 who had been discharged from a hospital during a five-month period in 1991; another group of similar patients received a general health mailing. In the first group, 18.5 percent completed the form; in the second, 0.4 percent. The authors concluded that patient education about advance directives should be encouraged.

Sass, Hans-Martin, and Rita Kielstein. 1993. "Wertanamnese und Betreuungsverfügung: Instrumente zur Selbstbestimmung des Patienten und zur Entscheidungshilfe des Arztes und Betreuers." *Medizinethische Materialien des Zentrum für Medizinische Ethik* 81.

Schreiber, Hans-Ludwig. 1993. "Tötung auf Verlangen." *Zeitschrift für ärztliche Fortbildung* 87:31–54.

The author discusses recent legal proposals to change the German Penal Code in order to allow for "killing on request."

Silberfield, Michel, Kevin V. Madigan, and Bernard M. Dickens. 1994. "Liability Concerns about the Implementation of Advance Directives." *Canadian Medical Association Journal* 151 (3): 285–89.

The authors address the legal status and liability associated with advance directives in Ontario law, discussing two case decisions that seem to indicate that current legislation can cause uncertainty for physician decision making.

Silberfeld, Michel, Carol Nash, and Peter A. Singer. 1993. "Capacity to Complete an Advance Directive." *Journal of the American Geriatrics Society* 41 (10): 1141–43.

Pointing out that advance directive choices are in the future, the authors state the importance of the patient's having the capability to understand that such choices will be acted on only if the patient becomes incapacitated. They offer guidelines to approach the issue and to obtain consent for competency assessment as well as ways to discuss the nature of advance directives.

Silverman, Henry J., Sara T. Fry, and Niti Armistead. 1994. "Nurses' Perspectives on Implementation of the Patient Self-determination Act." *Journal of Clinical Ethics* 5 (1): 30–37.

Medical Systems posed six questions about advance directives to hospital patients during a two-month period in 1992. The interviewers report that such questions caused anxiety or suspicion in many of the patients and noted little general interest in the topic. The nurses involved in the project thought that nurses should educate and have a major role in ensuring that patients understand the purposes and implications of advance directives, but that the best time for any discussion may not be at admission to the hospital.

Sugarman, Jeremy. 1994. "Outcomes Research and Advance Directives." *Journal of Clinical Ethics* 5 (1): 60–61.

Based on his conclusion that the Teno study "casts some doubt of the efficacy of formal advance directives," Sugarman says future studies must assess caregivers' knowledge of a patient's advance directive as well as communication with the patient about any directive and the resulting care decisions.

Sugarman, Jeremy, Nancy E. Kass, Ruth R. Faden, and S. N. Goodman. 1994. "Catalysts for Conversations about Advance Directives: The Influence of Physician and Patient Characteristics." *Journal of Law, Medicine and Ethics* 22 (1): 29–35.

SUPPORT Principle Investigators: Alfred F. Connors, Neal V. Dawson, Norman A. Desbiens, William J. Fulkerson, Lee Goldman, William A. Knaus, Joanne Lynn, and Robert K. Oye. 1995. "A Controlled Trial to Improve Care for Seriously Ill Hospitalized Patients: The Study to Understand Prognoses and Preferences for Outcomes and Risks of Treatments (SUPPORT)." *Journal of the American Medical Association* 274 (20): 1591–98.

Over 9,000 adult hospitalized patients who were seriously ill or dying were observed with a view to improving end-of-life decision making and reduction of the frequency of mechanically supported, painful, and prolonged process of dying. The study found that there were serious shortcomings in communication between physicians and patients or family members. Physicians either ignored DNR requests or did not write them until a few days before death, and often patients reported severe pain. The authors concluded that "the picture we describe of the care of seriously ill or dying persons is not attractive." They think family and patient should be included in discussion, realistic estimate of outcome valued, pain should be treated, and dying should not be prolonged.

Teno, Joan M., Joanne Lynn, Russell S. Phillips, Donald Murphy, Stuart J. Youngner, Paul Bellamy, Alfred F. Conners, Norman A. Desbiens, William Fulkerson, and William A. Knaus. 1994. "Do Formal Advance Directives Affect Resuscitation Decisions and the Use of Resources for Seriously Ill Patients?" *Journal of Clinical Ethics* 5 (1): 23–30.

The study of 3,058 seriously ill adults at five major American teaching hospitals looked at information on advance directives and patient resuscitation preferences. The use of advance directives appeared to have no effect on resuscitation decisions or use of resources as reflected in the hospital charges, therapy, or length of stay. The authors state that "advance directives were irrelevant to decision making." (The two-year study was conducted just before implementation of the Patient Self-determination Act.)

Uhlenbruck, Wilhelm. 1978. "Der Patientenbrief: die privatautonome Gestaltung des Rechts auf einen menschenwürdigen Tod." *Neue juristische Wochenschrift* 31:566–70.

Presents and discusses an advance directive form called a "patient's letter."

Virmani, Jaya, Lawrence J. Schneiderman, and Robert M. Kaplan. 1994. "Relationship of Advance Directives to Physician-Patient Communication." *Archives of Internal Medicine* 154 (8): 909–13.

The authors interviewed 115 seriously ill cancer patients and 22 of their physicians, finding that physicians were often unaware that patients had advance directives and that only 30 percent of patients had any discussion of treatment decisions with their physicians. They concluded that there was little evidence that advance directives improved patient and physician communication about end-of-life treatment decisions.

Weeks, William B. 1994. "Advance Directives and the Cost of Terminal Hospitalization." *Archives of Internal Medicine* 154 (18): 2077–83.

The authors studied 242 patients without advance directives and 66 with them who had died in a hospital. They found that patients without advance directives had higher terminal charges ($49,900) than those with directives ($31,200).

Wenger, Neil S., and Jodi Halpern. 1994. "The Physician's Role in Completing Advance Directives: Ensuring Patients' Capacity to Make Healthcare Decisions in

Advance." *Journal of Clinical Ethics* 5 (4): 320–22. [See above, commentaries by Harold Bursztajn and Archie Brodsky, Linda Emanuel, and Linda Ganzini et al.]

A case is presented where the patient's advance directive made it more difficult for the physician to understand the preferences of the psychiatrically impaired patient. The authors suggest that physicians should be involved in preparation of the documents to reflect authentic preferences.

Audiovisuals

Advance Directives: Guaranteeing Health Care Rights. 1991. VHS, 10 minutes, color. American Hospital Association, 840 N. Lake Shore Drive, Chicago, Ill. 60611, 312-280-6000.

This brief patient learning film clearly explains living wills and durable powers of attorney.

In Your Hands: The Tools for Preserving Personal Autonomy. 1987. VHS, 16 minutes, color. Produced by the American Bar Association. Distributed by Modern Talking Picture Service, 5000 Park St. N., St. Petersburg, Fla. 33709, 800-237-4599.

Actress Helen Hayes discusses personal finances, aging, and estate planning for women. She urges them to talk with their attorney about living wills and durable powers of attorney. Lawyer Peter Strauss describes them as a means to insure personal choices in decision making.

Living Choices. 1991. VHS, 16 minutes, color. Baxley Media Group, 110 W. Main Street, Urbana, Ill. 61801-2700, 217-384-4838.

Using different formats, this brief film explains the Patient Self-determination Act: a woman reads the law and explains it, various possible "users" discuss their feelings about living wills and durable powers of attorney, a physician talks about doctor-patient communication, and then all participate in a question-and-answer segment.

Partners in Health Care. 1991. VHS, 15 minutes, color. California Health Decisions, 505 S. Main Street, Suite 400, Orange, Calif. 92668, 714-647-4920.

A short drama oriented to patients, this film features discussions between family members about health care decisions, advance directives, and surrogate decision making.

Index

Library of Congress Cataloging-in-Publication Data

Advance directives and surrogate decision making in health care : United States, Germany, and Japan / edited by Hans-Martin Sass, Robert M. Veatch, and Rihito Kimura.

p. cm.

Includes bibliographical references and index.

ISBN 0-8018-5831-3 (alk. paper)

1. Advance directives (Medical care)—United States. 2. Advance directives (Medical care)—Germany. 3. Advance directives (Medical care)—Japan. 4. Advance directives (Medical care)—Cross-cultural studies. I. Sass, Hans-Martin. II. Veatch, Robert M. III. Kimura, Rihito, 1934– .

[DNLM: 1. Advance Directives—United States. 2. Advance Directives—Germany. 3. Advance Directives—Japan. 4. Patient Advocacy. 5. Ethics, Medical. 6. Cross-cultural comparison. W 85.5 A245 1998]

R726.2.A38 1998

174'.24—dc21

DNLM/DLC 98-2598

for Library of Congress CIP